Takotsubo (Stress) Cardiomyopathy

Editors

EDUARDO BOSSONE
RAIMUND ERBEL

HEART FAILURE CLINICS

www.heartfailure.theclinics.com

Consulting Editors
MANDEEP R. MEHRA
JAVED BUTLER

Founding Editor
JAGAT NARULA

April 2013 • Volume 9 • Number 2

ELSEVIER

1600 John F. Kennedy Boulevard • Suite 1800 • Philadelphia, Pennsylvania, 19103-2899

http://www.theclinics.com

HEART FAILURE CLINICS Volume 9, Number 2
April 2013 ISSN 1551-7136, ISBN-13: 978-1-4557-7099-1

Editor: Barbara Cohen-Kligerman

Developmental Editor: Teia Stone

Heart Failure Clinics (ISSN 1551-7136) is published quarterly by Elsevier Inc., 360 Park Avenue South, New York, NY 10010-1710. Months of publication are January, April, July, and October. Business and editorial offices: 1600 John F. Kennedy Boulevard, Suite 1800, Philadelphia, PA 19103-2899. Periodicals postage paid at New York, NY, and additional mailing offices. Subscription prices are USD 224.00 per year for US individuals, USD 361.00 per year for US institutions, USD 76.00 per year for US students and residents, USD 268.00 per year for Canadian individuals, USD 413.00 per year for Canadian institutions, USD 285.00 per year for international individuals, USD 413.00 per year for international institutions, and USD 96.00 per year for Canadian and foreign students/residents. To receive student and resident rate, orders must be accompanied by name of affiliated institution, date of term, and the *signature* of program/residency coordinator on institution letterhead. Orders will be billed at individual rate until proof of status is received. Foreign air speed delivery is included in all *Clinics* subscription prices. All prices are subject to change without notice. **POSTMASTER:** Send address changes to *Heart Failure Clinics*, Elsevier Health Sciences Division, Subscription Customer Service, 3251 Riverport Lane, Maryland Heights, MO 63043. **Customer Service: 1-800-654-2452 (US and Canada). From outside of the US and Canada, call 314-447-8871. Fax: 314-447-8029. For print support, e-mail: JournalsCustomerService-usa@elsevier.com. For online support, e-mail: JournalsOnlineSupport-usa@elsevier.com.**

Reprints. For copies of 100 or more of articles in this publication, please contact the Commercial Reprints Department, Elsevier Inc., 360 Park Avenue South, New York, NY 10010-1710. Tel.: 212-633-3812; Fax: 212-462-1935; E-mail: reprints@elsevier.com.

Heart Failure Clinics is covered in *MEDLINE/PubMed (Index Medicus)*.

Printed and bound by CPI Group (UK) Ltd, Croydon, CR0 4YY

Transferred to digital print 2012

Contributors

CONSULTING EDITORS

MANDEEP R. MEHRA, MD
Professor of Medicine, Harvard Medical School; Co-Director, BWH Cardiovascular; and Executive Director, Center for Advanced Heart Disease, Brigham and Women's Hospital, Boston, Massachusetts

JAVED BUTLER, MD, MPH
Professor of Medicine; Director, Heart Failure Research, Emory University, Atlanta, Georgia

EDITORS

EDUARDO BOSSONE, MD, PhD, FESC, FCCP, FACC
Director, Cardiology Division, Cava de' Tirreni and Amalfi Coast Hospital, Heart Department, University of Salerno; Consultant, Cardiac Surgery Department, IRCCS Policlinico San Donato, Milan, Italy

RAIMUND ERBEL, MD, FAHA, FESC, FACC, FASE
Professor of Medicine/Cardiology, Department of Cardiology, West-German Heart Center, University Duisburg-Essen, Essen, Germany

AUTHORS

KENICHI AIZAWA, MD, PhD
Department of Cardiovascular Medicine, Graduate School of Medicine, The University of Tokyo, Bunkyo-ku, Tokyo, Japan

YOSHIHIRO J. AKASHI, MD
Division of Cardiology, Department of Internal Medicine, St. Marianna University School of Medicine, Kawasaki-city, Japan

ANASTASIOS ATHANASIADIS, MD
Department of Cardiology, Robert-Bosch-Krankenhaus, Stuttgart, Germany

ALEX J. AUSEON, DO, FACC, FASE, FASNC
Associate Professor of Clinical Medicine, Associate Division Director for Education, Director, Fellowship Training Program, Division of Cardiovascular Medicine, Davis Heart and Lung Research Institute, The Ohio State University Medical Center, Columbus, Ohio

RAYMOND BIETRY, MD
Cardiology Fellow, Leon H. Charney Division of Cardiology, Department of Medicine, NYU Langone Medical Center, New York, New York

EDUARDO BOSSONE, MD, PhD, FESC, FCCP, FACC
Director, Cardiology Division, Cava de' Tirreni and Amalfi Coast Hospital, Heart Department, University of Salerno; Consultant, Cardiac Surgery Department, IRCCS Policlinico San Donato, Milan, Italy

PAOLO CALABRÒ, MD, PhD, FESC
Cardiologia SUN, Monaldi Hospital, AO Colli, Second University of Naples, Naples, Italy

RAFFAELE CALABRÒ, MD
Cardiologia SUN, Monaldi Hospital, AO Colli, Second University of Naples, Naples, Italy

RODOLFO CITRO, MD, FESC
Department of Heart Sciences, Circolo
Hospital and Macchi Foundation, University
of Insubria, Varese, Italy; Heart Department,
University Hospital San Giovanni di Dio e Ruggi
d'Aragona, University Hospital Scuola Medica
Salernitana, Salerno, Italy

ANTONIO CITTADINI, MD, PhD
Department of Medical Translational Sciences,
Federico II University, Naples, Italy

RAFFAELLA D'ALESSANDRO, DSc
Genomic and Cellular Lab, Monaldi Hospital,
AO Colli, Second University of Naples, Naples,
Italy

**PERRY MARK ELLIOTT, FRCP, MD,
FESC, FACC**
The Inherited Cardiac Diseases Unit, The Heart
Hospital/University College London, London,
United Kingdom

FABIO FABBIAN, MD
Assistant Professor, Clinica Medica,
Department of Medicine, General and University
Hospital of Ferrara, Cona, Ferrara, Italy

FRANCESCO FERRARA, MD
Department of Cardiology and Cardiac
Surgery, University Hospital Scuola Medica
Salernitana, Salerno, Italy; Department of
Medical Translational Sciences, Federico II
University, Naples, Italy

MASSIMO GALLERANI, MD
Chief, First Internal Unit of Internal Medicine,
Department of Medicine, General and University
Hospital of Ferrara, Cona, Ferrara, Italy

JUDITH Z. GOLDFINGER, MD
Cardiology Fellow, Cardiovascular Institute,
Mount Sinai Medical Center, New York,
New York

CHRISTIAN W. HAMM, MD
Department of Cardiology, Kerckhoff Heart
and Thorax Center, Bad Nauheim, Germany;
Medical Department I, Cardiology, University
of Giessen, Giessen, Germany

YASUKATSU IZUMI, MD, PhD
Department of Pharmacology, Osaka City
University Medical School, Osaka, Japan

STUART D. KATZ, MD, MS
Helen L. and Martin S. Kimmel Professor of
Advanced Cardiac Therapeutics, Leon H.
Charney Division of Cardiology, Department of
Medicine, NYU Langone Medical Center,
New York, New York

**GIUSEPPE LIMONGELLI, MD, PhD,
FESC, FAHA**
Department of Cardiology, Monaldi Hospital, AO
Colli, Second University of Naples, Naples, Italy

ALEXANDER R. LYON, MD, PhD
BHF Senior Lecturer and Consultant
Cardiologist, Myocardial Function Section,
National Heart and Lung Institute, Imperial
College London; Cardiovascular Biomedical
Research Unit, Royal Brompton Hospital,
London, United Kingdom

VALERIA MADDALONI, DSc
Genomic and Cellular Lab, Monaldi Hospital,
AO Colli, Second University of Naples, Naples,
Italy

FABIO MANFREDINI, MD
Assistant Professor, Vascular Diseases Center,
University of Ferrara, Ferrara, Italy

ROBERTO MANFREDINI, MD
Associate Professor of Medicine and Chief,
Section of Clinica Medica, Department of
Clinical and Experimental Medicine, General
and University Hospital of Ferrara, Cona,
Ferrara, Italy

DANIELE MASARONE, MD
Cardiologia SUN, Monaldi Hospital, AO Colli,
Second University of Naples, Naples, Italy

ROSALBA MINISINI, PhD
University of Eastern Piedmont Amedeo
Avogadro, Department of Translational
Medicine, Novara, Italy

HELGE MÖLLMANN, MD
Department of Cardiology, Kerckhoff Heart
and Thorax Center, Bad Nauheim, Germany;
Medical Department I, Cardiology, University
of Giessen, Giessen, Germany

SUSANNA MOSCA, MD
Department of Advanced Biomedical
Sciences, Federico II University, Naples, Italy

FRANCESCA MUSELLA, MD
Department of Advanced Biomedical
Sciences, Federico II University, Naples, Italy

AJITH NAIR, MD
Cardiovascular Institute, Mount Sinai Medical
Center, New York, New York

HOLGER M. NEF, MD
Department of Cardiology, Kerckhoff Heart
and Thorax Center, Bad Nauheim, Germany;
Medical Department I, Cardiology, University
of Giessen, Giessen, Germany

GIUSEPPE PACILEO, MD
Cardiologia SUN, Monaldi Hospital, AO Colli,
Second University of Naples, Naples, Italy

GUIDO PARODI, MD
Division of Cardiology, Careggi Hospital,
Florence, Italy

PASQUALE PERRONE FILARDI, MD, PhD
Department of Advanced Biomedical
Sciences, Federico II University, Naples, Italy

FEDERICO PISCIONE, MD
Professor of Cardiology, Department of
Medicine and Surgery, University of Salerno,
Salerno, Italy

**ABHIRAM PRASAD, MD, FRCP,
FESC, FACC**
Professor of Medicine, Division of
Cardiovascular Diseases, Department of
Internal Medicine, Mayo Clinic and Mayo
Foundation, Rochester, Minnesota

ALEX REYENTOVICH, MD
Assistant Professor of Medicine, Leon H.
Charney Division of Cardiology, Department
of Medicine, NYU Langone Medical Center,
New York, New York

MARIA GIOVANNA RUSSO, MD
Cardiologia SUN, Monaldi Hospital, AO Colli,
Second University of Naples, Naples, Italy

JORGE SALERNO-URIARTE, MD
Professor of Cardiology, Department of Heart
Sciences, Circolo Hospital and Macchi
Foundation, University of Insubria,
Varese, Italy

RAFFAELLA SALMI, MD
Second Internal Unit of Internal Medicine,
Department of Medicine, General and
University Hospital of Ferrara, Cona,
Ferrara, Italy

GIANLUIGI SAVARESE, MD
Department of Advanced Biomedical
Sciences, Federico II University, Naples, Italy

BIRKE SCHNEIDER, MD
Medizinische Klinik II, Department of
Cardiology, Sana Kliniken Lübeck GmbH,
Lübeck, Germany

BRETT A. SEALOVE, MD, FACC, RPVI
Monmouth Cardiology Associates, LLC,
Ocean, New Jersey

UDO SECHTEM, MD
Department of Cardiology, Robert-Bosch-
Krankenhaus, Stuttgart, Germany

SCOTT W. SHARKEY, MD
Cardiovascular Research Division, Minneapolis
Heart Institute Foundation, Minneapolis,
Minnesota

MARKUS B. SIKKEL, MD
Clinical Research Fellow, Myocardial
Function Section, National Heart and Lung
Institute, Imperial College London, London,
United Kingdom

SAKIMA A. SMITH, MD
Fellow, Advanced Heart Failure and
Transplantation, Division of Cardiovascular
Medicine, Davis Heart and Lung Research
Institute, The Ohio State University Medical
Center, Columbus, Ohio

MATTHEW R. SUMMERS, MD
Department of Internal Medicine, Duke
University Medical Center, Durham,
North Carolina

TORU SUZUKI, MD, PhD
Departments of Cardiovascular Medicine and
Ubiquitous Preventive Medicine, Graduate
School of Medicine, The University of Tokyo,
Bunkyo-ku, Tokyo, Japan

SEBASTIAN SZARDIEN, MD
Department of Cardiology, Kerckhoff Heart
and Thorax Center, Bad Nauheim, Germany

MATTHEW H. TRANTER, MRes
Myocardial Function Section, National Heart and Lung Institute, Imperial College London, London, United Kingdom

OLGA VRIZ, MD
Department of Cardiology and Emergency, Ospedale San Antonio, San Daniele del Friuli, Udine, Italy

MATTHIAS WILLMER, MD
Department of Cardiology, Kerckhoff Heart and Thorax Center, Bad Nauheim, Germany

PETER T. WRIGHT, MRes
Myocardial Function Section, National Heart and Lung Institute, Imperial College London, London, United Kingdom

Contents

Takotsubo cardiomyopathy (TTC) is an increasingly recognized, reversible cardiomyopathy with a clinical presentation that mimics an acute coronary syndrome but without evidence of obstructive coronary lesions. Typical presentation involves chest pain and/or dyspnea, transient ST-segment elevation on the electrocardiogram, and a modest increase in cardiac troponin. Cardiac imaging demonstrates wall-motion abnormalities that extend beyond the territory of a single epicardial coronary artery, and the absence of obstructive coronary lesions. Supportive treatment leads to spontaneous, rapid recovery of ventricular function, but about 10% of patients have recurrent events. This article reviews the defining features and clinical profile of TTC.

This article provides a comprehensive review of the clinical features of takotsubo (stress) cardiomyopathy. The author discusses key features that distinguish this cardiomyopathy from acute coronary syndrome. This review includes detail of characteristic findings on electrocardiogram, biochemical testing, and cardiac imaging, as well as complications including congestive heart failure, arrhythmia, ventricular thrombi, and left ventricular outflow obstruction. The review concludes with a discussion of the proper treatment, long-term survival, and proposed pathophysiology.

Takotsubo cardiomyopathy (TTC) predominantly occurs in elderly women. Men comprise 10% of the patients, with a similar clinical profile. In contrast to myocardial infarction, age distribution; symptoms, such as angina; and prehospital delay in TTC are not different between genders. In men, physical stress as a triggering event and shock or cardiac arrest on presentation are more frequent. Gender-related differences in TTC need to be carefully investigated at the clinical and experimental levels to explain the evident gender discrepancy in the prevalence of TTC, to clarify the pathogenetic background, and to develop preventive and therapeutic means against this life-threatening disease.

A considerable amount of evidence has shown that the major acute cardiovascular diseases, ie, myocardial infarction, sudden cardiac death, stroke, pulmonary embolism, and rupture or dissection of aortic aneurysms do not occur randomly in time, but exhibit specific temporal patterns in their onset, according to time of day, month or season, and day of the week. This contributes to the definition of "chronorisk", where several factors, not harmful if taken alone, are capable of triggering unfavorable events when presenting all together within the same temporal window. This article reviews the actual knowledge about time of onset of takotsubo cardiomyopathy.

Takotsubo cardiomyopathy (TTC) is characterized by transient and reversible left ventricular (LV) systolic dysfunction due to extended myocardial stunning. Despite a good long term prognosis, approximately one-third of patients with TTC experience life-threatening complications during the acute phase. Echocardiography is the first imaging modality for an early evaluation of LV systolic and diastolic function in patients with TTC. Moreover, echocardiography allows the detection of specific findings associated with TTC, such as LV outflow tract obstruction, mitral regurgitation, and right ventricular involvement, providing crucial information for clinical management and therapy and for monitoring myocardial function recovery during the follow-up.

Cardiac MRI (CMR) has become an important tool in the diagnosis of cardiomyopathies. CMR is a unique tool for further evaluating and characterizing patients with takotsubo cardiomyopathy (TTC) and studying the underlying causes and pathophysiologic mechanisms of TTC. Using CMR, regional wall motion abnormalities, right ventricular involvement, intraventricular thrombi, and reversible myocardial injury (inflammation or ischemic edema) or irreversible myocardial injury (necrosis or fibrosis) can be detected in patients presenting with TTC. CMR imaging can distinguish between acute myocardial infarction and TTC.

The clinical management of takotsubo cardiomyopathy is challenging. Its diagnosis must be made on clinical grounds and differentiated from alternative diagnoses with echocardiography, serum biomarkers, cardiac catheterization, and cardiac magnetic resonance imaging. Acute therapy includes supportive care, targeting the precipitating trigger if known, b-blockade, inhibitors of the renin-angiotensin system, and consideration of systemic anticoagulation in all patients. Recovery of left ventricular function to normal is expected regardless of early therapy. Although the prognosis is generally favorable, monitoring for early dangerous complications is essential. There is no evidence to support use of long-term medical therapy to reduce the risk of recurrence.

Takotsubo cardiomyopathy (TTC) is an acute heart failure syndrome classically characterized by hypocontractile apical and midventricular regions of the left ventricle, with a compensatory hypercontractile base. Available data support the hypothesis that TTC and atypical TTC-like disorders are primarily induced by catecholaminergic overstimulation, with epinephrine playing a crucial role. Knowledge from the available preclinical models should be used to guide the development of potential clinical trials in the most severe cases, where rates of acute morbidity and mortality are highest, and also to prevent recurrence in susceptible individuals.

Stress cardiomyopathy is a form of reversible systolic dysfunction of the mid and apical left ventricle with pathologic changes of the electrocardiogram in the absence of an obstructive coronary artery disease. The prevalence of stress cardiomyopathy among patients with symptoms suggestive of myocardial infarction is 0.7% to 2.5%, and it is found predominantly in postmenopausal women (90%). No large studies have confirmed the cause of stress cardiomyopathy. Published data suggest that substantially elevated plasma catecholamine levels, due to emotional or physical stress, may be relevant.

Takotsubo cardiomyopathy (TTC) is an enigmatic disease with a multifactorial and still unresolved pathogenesis. Recent experimental and clinical observation has suggested a role for genetics in the pathogenesis of TTC. Ethnic as well as seasonal variation in the prevalence of TTC is well described, but it is only recently that familial cases of TTC have been reported. In recent years technological advances in exome capture and DNA sequencing have offered clinicians a new opportunity to discover genetics-related disease. This article explores the role of genetic mechanisms that might explain or modulate the pathogenesis of TTC.

Takotsubo cardiomyopathy is classically stress induced and characterized by regional wall motion abnormalities in the absence of coronary occlusion. It predominantly affects postmenopausal women; emotional and physical stressors can trigger the classic cardiomyopathic findings. These changes are likely mediated by catecholamines, which cause a distinctive pattern of ventricular dysfunction with a unique pathologic phenotype of apical ballooning. Underlying mood disorders increase the risk for developing takotsubo cardiomyopathy after a triggering event. Takotsubo cardiomyopathy is one of several brain-heart disorders; its unique pathology can shed light on the complex interactions between the brain, sympathetic nervous system, and the cardiovascular system.

Takotsubo cardiomyopathy (TTC), also known as stress cardiomyopathy, is an increasingly recognized clinical syndrome of acute reversible left ventricular dysfunction precipitated by intense emotional or physical stress. Excessive sympa-thetic stimulation is believed to be central to the pathogenesis of this condition; thus, drugs with sympathetic effect could precipitate TTC. This review outlines previous reports regarding drugs that may induce TTC. Some reports link the use of the drug—primarily associated with sympathetic overstimulation—with the develop-ment of TTC Consequently, drug-induced TTC should be considered in patients diagnosed with TTC.

Stress cardiomyopathy, also known as takotsubo cardiomyopathy, is a rapidly reversible form of acute heart failure classically triggered by stressful events. It is associated with a distinctive left ventricular contraction pattern described as apical akinesis/ballooning with hyperdynamic contraction of the basal segments in the absence of obstructive coronary artery disease. The traditional paradigm has ex-panded to include other causes, in particular chemotherapeutic drugs. The literature increasingly suggests an association between cancer, chemotherapeutic drugs, and stress cardiomyopathy. Chemotherapy-induced takotsubo cardiomyopathy is a relatively new phenomenon, but one that merits detailed attention to the elucidation of possible mechanistic links.

Takotsubo cardiomyopathy is likely induced by stress, and postmenopausal women account for the majority of patients. Several questions about takotsubo cardiomyop-athy remain unanswered, including why it is induced by stress, what differentiates the stress that induces this disease from other types of stress that do not induce it, why women are more likely to develop this disease, why the apical part of the heart is affected, and how it is different from the subtype in which the base and mid-dle parts are affected. Although takotsubo cardiomyopathy is uncommon, clinicians should be aware that this disease can develop in wider areas.

Takotsubo cardiomyopathy (TTC) is a unique acute syndrome characterized by tran-sient left ventricular systolic dysfunction in the absence of significant coronary artery disease, occurring mostly in postmenopausal women after emotional and/or phys-ical stress. Given the nonspecific symptoms and signs, a high clinical index of sus-picion is necessary to detect the disease in different clinical settings and scenarios. Noninvasive multimodality imaging may be useful to distinguish this cardiomyopathy from other acute cardiac and thoracic diseases. Coronary angiography remains, however, mandatory to differentiate TTC from acute coronary syndromes. This article reviews the clinical features and management of TTC and some new insights.

HEART FAILURE CLINICS

Preface

The "Takotsubo Syndrome": From Legend to Science

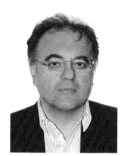

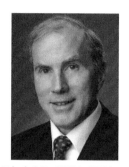

Eduardo Bossone, MD, PhD, FESC, FCCP, FACC   Raimund Erbel, MD, FAHA, FESC, FACC, FASE

Editors

Takotsubo cardiomyopathy (TC), also known as "stress cardiomyopathy," transient left ventricular (LV) "apical ballooning syndrome," or "broken heart syndrome," is a clinical condition mimicking an acute myocardial infarction usually occurring in postmenopausal women after an emotional and/or physical stress (**Fig. 1**).[1–18]

The historical term "tako-tsubo" was first used by Sato et al in 1990 because of similarities between LV morphologic features and the shape of a ceramic fishing pot (with a round bottom and a narrow neck) used since ancient times in Japan for trapping octopuses.[1,2,19] In fact, TC is usually characterized by transient LV systolic dysfunction with apical akinesis and compensatory hyperkinesis of the basal segments (typical form) in the absence of obstructive coronary artery disease or angiographic evidence of coronary luminal narrowing or complex lesions suggestive of plaque rupture.[8] In this regard, it is worth noting that recent data from the Tako-tsubo Italian Network reported a substantial number of patients (up to 10%) with critical stenosis ($\geq$50%) in the epicardial coronary arteries not supplying the dysfunctional

myocardium. It is not known if this represents a subgroup of the TC or another form of disease. More invasive studies, including intravascular ultrasound and optical coherence tomography, are needed in this respect.[20,21] In addition, TC has also recently been shown to be associated with variable but significant in-hospital (0%–8%) and long-term mortality (0%–17%) along with non-negligible recurrence rates (0%–11.4%).[22]

Although the pathophysiologic mechanisms remain unknown, increasing evidence suggests that sympathetic mediated transient myocardial dysfunction may occur in the presence of specific risk factors, such as estrogen deficiency, mood disorders, or endothelial dysfunction.[23] In recent years, technological advances in exome capture and DNA sequencing have opened new horizons for understanding a potential genetic role.[24] Thus, an international multidisciplinary effort is needed to identify specific TC patient cohorts in a 3-dimensional "Cartesian model" of demographics (gender, race, age), stressors (physical, emotional), and morphofunctional variants (typical vs atypical).

Heart Failure Clin 9 (2013) xiii–xv
http://dx.doi.org/10.1016/j.hfc.2013.01.001
1551-7136/13/$ – see front matter © 2013 Published by Elsevier Inc.

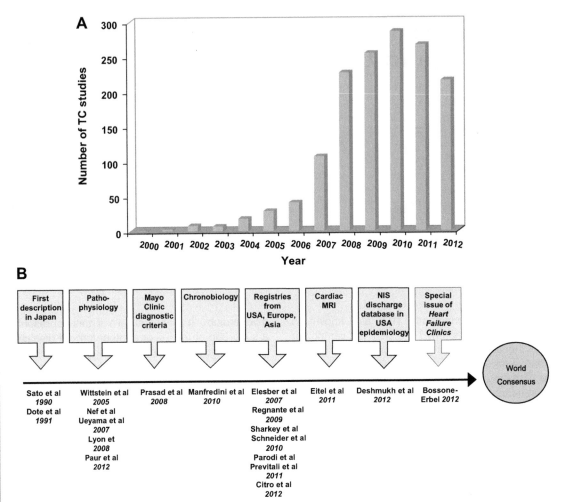

Fig. 1. (*A*) Number of TC studies available in the literature, 2000-2012. (*B*) Time line of reports in the literature. MRI, magnetic resonance imaging; NIS, nationwide inpatient sample.

Eduardo Bossone, MD, PhD, FESC, FCCP, FACC
Cardiology Division
"Cava de' Tirreni and Amalfi Coast" Hospital
Heart Department, University of Salerno
Via De Marinis
84013 Cava de' Tirreni (SA), Italy

Cardiac Surgery Department
IRCCS Policlinico San Donato
Piazza Edmondo Malan 1
20097 San Donato Milanese, Italy

Raimund Erbel, MD, FAHA, FESC, FACC, FASE
Department of Cardiology
West-German Heart Center
University Duisburg-Essen
Hufelandstr 55
D-45122 Essen, Germany

E-mail addresses:
ebossone@hotmail.com (E. Bossone)
erbel@uk-essen.de (R. Erbel)

REFERENCES

1. Sato H, Taiteishi H, Uchida T. Takotsubo-type cardio-myopathy due to multivessel spasm. In: Kodama K, Haze K, Hon M, editors. Clinical aspect of myocardial injury: from ischemia to heart failure. Tokyo: Kagaku-hyouronsha; 1990. p. 56–64.

2. Dote K, Sato H, Tateishi H, et al. Myocardial stunning due to simultaneous multivessel coronary spasms: a review of 5 cases. J Cardiol 1991;21:203–14.

3. Wittstein IS, Thiemann DR, Lima JA, et al. Neurohu-moral features of myocardial stunning due to sudden emotional stress. N Engl J Med 2005;352: 539–48.

4. Nef HM, Mollmann H, Kostin S, et al. Tako-Tsubo cardiomyopathy: intraindividual structural analysis in the acute phase and after functional recovery. Eur Heart J 2007;28:2456–64.

5. Ueyama T, Ishikura F, Matsuda A, et al. Chronic estrogen supplementation following ovariectomy improves the emotional stress-induced cardiovascular responses by indirect action on the nervous system and by direct action on the heart. Circ J 2007;71:565–73.

6. Lyon AR, Rees PS, Prasad S, et al. Stress (Takotsubo) cardiomyopathy––a novel pathophysiological hypothesis to explain catecholamine-induced acute myocardial stunning. Nat Clin Pract Cardiovasc Med 2008;5:22–9.

7. Paur H, Wright PT, Sikkel MB, et al. High levels of circulating epinephrine trigger apical cardiodepression in a β2-adrenergic receptor/Gi-dependent manner: a new model of Takotsubo cardiomyopathy. Circulation 2012;126:697–706.

8. Prasad A, Lerman A, Rihal CS. Apical ballooning syndrome (Tako-Tsubo or stress cardiomyopathy): a mimic of acute myocardial infarction. Am Heart J 2008;155:408–17.

9. Manfredini R, Citro R, Previtali M, et al, Takotsubo Italian Network Investigators. Monday preference in onset of takotsubo cardiomyopathy. Am J Emerg Med 2010;28:715–9.

10. Elesber AA, Prasad A, Lennon RJ, et al. Four-year recurrence rate and prognosis of the apical ballooning syndrome. J Am Coll Cardiol 2007;50: 448–52.

11. Regnante RA, Zuzek RW, Weinsier SB, et al. Clinical characteristics and four-year outcomes of patients in the Rhode Island Takotsubo Cardiomyopathy Registry. Am J Cardiol 2009;103:1015–9.

12. Sharkey SW, Windenburg DC, Lesser JR, et al. Natural history and expansive clinical profile of stress (tako-tsubo) cardiomyopathy. J Am Coll Cardiol 2010;55:333–41.

13. Schneider B, Athanasiadis A, Schwab J, et al. Clinical spectrum of tako-tsubo cardiomyopathy in Germany: results of the tako-tsubo registry of the Arbeitsgemeinschaft Leitende Kardiologische Krankenhausärzte (ALKK). Dtsch Med Wochenschr 2010;135:1908–13 [in German].

14. Parodi G, Bellandi B, Del Pace S, et al, Tuscany Registry of Tako-Tsubo Cardiomyopathy. Natural history of tako-tsubo cardiomyopathy. Chest 2011; 139:887–92.

15. Previtali M, Repetto A, Camporotondo R, et al. Clinical characteristics and outcome of left ventricular ballooning syndrome in a European population. Am J Cardiol 2011;107:120–5.

16. Citro R, Rigo F, Previtali M, et al. Differences in clinical features and in-hospital outcomes of older adults with tako-tsubo cardiomyopathy. J Am Geriatr Soc 2012;60:93–8.

17. Eitel I, von Knobelsdorff-Brenkenhoff F, Bernhardt P, et al. Clinical characteristics and cardiovascular magnetic resonance findings in stress (takotsubo) cardiomyopathy. JAMA 2011;306:277–86.

18. Deshmukh A, Kumar G, Pant S, et al. Prevalence of Takotsubo cardiomyopathy in the United States. Am Heart J 2012;164:66–71.e1.

19. Aizawa K, Suzuki T. Takostubo cardiomyopathy: Japanese perspective. Heart Fail Clin 2013, in press.

20. Parodi G, Citro R, Bellandi B. on the behalf of the Tako-tsubo Italian Network (TIN). Tako-tsubo cardiomyopathy and coronary artery disease: a possible association [abstract]. J Am Coll Cardiol 2012; 60(17 Suppl B):B142.

21. Alfonso F, Núñez-Gil IJ, Hernández R. Optical coherence tomography findings in Tako-Tsubo cardiomyopathy. Circulation 2012;126(13):166.

22. Bossone E, Savarese G, Ferrara F, et al. Takotsubo cardiomyopathy: overview. Heart Fail Clin 2013, in press.

23. Wittstein IS. Stress cardiomyopathy: a syndrome of catecholamine-mediated myocardial stunning? Cell Mol Neurobiol 2012;32:847–57.

24. Limongelli G, D'Alessandro R, Masarone D, et al. Takotsubo cardiomyopathy. Does genetics matter? Heart Fail Clin 2013, in press.

Takotsubo Cardiomyopathy
Definition and Clinical Profile

Matthew R. Summers, MD[a],
Abhiram Prasad, MD, FRCP, FESC[b],*

KEYWORDS

- Apical ballooning syndrome • Takotsubo cardiomyopathy • Stress cardiomyopathy

KEY POINTS

- Takotsubo cardiomyopathy (TTC) is an increasingly recognized, reversible cardiomyopathy with a clinical presentation that mimics an acute coronary syndrome (ACS).
- TTC is estimated to represent 1% to 2% of patients presenting with suspected ACS, most commonly manifests in postmenopausal women, and is precipitated by emotional or physical stressors in a majority of cases.
- Typical presentation involves chest pain and/or dyspnea, transient ST-segment elevation on the electrocardiogram, and a modest increase in cardiac troponin.
- Cardiac imaging demonstrates wall-motion abnormalities that generally extend beyond the territory of a single epicardial coronary artery, and the absence of obstructive coronary lesions.
- Supportive treatment typically leads to spontaneous, rapid recovery of ventricular function within weeks.

INTRODUCTION

Takotsubo cardiomyopathy (TTC), also known as stress-induced cardiomyopathy, apical ballooning syndrome, and broken heart syndrome, is an increasingly recognized transient condition that results in a characteristic pattern of ventricular systolic dysfunction frequently precipitated by a stressful event.[1–4] The syndrome was initially reported in Japan in 1991 and was named "takotsubo" after the round-bottomed and narrow-necked octopus trap that resembles the apical ballooning systolic morphology of the left ventricle in the classic form of TTC.[5] Since then there have been several case series reported from North America,[6–13] Europe,[14–17] Asia,[18–20] and Australia,[21] and TTC is now recognized as a primary acquired cardiomyopathy in the American Heart Association scientific statement on the classification of cardiomyopathies.[22] In the typical form of TTC, the systolic contractile dysfunction involves the mid and apical segments of the left ventricle with compensatory basal wall hyperkinesis.[2] Atypical forms involving basal or midventricular hypokinesis with apical sparing have been reported less commonly.[14,15,21,23–25] TTC is unique in that it disproportionately occurs in postmenopausal women,[4,7,14,20] and in a majority of cases is preceded by an acute physical or emotional stressor.[4,7,9,17,20] The pathophysiology of TTC is not well understood, but postulated mechanisms include catecholamine excess, either with direct myocardial toxicity or through induction of microvascular dysfunction or coronary spasm.[26,27]

Although there has been increasing recognition of this unique syndrome, TTC is often misdiagnosed

Conflicts of interest and financial disclosure: None.
[a] Department of Internal Medicine, Duke University Medical Center, 2301 Erwin Road, Durham, NC 27710, USA; [b] Division of Cardiovascular Diseases, Department of Internal Medicine, Mayo Clinic and Mayo Foundation, 200 First Street Southwest, Rochester, MN 55905, USA
* Corresponding author.
E-mail address: prasad.abhiram@mayo.edu

Heart Failure Clin 9 (2013) 111–122
http://dx.doi.org/10.1016/j.hfc.2012.12.007

as an acute coronary syndrome (ACS) given the similarities in the clinical presentation, electrocardiographic features, and cardiac biomarker profile; however, the cardiomyopathy virtually always occurs in the absence of flow-limiting coronary atherosclerosis. Thus it is an important differential diagnosis of acute myocardial infarction, and is estimated to represent approximately 1% to 2% of patients presenting with suspected ACS.[2,4,19,28] In a recent analysis from the Nationwide Inpatient Sample discharge records in the United States for the year 2008 using the *International Classification of Diseases, Ninth Revision*, code 429.83, the incidence of TTC among all hospitalizations in the United States was estimated to be approximately 0.02%.[29]

CLINICAL CHARACTERISTICS
Patient Demographics and Associated Factors

Most patients with TTC (80%–100%) are postmenopausal women with a mean age of 61 to 76 years, based on published case series.[4,7,14,27,30] TTC is uncommonly (<3%) reported in individuals who are younger than 50 years.[27] The exact incidence of TTC is unclear given the similarity to and misdiagnosis as ACS, but is estimated to account for 1.7% to 2.2% of cases presenting with suspected ACS.[27] A preceding emotional or physical stress is a unique feature of TTC, with approximately two-thirds of cases having associated, identifiable acute stressors.[10,27,31] A variety of emotional stressors has been reported, including the death of a loved one, natural disasters, financial loss, and domestic violence.[10,27] Physical stressors reported include acute critical illness (intensive care unit population without known cardiac diagnosis), postoperative state, severe pain, exacerbations of chronic obstructive pulmonary disease or asthma, as well as central nervous system disorders such as seizures, subarachnoid hemorrhage, and posterior reversible encephalopathy syndrome.[7,27,32–36] A comprehensive list of associated triggers are detailed in **Box 1**. Of importance, the absence of a precipitating stressor does not preclude a diagnosis of TTC, as up to one-third of patients do not have identifiable preceding triggers.

A genetic predisposition has been implicated with the report of familial cases of TTC.[107,108] Compared with the general population, TTC patients are more likely to have a chronic anxiety disorder or have a family history of psychiatric disease, thus implicating premorbid psychiatric disease as a possible predisposing factor.[109] The reason for a predominance of postmenopausal female patients is unknown. One study noted that compared with women, men more often developed TTC during or immediately after receiving medical therapy or an examination for a noncardiac medical illness (ie, in response to a physical trigger), suggesting sex differences in the types of TTC-provoking events.[110] Another study found higher concentrations of estradiol in postmenopausal TTC patients than in women with acute myocardial infarction and women with normal coronary arteries, with the investigators postulating that estradiol in these women exerts an atheroprotective effect diverting stress responses from ACS to TTC.[111]

Presenting Symptoms and Complications

Chest pain, which has the characteristics of angina, is the most common presenting symptom and has been reported in as many as 60% to 100% of patients among published series of patients.[10,31,35] Dyspnea is also a common symptom, and less frequently patients present with other symptoms such as syncope or cardiac arrest. A small proportion of asymptomatic patients are identified after ischemic changes on the electrocardiogram (ECG) or when cardiac biomarker elevations are noted during hospitalization for a noncardiac illness.[10,31,35]

Acute heart failure, manifesting as pulmonary edema, occurs in up to 45% of patients, and cardiogenic shock necessitating intra-aortic balloon counterpulsation (IABP) occurs in up to 20% of cases.[30,112] Other complications include dynamic left ventricular outflow tract obstruction (~10%–15%) and acute mitral regurgitation caused by transient valve dysfunction.[10,27,113,114] Rare complications include thrombus formation along the dyskinetic ventricular walls (typically seen in <5% of patients)[10] and cardiac rupture.[115]

Electrocardiogram

ECG changes of ischemia or injury are the most common clinical finding in TTC, with transient ST-segment elevation present on the initial ECG in 30% to 50% of patients.[10,18–20,31,37,116–118] The transient ST-segment elevation attributable to TTC cannot be distinguished from the findings in patients with an ST-segment elevation myocardial infarction, and most commonly involves the precordial leads.[119] Reported ECG diagnostic criteria for distinguishing the 2 conditions have not been validated and have limited diagnostic accuracy.[119–121] The extent and magnitude of ST-segment elevation on the electrocardiogram may be correlated with the likelihood of in-hospital complications.[122] Widespread, deep T-wave inversions in the precordial leads are noted at presentation in some patients, and develop over the course of 2 to 3 days in others (**Fig. 1**).

Box 1
Stressors associated with takotsubo cardiomyopathy

Emotional Stress[4,27,37]

- Death, severe illness, or injury involving a family member, friend, or pet[38]
- Receiving bad news (major medical diagnosis, daughter's divorce, spouse leaving for war)
- Severe argument
- Assault[39]
- Public speaking
- Involvement in legal proceedings
- Financial loss (business, gambling)
- Car accident[40]
- Surprise party
- Move to a new residence
- Natural disasters (eg, earthquakes[41])
- After adulterous intercourse[42]

Physical Stress[4,27,37]

Noncardiac surgeries or procedures

- Cholecystectomy, hysterectomy, rhinoplasty,[43] cesarean section,[44] radiofrequency liver ablation,[45] radiotherapy,[46] colonoscopy,[47] difficult urinary catheterization,[48] electroconvulsive therapy,[49] canalith repositioning,[50] carotid endarterectomy[51]

Cardiac procedures

- Radiofrequency arrhythmia ablation,[52] pacemaker implantation,[53] electrical cardioversion for atrial fibrillation[54]

Medical conditions

- Respiratory: exacerbation of asthma or chronic obstructive pulmonary disease,[55] pneumothorax, pulmonary embolism
- Rheumatologic: connective-tissue disorders
- Gastrointestinal: acute cholecystitis or biliary colic,[56] pseudomembranous colitis, acute pancreatitis,[57] severe vomiting,[58] acute diarrhea,[59] peritonitis[60]
- Infectious diseases: sepsis,[61,62] babesiosis[63]
- Endocrine: pheochromocytoma,[64] multiple endocrine neoplasia 2A syndrome,[65] hyperglycemic hyperosmolar state,[66] hyponatremia,[67] syndrome of inappropriate secretion of antidiuretic hormone,[68] endogenous thyrotoxicosis,[69] iatrogenic thyrotoxicosis,[70] severe hypothyroidism,[71] Addison disease,[72] adrenocorticotropin hormone deficiency,[73] autoimmune polyendocrine syndrome II[74]
- Hematologic and renal: thrombotic thrombocytopenic purpura,[75] blood transfusions,[76] hemodialysis[77]
- Neurologic: myasthenia gravis,[78] seizures,[79] limbic encephalitis,[80] spinal cord injury,[81] ischemic stroke,[82] Guillain-Barré syndrome,[83] posterior reversible encephalopathy syndrome,[34] subarachnoid hemorrhage,[32] Opiate withdrawal,[84] alcohol withdrawal[85]

Medications and illicit drugs

- Cocaine abuse,[86] Adderall,[87] nortriptyline overdose,[88] venlafaxine overdose,[89] albuterol,[90] flecanide,[91] metoprolol withdrawal,[92] epinephrine,[93,94] 5-fluorouracil,[95] duloxetine[96]

Stress tests

- Dobutamine stress echo,[97] dipyridamole stress test,[98] exercise stress test[99]

Other

- Lightning strike,[100] jellyfish sting,[101] near drowning,[102] severe burns,[103] multiple trauma,[104] car accident, heat stroke,[105] consumption of energy drinks[106]

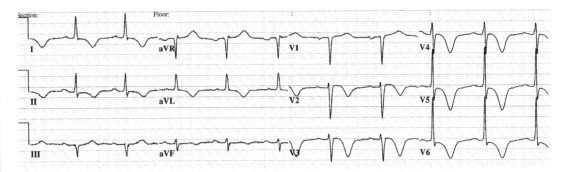

Fig. 1. Diffuse T-wave inversion with QT prolongation. (*Reproduced from* Prasad A, Lerman A, Rihal CS. Apical ballooning syndrome (Tako-Tsubo or stress cardiomyopathy): a mimic of acute myocardial infarction. Am Heart J 2008;155:409; with permission.)

Abnormal Q waves are rarely observed. Nonspecific T-wave abnormalities or a normal ECG may be present in up to 35% of patients.[117] Prolongation of the corrected QT interval occurs frequently but, paradoxically, malignant arrhythmias occur in only 5% of patients.[123] Based on a recent systematic review, ventricular fibrillation or sustained ventricular tachycardia are present in only 1.8% and 0.5% of published cases, respectively.[124] Atrial arrhythmias and conduction abnormalities are relatively uncommon as is atrial fibrillation, with sinus or atrioventricular nodal dysfunction occurring in fewer than 5% of cases.[124]

Cardiac Biomarkers and Laboratory Data

Nearly all patients have elevated levels of serum cardiac troponin, especially when contemporary assays are used. Creatine kinase–MB fraction and B-type natriuretic peptide (BNP) are elevated in the great majority.[27,125–127] Troponin-T peaks at modest levels in TTC, distinguishing it from the higher levels seen in ST-segment elevation myocardial infarction, but similar than that seen in non–ST-segment elevation myocardial infarction (**Fig. 2**).[1,126,127] Conversely, BNP levels are frequently higher in patients with apical ballooning syndrome than in those with ST-segment elevation myocardial infarction.[125–127] BNP levels increase over the first 24 hours and remain elevated for several days.[128] In TTC, BNP levels do not appear to correlate with troponin-T peaks or hemodynamic parameters such as ejection fraction and end-diastolic pressure.[126] Plasma catecholamine levels have been reported to be higher in TTC patients than in patients with acute myocardial infarction,[9] but this was not validated when 24-hour urine metanephrines and catecholamines were measured in another study.[127]

Cardiac Catheterization

In general, coronary angiography in patients with TTC demonstrates normal coronary arteries or nonobstructive (luminal stenosis <50%) coronary artery disease (CAD). Coronary angiography is usually necessary in suspected cases of TTC to differentiate it from an ACS with plaque rupture, thrombus, or embolism as the cause of the ventricular dysfunction. Given the high prevalence of CAD in the at-risk postmenopausal population that TTC predominantly affects, obstructive CAD may be coexistent, and a diagnosis should be made with caution in these patients.[13,129] In fact, one hypothesis is that TTC is not a distinct clinical entity, but rather the result of a transient occlusion and then spontaneous thrombolysis in a long

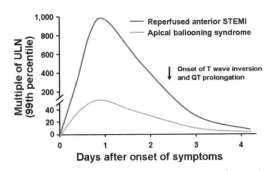

Fig. 2. Kinetics of cardiac troponin-T release in patients with apical ballooning syndrome versus acute anterior ST-segment elevation myocardial infarction (STEMI) treated with mechanical reperfusion within 3 hours of symptom onset. ULN, upper limit of normal. (*Reproduced from* Prasad A, Lerman A, Rihal CS. Apical ballooning syndrome (Tako-Tsubo or stress cardiomyopathy): a mimic of acute myocardial infarction. Am Heart J 2008;155:409; with permission.)

"wrap-around" left anterior descending artery that causes resultant myocardial stunning. The prevalence of this left anterior descending artery anatomy in TTC patients, however, is low (27%) and similar to that of patients with a diagnosis of anterior myocardial infarction, making this hypothesis unlikely.[13]

Echocardiography

The characteristic wall-motion abnormalities with hypokinesis or akinesis of the apex and/or mid segments of the left ventricle and hyperkinesis of the basal walls can be imaged by echocardiography.[4,7,14,17] This left ventricular dysfunction extends beyond the territory of any one epicardial coronary artery and yields the octopus-trap configuration after which the syndrome was named. The characteristic appearance is most frequently identified during left ventricular angiography at centers where access to a cardiac catheterization facility is routinely available. The reduction in left ventricular ejection fraction that accompanies the wall-motion abnormalities on presentation is transient, and complete recovery of systolic function usually occurs over the first 6 to 8 weeks following the onset but can resolve as early as within 2 to 3 days.[4,10,14,17] The apical ballooning or typical variant is the most common (**Fig. 3**), but 17% to 41% of reported TTC cases have preserved apical function with midventricular akinesis or hypokinesis instead.[14,15,23,24] These forms have been termed atypical variant, apical sparing variant, or midventricular ballooning syndrome (**Fig. 4**). The least common variant is known as the inverted/reverse TTC, whereby the basal segments are hypokinetic/akinetic and the function of apex is preserved. Although they have a different morphology, these variant forms of TTC have clinical characteristics and prognosis similar to those of the typical form.[24] The right ventricle, in particular the apex, is involved in 26% to 34% of patients and is associated with lower left ventricular ejection fraction when compared with patients with normal right ventricular function.[130,131] Moreover, right ventricular regional wall-motion abnormalities typically resolve on follow-up.[130,131] In one study, patients with TTC were found to have better left ventricular diastolic function, but worse systolic function and higher systolic strain, in comparison with a control group of patients with ST-segment elevation myocardial infarction.[132]

Cardiac Magnetic Resonance Imaging

Cardiac magnetic resonance imaging (MRI) is helpful in differentiating TTC from acute myocardial infarction and myocarditis. Typically the cardiac MRI in TTC patients does not demonstrate delayed gadolinium enhancement, whereas intense subendocardial or transmural hyperenhancement is seen in acute myocardial infarction.[12,15,25,133] Likewise, myocarditis may result in patchy, delayed gadolinium hyperenhancement. Cardiac MRI may also be more sensitive than echocardiography and left ventriculography for detecting thrombus in the left or right ventricle.[10]

DIAGNOSTIC CRITERIA

The diagnosis of TTC should be a consideration in patients presenting with features of an acute myocardial infarction and reduced left ventricular function in the absence of significant CAD. The lack of a diagnostic test and the variability in clinical presentations necessitates the use of diagnostic criteria that encompass the broadest defining features of TTC. The Mayo Clinic diagnostic criteria for TTC have been widely used and are based on

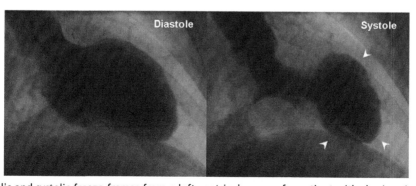

Fig. 3. Diastolic and systolic freeze frames from a left ventriculogram of a patient with classic apical ballooning syndrome illustrating hyperdynamic basal contraction, but akinesis of the mid and apical segments (*arrowheads*). (*Reproduced from* Prasad A, Lerman A, Rihal CS. Apical ballooning syndrome (Tako-Tsubo or stress cardiomyopathy): a mimic of acute myocardial infarction. Am Heart J 2008;155:410; with permission.)

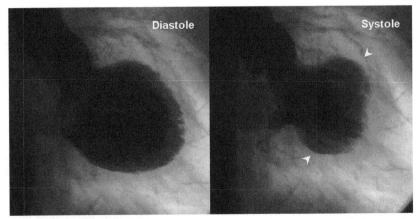

Fig. 4. Diastolic and systolic freeze-frames from a left ventriculogram of a patient with the apical sparing variant of apical ballooning syndrome. Function at the base and apex is preserved with akinesis of the mid segments (*arrowheads*). (*Reproduced from* Prasad A, Lerman A, Rihal CS. Apical ballooning syndrome (Tako-Tsubo or stress cardiomyopathy): a mimic of acute myocardial infarction. Am Heart J 2008;155:410; with permission.)

an expert consensus (**Box 2**).[1,4] It is important that age, gender, and the presence of a precipitating factor are not included in the criteria, as TTC can occur in younger women, men, and in the absence of a stressor. In addition, the reversibility of left ventricular systolic dysfunction is not included, given

> **Box 2**
> **Mayo Clinic diagnostic criteria for apical ballooning syndrome (takotsubo cardiomyopathy)**
>
> 1. Transient hypokinesis, akinesis, or dyskinesis of the left ventricular mid segments with or without apical involvement; the regional wall motion abnormalities extend beyond a single epicardial vascular distribution; a stressful trigger is often, but not always present[a]
>
> 2. Absence of obstructive coronary disease or angiographic evidence of acute plaque rupture[b]
>
> 3. New electrocardiographic abnormalities (either ST-segment elevation and/or T-wave inversion) or modest elevation in cardiac troponin
>
> 4. Absence of pheochromocytoma and/or myocarditis
>
> [a] There are rare exceptions to these criteria such as those patients in whom the regional wall-motion abnormality is limited to a single coronary territory.
> [b] It is possible that a patient with obstructive coronary atherosclerosis may also develop apical ballooning syndrome. However, this is very rare in the authors' experience and in the published literature, perhaps because such cases are misdiagnosed as an ACS.

this can take up to 8 weeks to occur. The diagnosis of TTC cannot be established before coronary angiography and imaging of the heart, and hence in patients with ST-segment elevation on the electrocardiogram that meets criteria for acute myocardial infarction, reperfusion therapy (ie, either proceeding to emergency coronary angiography with the intention of performing primary percutaneous coronary intervention, or administration of fibrinolytic therapy) should not be withheld. In cases with a high index of suspicion for TTC, administration of fibrinolytics may be deferred if immediate access to cardiac catheterization to differentiate the 2 conditions is feasible.

TREATMENT AND PROGNOSIS

There are inadequate published data for an evidence-based approach to the management of TTC. In general, patients are treated with standard heart-failure medications including angiotensin-converting enzyme inhibitors and β-receptor blockers. Angiotensin-converting enzyme inhibitors may be discontinued once there is complete recovery of systolic function, but it is reasonable to continue therapy with β-receptor blockers with the goal of preventing recurrence. Diuretics are used for treating pulmonary edema, and cases with severe cardiogenic shock may necessitate IABP or inotropic support. The presence of moderate to severe left ventricular outflow tract obstruction precludes the use of inotropes, as these can worsen the obstruction. Aspirin and statins are often prescribed if there is coexistent CAD.

The prognosis of TTC is generally very good, although there is some heterogeneity with respect to acute outcomes. Patients who are admitted to hospital with the primary diagnosis of TTC may be

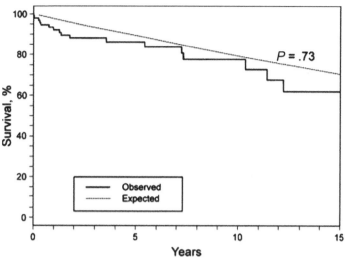

Fig. 5. Survival of patients with apical ballooning syndrome versus an age-matched and gender-matched population. Kaplan-Meier curves show observed and expected survival over time. (*Reproduced from* Elesber AA, Prasad A, Lennon RJ, et al. Four-year recurrence rate and prognosis of the apical ballooning syndrome. J Am Coll Cardiol 2007;50(5):451; with permission.)

risk stratified using the Mayo Clinic risk score.[112] This score determines the likelihood of acute heart failure developing as a consequence of left ventricular dysfunction. One point each is assigned for the presence of the following 3 variables: age older than 70 years, presence of a physical stressor, and left ventricular ejection fraction less than 40%. The likelihood of developing acute heart failure in development cohort for the model was less than 10%, 28%, 58%, and 85% in the presence of no, 1, 2, or 3 risk factors, respectively. In-hospital mortality rates range from 0% to 8%, and patients who survive the acute event generally recover normal left ventricular function over a matter of a few weeks.[4,7,30,37] Over a follow-up of about 5 years, 31% of patients will continue to experience chest pain and up to 10% of patients will have a recurrent episode of TTC.[31] Long-term survival for those discharged from hospital is similar to that expected in an age-matched and gender-matched population (**Fig. 5**).

REFERENCES

1. Prasad A, Lerman A, Rihal CS. Apical ballooning syndrome (Tako-Tsubo or stress cardiomyopathy): a mimic of acute myocardial infarction. Am Heart J 2008;155:408–17.

2. Prasad A. Apical ballooning syndrome: an important differential diagnosis of acute myocardial infarction. Circulation 2007;115:e56–9.

3. Bybee KA, Prasad A. Stress-related cardiomyopathy syndromes. Circulation 2008;118:397–409.

4. Bybee KA, Kara T, Prasad A, et al. Systematic review: transient left ventricular apical ballooning: a syndrome that mimics ST-segment elevation myocardial infarction. Ann Intern Med 2004;141: 858–65.

5. Dote K, Sato H, Tateishi H, et al. Myocardial stunning due to simultaneous multivessel coronary spasms: a review of 5 cases. J Cardiol 1991;21: 203–14 [in Japanese].

6. Bybee KA, Prasad A, Barsness GW, et al. Clinical characteristics and thrombolysis in myocardial infarction frame counts in women with transient left ventricular apical ballooning syndrome. Am J Cardiol 2004;94:343–6.

7. Sharkey SW, Lesser JR, Zenovich AG, et al. Acute and reversible cardiomyopathy provoked by stress in women from the United States. Circulation 2005; 111:472–9.

8. Hachamovitch R, Chang JD, Kuntz RE, et al. Recurrent reversible cardiogenic shock triggered by emotional distress with no obstructive coronary disease. Am Heart J 1995;129:1026–8.

9. Wittstein IS, Thiemann DR, Lima JA, et al. Neurohumoral features of myocardial stunning due to sudden emotional stress. N Engl J Med 2005;352:539–48.

10. Sharkey SW, Windenburg DC, Lesser JR, et al. Natural history and expansive clinical profile of stress (tako-tsubo) cardiomyopathy. J Am Coll Cardiol 2010;55:333–41.

11. Seth PS, Aurigemma GP, Krasnow JM, et al. A syndrome of transient left ventricular apical wall motion abnormality in the absence of coronary disease: a perspective from the United States. Cardiology 2003;100:61–6.

12. Mitchell JH, Hadden TB, Wilson JM, et al. Clinical features and usefulness of cardiac magnetic resonance imaging in assessing myocardial viability and prognosis in Takotsubo cardiomyopathy (transient left ventricular apical ballooning syndrome). Am J Cardiol 2007;100:296–301.

13. Hoyt J, Lerman A, Lennon RJ, et al. Left anterior descending artery length and coronary atherosclerosis in apical ballooning syndrome (Takotsubo/stress induced cardiomyopathy). Int J Cardiol 2009;145:112–5.

14. Kurowski V, Kaiser A, von Hof K, et al. Apical and midventricular transient left ventricular dysfunction syndrome (tako-tsubo cardiomyopathy): frequency, mechanisms, and prognosis. Chest 2007;132:809–16.

15. Haghi D, Fluechter S, Suselbeck T, et al. Cardiovascular magnetic resonance findings in typical versus atypical forms of the acute apical ballooning syndrome (Takotsubo cardiomyopathy). Int J Cardiol 2007;120:205–11.

16. El Mahmoud R, Mansencal N, Pilliere R, et al. Prevalence and characteristics of left ventricular outflow tract obstruction in Tako-Tsubo syndrome. Am Heart J 2008;156:543–8.

17. Desmet WJ, Adriaenssens BF, Dens JA. Apical ballooning of the left ventricle: first series in white patients. Heart 2003;89:1027–31.

18. Kurisu S, Sato H, Kawagoe T, et al. Tako-tsubo-like left ventricular dysfunction with ST-segment elevation: a novel cardiac syndrome mimicking acute myocardial infarction. Am Heart J 2002;143:448–55.

19. Akashi YJ, Musha H, Kida K, et al. Reversible ventricular dysfunction takotsubo cardiomyopathy. Eur J Heart Fail 2005;7:1171–6.

20. Abe Y, Kondo M, Matsuoka R, et al. Assessment of clinical features in transient left ventricular apical ballooning. J Am Coll Cardiol 2003;41:737–42.

21. Abdulla I, Kay S, Mussap C, et al. Apical sparing in tako-tsubo cardiomyopathy. Intern Med J 2006;36: 414–8.

22. Maron BJ, Towbin JA, Thiene G, et al. Contemporary definitions and classification of the cardiomyopathies: an American Heart Association Scientific Statement from the Council on Clinical Cardiology, Heart Failure and Transplantation Committee; Quality of Care and Outcomes Research and Functional Genomics and Translational Biology Interdisciplinary Working Groups; and Council on Epidemiology and Prevention. Circulation 2006; 113:1807–16.

23. Hurst RT, Askew JW, Reuss CS, et al. Transient midventricular ballooning syndrome: a new variant. J Am Coll Cardiol 2006;48:579–83.

24. Hahn JY, Gwon HC, Park SW, et al. The clinical features of transient left ventricular nonapical ballooning syndrome: comparison with apical ballooning syndrome. Am Heart J 2007;154:1166–73.

25. Eitel I, von Knobelsdorff-Brenkenhoff F, Bernhardt P, et al. Clinical characteristics and cardiovascular magnetic resonance findings in stress (takotsubo) cardiomyopathy. JAMA 2011;306:277–86.

26. Nef HM, Mollmann H, Kostin S, et al. Tako-Tsubo cardiomyopathy: intraindividual structural analysis in the acute phase and after functional recovery. Eur Heart J 2007;28:2456–64.

27. Gianni M, Dentali F, Grandi AM, et al. Apical ballooning syndrome or takotsubo cardiomyopathy: a systematic review. Eur Heart J 2006;27:1523–9.

28. Azzarelli S, Galassi AR, Amico F, et al. Clinical features of transient left ventricular apical ballooning. Am J Cardiol 2006;98:1273–6.

29. Deshmukh A, Kumar G, Pant S, et al. Prevalence of Takotsubo cardiomyopathy in the United States. Am Heart J 2012;164:66–71.e61.

30. Akashi YJ, Goldstein DS, Barbaro G, et al. Takotsubo cardiomyopathy: a new form of acute, reversible heart failure. Circulation 2008;118:2754–62.

31. Elesber AA, Prasad A, Lennon RJ, et al. Four-year recurrence rate and prognosis of the apical ballooning syndrome. J Am Coll Cardiol 2007;50: 448–52.

32. Lee VH, Connolly HM, Fulgham JR, et al. Takotsubo cardiomyopathy in aneurysmal subarachnoid hemorrhage: an underappreciated ventricular dysfunction. J Neurosurg 2006;105:264–70.

33. Lee VH, Oh JK, Mulvagh SL, et al. Mechanisms in neurogenic stress cardiomyopathy after aneurysmal subarachnoid hemorrhage. Neurocrit Care 2006;5:243–9.

34. Summers MR, Madhavan M, Chokka RG, et al. Coincidence of apical ballooning syndrome (takotsubo/stress cardiomyopathy) and posterior reversible encephalopathy syndrome: potential common substrate and pathophysiology? J Card Fail 2012;18:120–5.

35. Pilgrim TM, Wyss TR. Takotsubo cardiomyopathy or transient left ventricular apical ballooning syndrome: A systematic review. Int J Cardiol 2008;124:283–92.

36. Park JH, Kang SJ, Song JK, et al. Left ventricular apical ballooning due to severe physical stress in patients admitted to the medical ICU. Chest 2005;128:296–302.

37. Tsuchihashi K, Ueshima K, Uchida T, et al. Transient left ventricular apical ballooning without coronary artery stenosis: a novel heart syndrome mimicking acute myocardial infarction. Angina Pectoris-Myocardial Infarction Investigations in Japan. J Am Coll Cardiol 2001;38:11–8.

38. Mittal M, Needham E. Case report: Takotsubo cardiomyopathy in a recently widowed woman. Am Fam Physician 2009;80:908.

39. Stollberger C, Sporn R, Skala K, et al. Assault-induced Takotsubo cardiomyopathy associated

with persisting anterograde amnesia and myopathy. Int J Legal Med 2010;124:467–70.

40. Schutte F, Ebstein M, Rottmann M, et al. Nearly asymptomatic left ventricular apical ballooning after a hit-and-run accident. Int J Cardiol 2008; 128:439–41.

41. Vieweg WV, Hasnain M, Mezuk B, et al. Depression, stress, and heart disease in earthquakes and Takotsubo cardiomyopathy. Am J Med 2011; 124:900–7.

42. Brunetti ND, De Gennaro L, Correale M, et al. Les liaisons dangereuses: tako-Tsubo syndrome after an adulterous intercourse in an elderly male. Int J Cardiol 2011;149:e113–7.

43. Glamore M, Wolf C, Boolbol J, et al. Broken heart syndrome: a risk of teenage rhinoplasty. Aesthet Surg J 2012;32:58–60.

44. Zdanowicz JA, Utz AC, Bernasconi I, et al. "Broken heart" after cesarean delivery. Case report and review of literature. Arch Gynecol Obstet 2011; 283:687–94.

45. Joo I, Lee JM, Han JK, et al. Stress (tako-tsubo) cardiomyopathy following radiofrequency ablation of a liver tumor: a case report. Cardiovasc Intervent Radiol 2011;34(Suppl 2):S86–9.

46. Modi S, Baig W. Radiotherapy-induced Tako-tsubo cardiomyopathy. Clin Oncol (R Coll Radiol) 2009; 21:361–2.

47. Mohammad M, Patel AK, Koirala A, et al. Tako-tsubo cardiomyopathy following colonoscopy: insights on pathogenesis. Int J Cardiol 2011;147:e46–9.

48. Vidi V, Singh PP, Nesto RW. Tako-tsubo syndrome following a difficult urinary catheterization. Int J Cardiol 2009;134:247–9.

49. Serby MJ, Lantz M, Chabus BI, et al. Takotsubo cardiomyopathy and electroconvulsive treatments: a case study and review. Int J Psychiatry Med 2010;40:93–6.

50. Karatayli-Ozgursoy S, Lundy LB, Zapala DA, et al. Takotsubo cardiomyopathy and canalith repositioning procedure for benign paroxysmal positional vertigo. J Am Acad Audiol 2010;21:73–7 [quiz: 139–40].

51. Syed ON, Heyer EJ, Connolly ES Jr. Takotsubo syndrome after carotid endarterectomy. J Neurosurg Anesthesiol 2009;21:181–2.

52. Hasdemir C, Yavuzgil O, Simsek E, et al. Stress cardiomyopathy (Tako-Tsubo) following radiofrequency ablation in the right ventricular outflow tract. Europace 2008;10:1452–4.

53. Golzio PG, Anselmino M, Presutti D, et al. Takotsubo cardiomyopathy as a complication of pacemaker implantation. J Cardiovasc Med (Hagerstown) 2011; 12:754–60.

54. Eggleton S, Mathur G, Lambros J. An unusual precipitant of tako-tsubo cardiomyopathy. Heart Lung Circ 2008;17:512–4.

55. Stanojevic DA, Alla VM, Lynch JD, et al. Case of reverse takotsubo cardiomyopathy in status asthmaticus. South Med J 2010;103:964.

56. Dande AS, Fisher LI, Warshofsky MK. Inverted takotsubo cardiomyopathy. J Invasive Cardiol 2011;23:E76–8.

57. Cheezum MK, Willis SL, Duffy SP, et al. Broken pancreas, broken heart. Am J Gastroenterol 2010;105:237–8.

58. Awais M, Hernandez RA, Bach DS. Takotsubo cardiomyopathy triggered by severe vomiting. Am J Med 2008;121:e3–4.

59. Novo G, Ferro G, Fazio G, et al. Takotsubo cardiomyopathy after acute diarrhea. Intern Med 2010; 49:903–5.

60. Hassan S, Hassan F, Hassan D, et al. Takotsubo cardiomyopathy associated with peritonitis in peritoneal dialysis patient. Ren Fail 2011;33:904–7.

61. Geng S, Mullany D, Fraser JF. Takotsubo cardiomyopathy associated with sepsis due to Streptococcus pneumoniae pneumonia. Crit Care Resusc 2008;10:231–4.

62. Palacio C, Nugent K, Alalawi R, et al. Severe reversible myocardial depression in a patient with Pseudomonas aeruginosa sepsis suggesting tako-tsubo cardiomyopathy. Int J Cardiol 2009;135:e16–9.

63. Odigie-Okon E, Okon E, Dodson J, et al. Stress-induced cardiomyopathy complicating severe babesiosis. Cardiol J 2011;18:83–6.

64. Chia PL, Foo D. Tako-tsubo cardiomyopathy precipitated by pheochromocytoma crisis. Cardiol J 2011;18:564–7.

65. Gingles C, Leslie S, Harvey R. A case of Takotsubo's cardiomyopathy and multiple endocrine neoplasia 2A syndrome. Clin Endocrinol (Oxf) 2010;73:827–9.

66. Oe K, Mori K, Otsuji M, et al. Takotsubo cardiomyopathy with marked ST-segment elevation and electrical alternans complicated with hyperglycemic hyperosmolar state. Int Heart J 2008;49: 629–35.

67. AbouEzzeddine O, Prasad A. Apical ballooning syndrome precipitated by hyponatremia. Int J Cardiol 2010;145:e26–9.

68. Kawano H, Matsumoto Y, Arakawa S, et al. Takotsubo cardiomyopathy in a patient with severe hyponatremia associated with syndrome of inappropriate antidiuretic hormone. Intern Med 2010;50:727–32.

69. Cakir M. Takotsubo cardiomyopathy in thyrotoxicosis. Int J Cardiol 2010;145:499–500.

70. Kwon SA, Yang JH, Kim MK, et al. A case of Takotsubo cardiomyopathy in a patient with iatrogenic thyrotoxicosis. Int J Cardiol 2010;145:e111–3.

71. Micallef T, Gruppetta M, Cassar A, et al. Takotsubo cardiomyopathy and severe hypothyroidism. J Cardiovasc Med (Hagerstown) 2011;12:824–7.

72. Punnam SR, Gourineni N, Gupta V. Takotsubo cardiomyopathy in a patient with Addison disease. Int J Cardiol 2010;144:e34–6.

73. Ukita C, Miyazaki H, Toyoda N, et al. Takotsubo cardiomyopathy during acute adrenal crisis due to isolated adrenocorticotropin deficiency. Intern Med 2009;48:347–52.

74. Lim T, Murakami H, Hayashi K, et al. Takotsubo cardiomyopathy associated with autoimmune polyendocrine syndrome II. J Cardiol 2009;53:306–10.

75. Zhan H, Zheng H, Moliterno AR, et al. Acute cardiomyopathy in a patient with thrombotic thrombocytopenic purpura. Am J Med 2010;123:e3–4.

76. Wever-Pinzon O, Tami L. Takotsubo cardiomyopathy following a blood transfusion. Congest Heart Fail 2010;16:129–31.

77. Takemoto F, Chihara N, Sawa N, et al. Takotsubo cardiomyopathy in a patient undergoing hemodialysis. Kidney Int 2009;76:467.

78. Bansal V, Kansal MM, Rowin J. Broken heart syndrome in myasthenia gravis. Muscle Nerve 2011;44:990–3.

79. Schneider F, Kadel C, Pagitz M, et al. Takotsubo cardiomyopathy and elevated troponin levels following cerebral seizure. Int J Cardiol 2010;145:586–7.

80. Gelow J, Kruer M, Yadav V, et al. Apical ballooning resulting from limbic encephalitis. Am J Med 2009;122:583–6.

81. Morita S, Inokuchi S, Yamagiwa T, et al. Tako-tsubo-like left ventricular dysfunction with ST-segment elevation after central spinal cord injury: a case report. J Emerg Med 2010;39:301–4.

82. Scheitz JF, Mochmann HC, Witzenbichler B, et al. Takotsubo cardiomyopathy following ischemic stroke: a cause of troponin elevation. J Neurol 2012;259:188–90.

83. Martins RP, Barbarot N, Coquerel N, et al. Takotsubo cardiomyopathy associated with Guillain-Barre syndrome: a differential diagnosis from dysautonomia not to be missed. J Neurol Sci 2010;291:100–2.

84. Rivera JM, Locketz AJ, Fritz KD, et al. "Broken heart syndrome" after separation (from OxyContin). Mayo Clin Proc 2006;81:825–8.

85. Yazdan-Ashoori P, Nichols R, Baranchuk A. Tako-tsubo cardiomyopathy precipitated by alcohol withdrawal. Cardiol J 2012;19:81–5.

86. Arora S, Alfayoumi F, Srinivasan V. Transient left ventricular apical ballooning after cocaine use: is catecholamine cardiotoxicity the pathologic link? Mayo Clin Proc 2006;81:829–32.

87. Alsidawi S, Muth J, Wilkin J. Adderall induced inverted-Takotsubo cardiomyopathy. Catheter Cardiovasc Interv 2011;78:910–3.

88. De Roock S, Beauloye C, De Bauwer I, et al. Tako-tsubo syndrome following nortriptyline overdose. Clin Toxicol (Phila) 2008;46:475–8.

89. Christoph M, Ebner B, Stolte D, et al. Broken heart syndrome: Tako Tsubo cardiomyopathy associated with an overdose of the serotonin-norepinephrine reuptake inhibitor Venlafaxine. Eur Neuropsychopharmacol 2010;20:594–7.

90. Rennyson SL, Parker JM, Symanski JD, et al. Recurrent, severe, and rapidly reversible apical ballooning syndrome in status asthmaticus. Heart Lung 2010;39:537–9.

91. Gabriel L, Chenu P, Guedes A, et al. A possible association between takotsubo cardiomyopathy and treatment with flecainide. Int J Cardiol 2011;147:173–5.

92. Jefic D, Koul D, Boguszewski A, et al. Transient left ventricular apical ballooning syndrome caused by abrupt metoprolol withdrawal. Int J Cardiol 2008;131:e35–7.

93. Winogradow J, Geppert G, Reinhard W, et al. Tako-tsubo cardiomyopathy after administration of intravenous epinephrine during an anaphylactic reaction. Int J Cardiol 2011;147:309–11.

94. Manivannan V, Li JT, Prasad A, et al. Apical ballooning syndrome after administration of intravenous epinephrine during an anaphylactic reaction. Mayo Clin Proc 2009;84:845–6.

95. Basselin C, Fontanges T, Descotes J, et al. 5-Fluorouracil-induced Tako-Tsubo-like syndrome. Pharmacotherapy 2011;31:226.

96. Trohman RG, Madias C. Duloxetine-induced tako-tsubo cardiomyopathy: implications for preventing a broken heart. South Med J 2011;104:303–4.

97. Skolnick AH, Michelin K, Nayar A, et al. Transient apical ballooning syndrome precipitated by dobutamine stress testing. Ann Intern Med 2009;150:501–2.

98. Koh AS, Kok H, Chua T, et al. Takotsubo cardiomyopathy following dipyridamole pharmacologic stress. Ann Nucl Med 2010;24:497–500.

99. Dorfman T, Aqel R, Allred J, et al. Takotsubo cardiomyopathy induced by treadmill exercise testing: an insight into the pathophysiology of transient left ventricular apical (or midventricular) ballooning in the absence of obstructive coronary artery disease. J Am Coll Cardiol 2007;49:1223–5.

100. Dundon BK, Puri R, Leong DP, et al. Takotsubo cardiomyopathy following lightning strike. Emerg Med J 2008;25:460–1.

101. Bianchi R, Torella D, Spaccarotella C, et al. Mediterranean jellyfish sting-induced Tako-Tsubo cardiomyopathy. Eur Heart J 2011;32:18.

102. Citro R, Patella MM, Bossone E, et al. Near-drowning syndrome: a possible trigger of tako-tsubo cardiomyopathy. J Cardiovasc Med (Hagerstown) 2008;9:501–5.

103. Yokobori S, Miyauchi M, Eura S, et al. Takotsubo cardiomyopathy after severe burn injury: a poorly

recognized cause of acute left ventricular dysfunction. J Trauma 2010;68:E77–9.

104. Vergez M, Pirracchio R, Mateo J, et al. Tako Tsubo cardiomyopathy in a patient with multiple trauma. Resuscitation 2009;80:1074–7.

105. Chen WT, Lin CH, Hsieh MH, et al. Stress-induced cardiomyopathy caused by heat stroke. Ann Emerg Med 2012;60(1):63–6.

106. Kaoukis A, Panagopoulou V, Mojibian HR, et al. Reverse Takotsubo cardiomyopathy associated with the consumption of an energy drink. Circulation 2012;125:1584–5.

107. Pison L, De Vusser P, Mullens W. Apical ballooning in relatives. Heart 2004;90:e67.

108. Kumar G, Holmes DR Jr, Prasad A. "Familial" apical ballooning syndrome (Takotsubo cardiomyopathy). Int J Cardiol 2010;144:444–5.

109. Summers MR, Lennon RJ, Prasad A. Pre-morbid psychiatric and cardiovascular diseases in apical ballooning syndrome (tako-tsubo/stress-induced cardiomyopathy): potential pre-disposing factors? J Am Coll Cardiol 2011;55:700–1.

110. Kurisu S, Inoue I, Kawagoe T, et al. Presentation of Tako-tsubo cardiomyopathy in men and women. Clin Cardiol 2010;33:42–5.

111. Brenner R, Weilenmann D, Maeder MT, et al. Clinical characteristics, sex hormones, and long-term follow-up in Swiss postmenopausal women presenting with takotsubo cardiomyopathy. Clin Cardiol 2012;35:340–7.

112. Madhavan M, Rihal CS, Lerman A, et al. Acute heart failure in apical ballooning syndrome (TakoTsubo/ stress cardiomyopathy): clinical correlates and Mayo Clinic risk score. J Am Coll Cardiol 2011;57: 1400–1.

113. Villareal RP, Achari A, Wilansky S, et al. Anteroapical stunning and left ventricular outflow tract obstruction. Mayo Clin Proc 2001;76:79–83.

114. Shah BN, Curzen NP. Dynamic left ventricular outflow tract obstruction and acute heart failure in tako-tsubo cardiomyopathy. J Am Coll Cardiol 2011;58:1195–6 [author reply: 1196].

115. Kumar S, Kaushik S, Nautiyal A, et al. Cardiac rupture in takotsubo cardiomyopathy: a systematic review. Clin Cardiol 2011;34:672–6.

116. Sharkey SW, Lesser JR, Menon M, et al. Spectrum and significance of electrocardiographic patterns, troponin levels, and thrombolysis in myocardial infarction frame count in patients with stress (tako-tsubo) cardiomyopathy and comparison to those in patients with ST-elevation anterior wall myocardial infarction. Am J Cardiol 2008;101: 1723–8.

117. Dib C, Asirvatham S, Elesber A, et al. Clinical correlates and prognostic significance of electrocardiographic abnormalities in apical ballooning syndrome (Takotsubo/stress-induced cardiomyopathy). Am Heart J 2009;157:933–8.

118. Sato M, Fujita S, Saito A, et al. Increased incidence of transient left ventricular apical ballooning (so-called 'Takotsubo' cardiomyopathy) after the mid-Niigata Prefecture earthquake. Circ J 2006;70: 947–53.

119. Bybee KA, Motiei A, Syed IS, et al. Electrocardiography cannot reliably differentiate transient left ventricular apical ballooning syndrome from anterior ST-segment elevation myocardial infarction. J Electrocardiol 2007;40:38.e1–6.

120. Johnson NP, Chavez JF, Mosley WJ 2nd, et al. Performance of electrocardiographic criteria to differentiate Takotsubo cardiomyopathy from acute anterior ST elevation myocardial infarction. Int J Cardiol 2011. [Epub ahead of print].

121. Kosuge M, Ebina T, Hibi K, et al. Simple and accurate electrocardiographic criteria to differentiate takotsubo cardiomyopathy from anterior acute myocardial infarction. J Am Coll Cardiol 2010;55: 2514–6.

122. Takashio S, Yamamuro M, Kojima S, et al. Usefulness of SUM of ST-segment elevation on electrocardiograms (limb leads) for predicting in-hospital complications in patients with stress (takotsubo) cardiomyopathy. Am J Cardiol 2012;109:1651–6.

123. Dib C, Prasad A, Friedman PA, et al. Malignant arrhythmia in apical ballooning syndrome: risk factors and outcomes. Indian Pacing Electrophysiol J 2008;8:182–92.

124. Syed FF, Asirvatham SJ, Francis J. Arrhythmia occurrence with takotsubo cardiomyopathy: a literature review. Europace 2011;13:780–8.

125. Akashi YJ, Musha H, Nakazawa K, et al. Plasma brain natriuretic peptide in takotsubo cardiomyopathy. QJM 2004;97:599–607.

126. Ahmed KA, Madhavan M, Prasad A. Brain natriuretic peptide in apical ballooning syndrome (Takotsubo/ stress cardiomyopathy): comparison with acute myocardial infarction. Coron Artery Dis 2012;23: 259–64.

127. Madhavan M, Borlaug BA, Lerman A, et al. Stress hormone and circulating biomarker profile of apical ballooning syndrome (Takotsubo cardiomyopathy): insights into the clinical significance of B-type natriuretic peptide and troponin levels. Heart 2009;95: 1436–41.

128. Nguyen TH, Neil CJ, Sverdlov AL, et al. N-terminal pro-brain natriuretic protein levels in takotsubo cardiomyopathy. Am J Cardiol 2011;108: 1316–21.

129. Gaibazzi N, Ugo F, Vignali L, et al. Tako-Tsubo cardiomyopathy with coronary artery stenosis: a case-series challenging the original definition. Int J Cardiol 2009;133:205–12.

130. Elesber AA, Prasad A, Bybee KA, et al. Transient cardiac apical ballooning syndrome: prevalence and clinical implications of right ventricular involvement. J Am Coll Cardiol 2006;47:1082–3.

131. Haghi D, Athanasiadis A, Papavassiliu T, et al. Right ventricular involvement in Takotsubo cardiomyopathy. Eur Heart J 2006;27:2433–9.

132. Park SM, Prasad A, Rihal C, et al. Left ventricular systolic and diastolic function in patients with apical ballooning syndrome compared with patients with acute anterior ST-segment elevation myocardial infarction: a functional paradox. Mayo Clin Proc 2009;84:514–21.

133. Deetjen AG, Conradi G, Mollmann S, et al. Value of gadolinium-enhanced magnetic resonance imaging in patients with Tako-Tsubo-like left ventricular dysfunction. J Cardiovasc Magn Reson 2006; 8:367–72.

Takotsubo Cardiomyopathy
Natural History

Scott W. Sharkey, MD

KEYWORDS

- Takotsubo cardiomyopathy • Stress cardiomyopathy • Congestive heart failure

KEY POINTS

- Takotsubo (stress) cardiomyopathy is a recently recognized cardiomyopathy with acute onset, distinctive left ventricular (LV) contraction profile, and a predilection for women older than 50 years. It is often triggered by a stressful event and is typically completely reversible.
- At presentation, takotsubo cardiomyopathy resembles acute coronary syndrome with ischemic electrocardiogram changes and troponin elevation. Abnormal regional LV contraction is in a non-coronary distribution and occurs in the absence of acute coronary artery obstruction.
- A triggering stressful event, either physical or emotional, is frequent but not universal.
- Complications include congestive heart failure, ventricular arrhythmias, left ventricular outflow tract obstruction, and ventricular mural thrombi with the potential for embolization.
- Hospital rate of mortality is low but after hospital survival is less than the general population and rate of recurrence is 5% to 10%. Complete recovery of LV systolic function is a hallmark.

INTRODUCTION

Takotsubo (stress) cardiomyopathy (TTC) is a recently recognized cardiomyopathy with acute onset, characterized by a distinctive left ventricular (LV) contraction profile, a predilection for middle-aged and older women, which is triggered by a stressful event and typically completely reversible. The clinical presentation resembles that of acute coronary syndrome, yet this cardiomyopathy occurs in the absence of significant obstructive coronary artery disease.[1–6] Although uncommon, 5%–10% of women with suspected acute coronary syndrome are ultimately proven to have TTC.[7–10]

The first reports of this cardiomyopathy emerged from Japan in 1991 at which time Dote and colleagues[11] reported 5 patients with a novel acute cardiac condition characterized by distinctive LV dysfunction in the absence of atherosclerotic obstructive coronary artery disease. These and other investigators were intrigued by the unusual end-systolic LV shape (as captured on right anterior oblique left ventriculogram), which resembled the Japanese takotsubo, a pot with a narrow neck and round bottom used for the harvest of the octopus (Fig. 1). Consequently, the term takotsubo cardiomyopathy was introduced to describe this condition.[12,13]

For several years, recognition of TTC was confined to Japan and much of the early literature was written in the Japanese language. Beginning in the late 1990s, publications first emerged in the English literature; thereafter, TTC became widely recognized with greater than 1000 reports by 2011.[13–16] The condition is now recognized worldwide and during this process has acquired a variety of additional names (at least 75), the most common being stress cardiomyopathy and apical ballooning syndrome.[16] With this increased attention has come the recognition that TTC has

Disclosures/Conflict of Interest: None.
Cardiovascular Research Division, Minneapolis Heart Institute Foundation, 920 East 28th Street, Suite 620, Minneapolis, MN 55407, USA
E-mail address: scott.sharkey@allina.com

Heart Failure Clin 9 (2013) 123–136
http://dx.doi.org/10.1016/j.hfc.2012.12.006

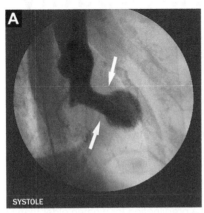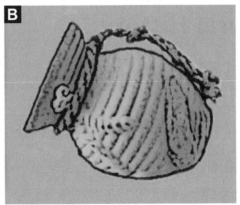

Fig. 1. (*A*) Left ventriculogram (right anterior oblique projection) at end-systole demonstrating classic apical ballooning pattern. Arrows depict demarcation between hypercontractile basal myocardium and dyskinetic ballooning apex. (*B*) The Japanese takotsubo has a shape that resembles the left ventricle.

a much more diverse clinical presentation than initially considered.[2,5,17–20]

ACUTE PRESENTATION

The clinical features of TTC are summarized in **Table 1**. Patients usually present to the emergency department with sudden onset of chest discomfort or shortness of breath, symptoms indistinguishable from acute coronary syndrome. In an important minority, TTC occurs during hospitalization for a noncardiac illness, in which case symptoms may be atypical or absent, and cardiac evaluation is triggered by hypotension, tachycardia, heart failure, abnormal electrocardiogram (ECG), or unexpected troponin elevation.[18] The ECG often shows ischemic changes, most frequently ST-segment elevation. Furthermore, the initial troponin is elevated in 90% of patients. By currently established guidelines, patients with TTC usually meet the definition for acute myocardial infarction.[21]

The clinician may suspect TTC because of its predilection for older women and its usual association with an antecedent stressful event. The average age at onset is 65 to 70 years, although the condition has been described in younger patients, including a 2-year-old girl.[2,17,22] Men comprise only 10% to 15% of patients.[2,5] The inciting stressor (**Table 2**) may be physical (40%–45% of patients), such as sepsis or acute respiratory failure, or emotional (40%–45% of patients), such as anger or grief from a death of a family member.[8,17] Questioning the patient and family is useful because some emotional stressors may be intensely private. It is now recognized that TTC also occurs spontaneously (in the absence of an overt stressor) in up to 30% of patients, consequently the term stress cardiomyopathy does not accommodate all patients.[2,8,17]

DIAGNOSIS

The hallmark is a reversible LV contraction abnormality extending beyond the geographic territory of a single epicardial coronary artery, occurring in the absence of significant obstructive coronary artery disease or acute plaque rupture (**Box 1**). An urgent coronary angiogram with left ventriculogram is necessary to differentiate TTC from acute coronary syndrome. It is not unusual to note reduced epicardial coronary artery flow rate (reduced thrombolysis in myocardial infarction frame count) despite absent obstruction, likely signifying microvascular dysfunction.[23–25] Until the diagnosis is verified, it is reasonable to treat the patient with suspected TTC as you would a patient with acute coronary syndrome (aspirin, heparin, β-blocker, and clopidogrel). A 2-dimensional echocardiogram is useful to assess LV outflow tract obstruction, mitral valve regurgitation, LV and right ventricular (RV) thrombus, and RV dysfunction.

LV AND RV CONTRACTION PATTERNS

Three distinct patterns of abnormal LV contraction (ballooning) characterize TTC.[2,8,17] The LV apical ballooning pattern was the first described pattern, currently the most common and observed in 70% to 80% of patients (**Fig. 2**). More recently, the mid-ventricular ballooning pattern has been defined[26] and is present in a substantial minority of patients (20%–30%) (**Fig. 3**). A third pattern, inverted ballooning, is rarely encountered (1%–2%) and seems to occur predominantly in younger women (**Fig. 4**).[27]

Each of these LV contraction patterns is, in general, unlike that caused by obstructive coronary artery disease and can be recognized by

Table 1
Clinical features of takotsubo cardiomyopathy

Attribute	Frequency
Acute onset	Very frequent
Chest pain	Frequent
Female sex	Very frequent[a]
Age ≥50	Very frequent
Antecedent physical stressor	Frequent[a]
Antecedent emotional stressor	Frequent[a]
Antecedent stressor absent	Infrequent
ST-segment elevation on initial electrocardiogram	Frequent
Evolution to T-wave inversion	Very frequent
Troponin release	Very frequent
Left ventricular ejection fraction <50%	Very frequent
Left ventricular ejection fraction ≤35%	Very frequent
Atypical (noncoronary) regional LV wall motion abnormality	Very frequent[a]
Apical ballooning	Very frequent[a]
Midventricular ballooning	Infrequent
Inverted ballooning	Rare
Cardiovascular MRI delayed hyperenhancement	Rare
Congestive heart failure	Frequent
Right ventricular involvement	Infrequent
Left ventricular outflow tract obstruction	Infrequent
Left or right ventricular thrombus	Rare
Hypotension requiring inotrope or intra-aortic balloon pump	Infrequent
Reversible left ventricular dysfunction (stunning)	Very frequent[a]
Hospital death	Rare
Recurrence	Infrequent
Cardiac arrest	Rare
Torsade de pointes	Rare

[a] Considered a hallmark of the condition.

Table 2
Diversity of triggers in TTC patients

Physical Events	Emotional Events
Acute respiratory failure (chronic obstructive pulmonary disease)	Anger or frustration
Malignancy or chemotherapy	Job-related stress
Infection (pneumonia, peritonitis, urosepsis, wound infection)	Anxiety, fear, panic
Central nervous system (stroke, seizure, migraine)	Interpersonal conflict
Diabetes related (gastroparesis)	Grief, loss, desperation
Therapeutic drug related (catecholamine administration, drug allergy)	Financial stress
Drug abuse (alcohol withdrawal, cocaine intoxication)	
Postsurgical (knee or hip arthroplasty, hysterectomy, discectomy)	

Box 1
Diagnostic features of takotsubo cardiomyopathy

1. Acute onset
2. Reversible[a] left ventricular contraction abnormality involving both apical and midventricular segments (apical ballooning), or midventricular segments (mid-ventricular ballooning), or basal ventricular segments (inverted ballooning), not corresponding to a typical coronary artery distribution
3. Absence of acute obstructive coronary artery disease (plaque rupture or severe stenosis) in a location that could be responsible for observed abnormal left ventricular contraction[b]
4. Ischemic ECG abnormality and/or troponin elevation[c]

[a] Requires demonstration of normal wall motion and ejection fraction at follow-up.
[b] Obstructive coronary artery disease does not exclude the diagnosis.
[c] Rarely, ECG and troponin are normal in TTC.

careful examination of imaging modalities including 2-dimensional echocardiography, left ventriculography, and cardiac magnetic resonance imaging (MRI). Given the variation in LV contraction patterns, the term apical ballooning syndrome is too restrictive. The apical ballooning pattern

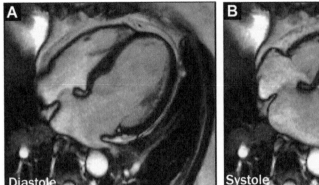
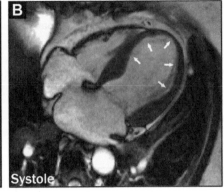

Fig. 2. Cardiac magnetic resonance images (horizontal long axis) demonstrate apical ballooning pattern. (*A*) End diastole. (*B*) End systole. Arrows depict dyskinetic mid and apical left ventricular segments with sparing of the basal segments.

resembles the wall motion abnormality caused by an acute coronary syndrome from a wrap-around left anterior descending coronary artery and the inverted ballooning pattern resembles the wall motion abnormality caused by acute myocarditis. In uncertain cases, a cardiac MRI with gadolinium contrast is valuable because late gadolinium enhancement (a marker for scar) is rarely present in TTC, yet frequently is present in a vascular distribution (acute coronary syndrome) or patchy distribution (acute myocarditis).

Abnormal RV contraction is present in about 25% of patients, usually involving the apical RV segments and best imaged with 2-dimensional echocardiography or cardiac MRI (**Fig. 5**). RV involvement can be present with either LV apical ballooning or midventricular ballooning and thrombus can form within abnormally contracting RV segments.[8,17] RV dysfunction is associated with more severe heart failure, longer hospital stay, lower LV ejection fraction, and greater hemodynamic instability.[28]

NUCLEAR IMAGING

Several nuclear imaging techniques have been used to evaluate TTC.[29,30] During the acute phase, perfusion imaging with thallium, tetrafosmin, or sestamibi demonstrates a defect extending beyond a single coronary artery distribution corresponding to the area of abnormal LV contraction. Serial imaging shows gradual resolution of the perfusion defect in association with improving LV ejection fraction (**Fig. 6**). Diminished perfusion may reflect either abnormal microvascular flow or myocyte injury (impaired cellular uptake of radioisotope). Regional perfusion defects have also been demonstrated with positron emission tomography with ammonia N-13.[31]

Metabolic imaging with ^{123}I-beta-methyl-iodophenylpentadecanoic acid or F-18 fluorodeoxyglucose demonstrates significant but reversible reduction in regional free fatty acid use and glucose transport in abnormally contracting LV segments. The size of the metabolic defect often exceeds that of the perfusion defect.[31,32]

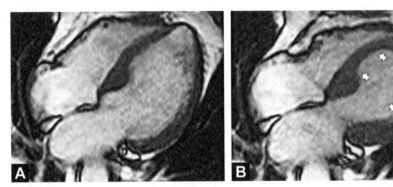

Fig. 3. Cardiac magnetic resonance images (horizontal long axis) demonstrate midventricular ballooning pattern. (*A*) End diastole. (*B*) End systole. Arrows depict dyskinetic mid left ventricular segments with sparing of the basal and apical segments.

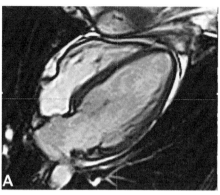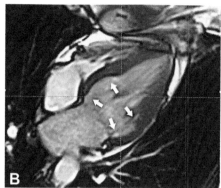

Fig. 4. Cardiac magnetic resonance images (horizontal long axis) demonstrate inverted ventricular ballooning pattern. (*A*) End diastole. (*B*) End systole. Arrows depict dyskinetic basal left ventricular segments with sparing of the mid and apical segments.

Cardiac sympathetic nerve activity imaging with the radioactive norepinephrine analogue ^{123}I-labeled *meta*-iodobenzylguanidine demonstrates reduced function in abnormally contracting myocardium, which may persist for several months.[33,34]

This constellation of abnormal perfusion, metabolism, sympathetic nerve activity, and LV contraction, each of which is reversible, likely represents myocardial stunning.[35] Whether any of these abnormalities have a cause-and-effect relationship to TTC or are merely a consequence of another process is unknown.

ECG

The initial ECG is abnormal in more than 90% of patients, usually with changes associated with myocardial ischemia.[17,23,36–40] Most common is ST-segment elevation, resembling acute anterior myocardial infarction owing to left anterior descending coronary artery occlusion, occurring in 40% to 50% of patients (**Fig. 7**). Some investigators have noted ST-segment elevation in TTC is more likely to be focused in leads V3–V6 (vs V1–V3 for acute anterior myocardial infarction); nonetheless, overlap is present.[39] Therefore, an urgent coronary angiogram is necessary to distinguish the 2 conditions reliably. Anterior Q waves may be present but generally resolve with resolution of abnormal LV wall motion. Other ECG findings include diffuse T-wave inversion, healed anterior infarction, nonspecific patterns, and left bundle branch block. Rarely (in 1%–2% of occurrences) the initial ECG is normal.[17]

An ECG hallmark is progressive and a sometimes dramatic T-wave inversion with QT interval prolongation evolving over the course of several days (**Fig. 8**).[38,41] These ECG changes may represent an electrophysiologic marker for myocardial

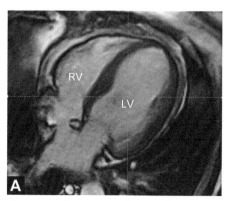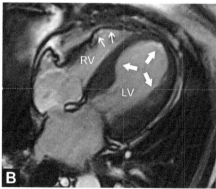

Fig. 5. Cardiac magnetic resonance images (horizontal long axis) demonstrate right ventricular apical dyskinesia and left ventricular apical ballooning pattern. (*A*) End diastole. (*B*) End systole. Small arrows depict dyskinetic right ventricular apical segments. Large arrows depict dyskinetic mid and apical left ventricular segments.

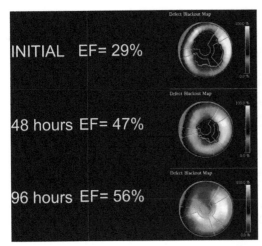

INITIAL   EF= 29%

48 hours EF= 47%

96 hours EF= 56%

Fig. 6. Serial SPECT LV perfusion polar maps with corresponding LV EF at 0, 48, and 96 hours in apical ballooning. The initial study demonstrates a large circumferential LV perfusion defect not corresponding to the distribution of a single coronary artery with LV EF 29%. At 48 hours, the perfusion defect is substantially smaller with LV EF 47%. At 96 hours, both LV perfusion and EF are normal. EF, ejection fraction; LV, left ventricle; SPECT, single-photon emission computed tomography.

stunning.[42,43] Although these changes can be visually alarming, LV contraction is usually improved during this time.

BIOMARKER PROFILE

Compared with acute coronary syndrome, TTC is characterized by lower peak levels of troponin, creatine kinase (CK), and CK-MB.[2,8,17,19,44] The initial troponin is abnormal in 90% of patients and the average peak troponin T is 0.6 ng/mL. The initial and peak levels of troponin are frequently similar; therefore, the troponin release pattern may be either a rise and fall pattern or a decreasing pattern. CK elevation is quite modest (100–500 U/L). The troponin release pattern using new high-sensitivity troponin assays is currently unknown. The disparity between minor troponin and CK release, in the presence of significant LV dysfunction, likely represents myocardial stunning rather than myocardial necrosis. Levels of brain natriuretic peptide are elevated (average 1000 pg/mL), often above those reported with acute coronary syndrome, and may reflect underlying congestive heart failure.[45] The average level of brain natriuretic peptide may be 3 to 4 times that observed in acute coronary syndrome and the peak may not occur until 48 hours after presentation.

CONGESTIVE HEART FAILURE

Congestive heart failure complicates TTC in a substantial number of patients and ranges in severity from radiographic pulmonary congestion to cardiogenic shock. A preliminary report documented evidence of congestive heart failure in 45% of patients, almost half of whom had Killip class IV heart failure.[45] Patients with heart failure were older and more likely to have a physical illness trigger, higher cardiac troponin, more frequent ST-segment elevation, and lower ejection fraction.

Several factors contribute to heart failure in TTC. Marked LV systolic dysfunction is typical (median LV ejection fraction is 30%) and significantly less than that observed in patients with acute coronary

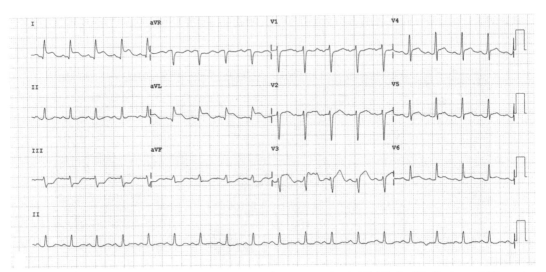

Fig. 7. Initial 12-lead ECG demonstrates ST-segment elevation in leads V3–V6, I, aVL. Reciprocal ST-segment depression is present in leads III, aVF. Emergency coronary angiography showed no coronary artery obstruction.

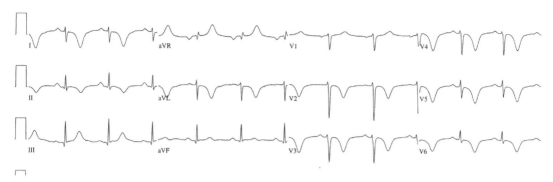

Fig. 8. Twelve-lead ECG from TTC patient recorded several days after admission demonstrates widespread T-wave inversion and QT interval lengthening typical of the ECG evolution in TTC. TTC, takotsubo cardiomyopathy.

syndrome.[2,5,17] The ejection fraction profile of TTC patients from the author's single-institution experience is shown in **Fig. 9**.

Myocardial edema within the abnormally contracting myocardium (best evaluated with cardiac MRI) is present in up to 80% of patients and may contribute to heart failure by reducing LV compliance and thereby increasing LV filling pressure.[8]

LV outflow tract obstruction owing to systolic anterior mitral valve leaflet motion occurs in

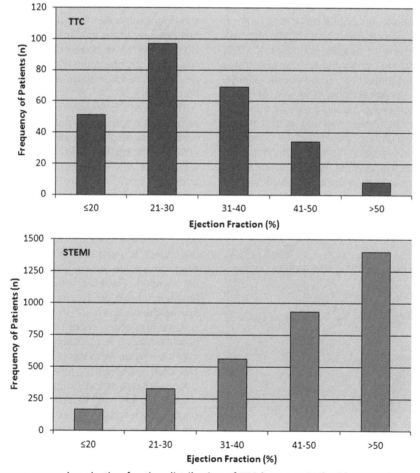

Fig. 9. Histograms comparing ejection fraction distribution of TTC (top, n = 259) with STEMI (bottom, n = 3391). Consecutive data from 2001 to 2012 (Minneapolis Heart Institute at Abbott Northwestern Hospital). STEMI, ST-segment elevation myocardial infarction; TTC, takotsubo cardiomyopathy.

10% to 20% of patients[17,46–48] and is an important factor to consider in the evaluation of heart failure (**Fig. 10**). This complication is more likely to occur in the subset of patients with the apical ballooning contraction pattern and may be exacerbated by the use of inotropic drugs used to support blood pressure. Systolic anterior mitral leaflet motion with LV outflow tract obstruction can lead to clinically important mitral valve regurgitation and the murmur of mitral valve regurgitation may be obscured by the murmur of LV outflow tract obstruction. A 2-dimensional echocardiogram is needed to evaluate this complication. Persistence of systolic anterior mitral leaflet motion and LV outflow tract obstruction after recovery should raise the possibility of coexisting hypertrophic cardiomyopathy.

LV systolic dysfunction of a magnitude requiring either intravenous vasopressor drugs or an intra-aortic balloon pump occurs in up to 20% of TTC patients and is associated with lower LV ejection fraction (median 25%), male sex, higher heart rate, greater troponin elevation, and the presence of physical stressor, but not LV ballooning pattern. These patients represent a particularly high-risk subset with a rate of hospital mortality of 20%. Most respond to intravenous catecholamine drugs, including dopamine, dobutamine, phenylephrine, and norepinephrine. The use of these drugs to support blood pressure may be concerning, because catecholamines are postulated to play a role in the pathophysiology of the condition. Nonetheless, in physiologic doses, catecholamine drugs are effective treatment for hypotension in this cardiomyopathy. Whether a noncatecholamine

drug such as vasopressin is superior is unknown. For more profound hemodynamic compromise, an intra-aortic balloon pump is effective. Some investigators were concerned that an intra-aortic balloon pump might create or worsen LV outflow tract obstruction by reducing LV cavity size, although this has not been a common problem.[49]

ARRHYTHMIA

Despite significant LV dysfunction, clinically important ventricular arrhythmias are uncommon.[2,5,17,50] Ventricular fibrillation is rare, unpredictable, and sometimes fatal. A recent survey noted ventricular fibrillation prevalence of 1.8% and life-threatening ventricular arrhythmia on presentation in about 1%.[50] Ventricular fibrillation or tachycardia at presentation may be a complication of the TTC event. It is conceivable, although unproven, that a cardiac arrest and subsequent resuscitation process could trigger a TTC event. Acute noncardiac events, such as intracranial hemorrhage, can present with both cardiac arrest and TTC. Postdischarge ventricular fibrillation, sometimes fatal, has been reported in a small number of patients. Current evidence does not support the routine use of a prophylactic implantable defibrillator, although individual patients may require special consideration.

The most common significant ventricular arrhythmia is torsade de pointes ventricular tachycardia, occurring in the setting of significant QT interval prolongation (**Fig. 11**). Even though the QT interval often exceeds 500 ms, torsade de pointes is rare.[51] Patients with bradycardia, heart block, and variable R-R intervals (as with atrial fibrillation), and men also seem to be more vulnerable.[51] Because QT interval lengthening is a delayed process, rhythm monitoring should be continued, at least until hospital discharge, and drugs known to prolong the QT interval should be avoided. Patients with marked QT interval lengthening and bradycardia require careful scrutiny before discharge.

Atrial fibrillation, either on admission or during hospitalization, is occasionally present (5%), as might be expected in this older aged population.[50] Standard treatment of atrial fibrillation is appropriate. Antiarrhythmic drugs that prolong the QT interval (such as ibutilide) should be used cautiously because the risk for torsade de pointes may be greater in these patients.

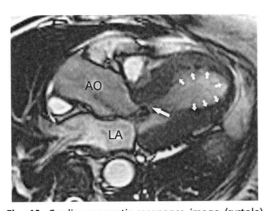

Fig. 10. Cardiac magnetic resonance image (systole) demonstrates left ventricular outflow tract obstruction following administration of an inotropic agent for hypotension. Outflow tract obstruction is caused by systolic anterior mitral leaflet motion with septal contact (*large arrow*) in this patient with apical ballooning (*small arrows*). AO, aorta; LA, left atrium.

VENTRICULAR THROMBUS

Akinetic segments within the LV or RV provide a substrate for thrombus formation (**Fig. 12**).

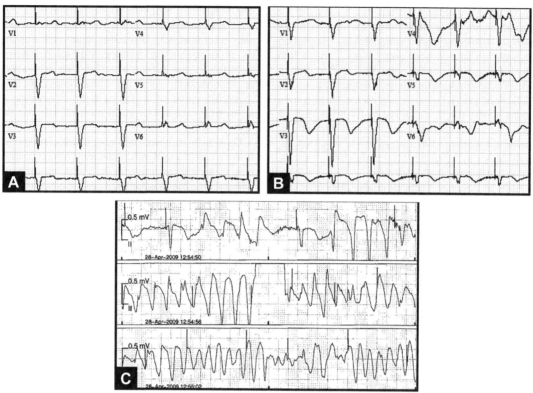

Fig. 11. Occurrence of torsade de pointes ventricular tachycardia. (*A*) Admission 6-lead ECG (V1–V6) demonstrates ventricular pacing and underlying atrial fibrillation. (*B*) Follow-up 6-lead ECG demonstrates deep T-wave inversion and QT interval lengthening. (*C*) Lead II rhythm strip demonstrates torsade de pointes ventricular tachycardia, which required cardioversion for termination.

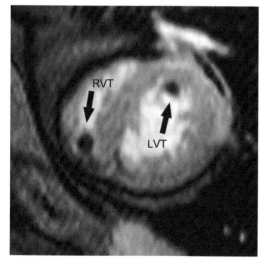

Fig. 12. Cardiac magnetic resonance image (horizontal short axis). Arrows identify left ventricular thrombus (LVT), and right ventricular thrombus (RVT). Pulmonary embolism occurred in this patient, presumably from RVT.

Thrombi can be multiple and can be located distinctly from those observed in acute myocardial infarction caused by coronary artery occlusion. These thrombi can be the source of both systemic and pulmonary embolism.[2,17] Cardiac MRI is probably more sensitive than 2-dimensional echocardiography for the detection of ventricular thrombus.

HOSPITAL MANAGEMENT

During the first 24 hours, the patient should be confined to an intensive care unit or telemetry unit depending on the hemodyamic status and comorbid illnesses. Traditionally, TTC patients have been treated with a β-blocker and an angiotensin converting enzyme inhibitor, analogous to the patient with acute coronary syndrome and LV dysfunction. Whether these drugs actually improve the natural history of this acute cardiomyopathy remains unknown, because LV function usually improves spontaneously. β-blockers and angiotensin converting enzyme inhibitors (in standard doses) do not prevent the occurrence or recurrence of TTC. In fact, about 20% of patients are receiving these drugs at presentation (usually as treatment for hypertension). It is reasonable to treat patients with a β-blocker and angiotensin converting enzyme inhibitor at least until LV ejection fraction has returned to normal (generally 1–3 months). Aspirin and clopidogrel are not necessary because TTC is not caused by an acute epicardial coronary event. In the presence of RV or LV thrombus, or high-risk apical akinesia, intravenous heparin followed by warfarin anticoagulation is appropriate, until abnormal myocardial contraction has resolved or substantially improved.

Rate of hospital mortality is low (2%–3%) and may be either cardiac (cardiogenic shock, systemic embolization, ventricular fibrillation) or noncardiac from a comorbid condition such as malignancy or severe lung disease.[2,5,8,17,20] Death due to cardiac rupture has been reported.[52] As experience with TTC broadens, recognized complications and rate of mortality will likely increase.

AFTER HOSPITAL MANAGEMENT

Complete recovery of LV systolic function is a hallmark and persistent LV dysfunction should raise concern for a different or coexisting cardiomyopathy.[2,5,8,17] While rapid normalization of LV systolic function (within days) can occur, it is sometimes delayed for 1 to 3 months. Follow-up echocardiography should be performed at 1 to 3 months postdischarge in those patients with abnormal LV systolic dysfunction at hospital discharge. The ECG may be abnormal for several weeks with persistent T-wave inversion and lengthened QT interval despite normal LV systolic function. In general these ECG abnormalities are not cause for alarm.

Postdischarge pharmacologic treatment is empiric. It is reasonable to continue β-blocker and angiotensin converting inhibitor drugs until return of normal LV ejection fraction. Whether these drugs provide long-term benefit is not established. Other drugs directed at sympathetic nervous system blockade (reserpine, clonidine) have not been evaluated. Warfarin anticoagulation (most appropriate for patients with apical ballooning) can be discontinued once LV systolic dysfunction has resolved.

The rate of recurrence is 5% to 10% during the 5 years following the initial event.[2,5,17,20] Recurrences are often similar to the index event and can be early (weeks) or late (years). Multiple recurrences have been reported. The recurrent TTC event may be life threatening, for example, when complicated by ventricular fibrillation. To date, no clinical or demographic features distinguish patients with/without recurrent events. Recurrences are not prevented by β-blocking agents and no published data are available to guide treatment in patients with recurrence.[17] Reports have documented recurrent events with a ballooning pattern different from that of the initial event.[53,54] This observation is inconsistent with the hypothesis of fixed anatomic variation in sympathetic innervation or adrenergic receptor density/sensitivity as a mechanism of TTC.

Long-term survival data on patients are limited. Survival at 3 years is significantly reduced when compared with an age-matched and sex-matched general population with the excess mortality occurring predominantly in the first year after diagnosis (standardized mortality ratio 6.8) and usually is due to a noncardiac illness such as malignancy.[17] To date, no study has examined whether an initial TTC event predisposes the patient to a later cardiomyopathic process, although current experience suggests this is not an issue.

PATHOPHYSIOLOGY

Thus far, the pathophysiology of TTC has defied explanation. Features that require reconciliation include acute onset, association with a triggering stressor, female predilection, unique noncoronary LV contraction abnormality, and reversibility. Takotsubo cardiomyopathy and acute coronary syndrome share many clinical features and myocardial ischemia due to transient epicardial coronary artery spasm or plaque rupture in the left anterior descending coronary artery have been proposed as mechanisms.[11,55] Neither seems likely given the unusual geographic profile of abnormal LV contraction. The midventricular ballooning and inverted ballooning patterns do not match the distribution of an epicardial coronary artery. Although the apical ballooning pattern matches the distribution of a wrap-around left anterior descending coronary artery, this ballooning pattern is also present in other anatomic left anterior descending variants including those that do not reach the LV apex. The frequent occurrence of segmental RV akinesia is not typical of left anterior descending ischemic events. Furthermore, the chronobiological patterns of TTC onset are distinct from those of acute coronary syndrome.[56]

Microvascular ischemia, in the absence of significant epicardial coronary obstruction, has been proposed as a potential mechanism but is difficult to study given current spatial resolution of coronary angiography.

A substantial body of indirect evidence points to catecholamine excess in TTC pathophysiology.[2,4,5] The acute onset and association with an inciting stressor implicate the sympathetic nervous system. A frequently cited study demonstrated several-fold elevation in epinephrine, norepinephrine, and dopamine in TTC patients and these levels were significantly greater than among patients with Killip class III acute myocardial infarction.[4] Furthermore, TTC can be provoked by accidental or intentional overdose of catecholamine drugs and is sometimes observed as a complication of pheochromocytoma or paraganglioma.[2,57] Histologic examination of myocardium obtained by endomyocardial biopsy during acute TTC has shown contraction band necrosis and leukocytic inflammatory response, findings that have been reported with catecholamine cardiotoxicity.[58] A TTC-like condition has been provoked in rats stressed by immobilization, with occurrence prevented by pretreatment with amosulolol, an α-adrenergic and β-adrenergic receptor antagonist.[59]

Although catecholamine excess is an attractive hypothesis, the mechanism for causing reversible myocardial injury in geographic patterns observed in TTC is not obvious. To account for these findings, it is necessary to postulate regional differences in myocardial sympathetic innervation or adrenergic receptor behavior. Limited data suggest anatomic variability in adrenergic receptor density is present in the human heart.[60] Functional polymorphisms of the B1-adrenergic and α2c-adrenergic receptors have been linked to sympathetic nervous system overactivity, but the frequency distribution is similar in TTC and non-TTC patients, making this an unlikely mechanism for excessive sympathetic nervous system activity.[61] Catecholamines might interact with the coronary microvasculature to produce intense vasoconstriction and subsequent transient myocardial ischemia. Contraction band necrosis is observed in both catecholamine toxicity and ischemia-reperfusion myocardial injury.[62] Despite substantial evidence in support of a catecholamine hypothesis, some investigators have been unable to reproduce the findings of elevated catecholamines in TTC patients.[44]

An intriguing feature of TTC is the striking predilection for older women. Reports have consistently noted nearly 90% of patients are women and usually more than 50 years of age. Naturally, these observations have generated speculation regarding the role of reduced levels of estrogen and progesterone in promoting an older female vulnerability. There is evidence that estrogen may influence the release of epinephrine in the presynaptic cardiac sympathetic nerves.[63] It is also possible that sympathetic nervous system responsiveness is biologically different in men and women independent of levels of sex hormone.

SUMMARY

Takotsubo cardiomyopathy is now recognized as a unique acute and reversible cardiomyopathy.[64] Distinguishing features include LV systolic dysfunction in a noncoronary pattern, occurrence without acute coronary artery disease, reversibility, predilection for older women, and an association with triggering stressful event. However, TTC also occurs in men and younger individuals and without a stress trigger. Future investigation may establish a link between TTC and other conditions, such as acute brain injury and stress-associated sudden death.[65,66] Complications include congestive heart failure, arrhythmia, mural thrombi, and LV outflow tract obstruction. Although initial hospital mortality rate is low, longer term survival is substantially less than the general population, predominantly owing to comorbid conditions. Recurrence is infrequent, not necessarily prevented by β-blockers, and occasionally complicated by significant ventricular arrhythmia. Current evidence favors catecholamine myocardial toxicity and/or microvascular ischemia in TTC pathophysiology.

ACKNOWLEDGMENTS

Victoria Pink, RN, CCRC and Ross Garberich, MS provided professional assistance in the preparation of this article.

REFERENCES

1. Sharkey SW, Lesser JR, Zenovich AG, et al. Acute and reversible cardiomyopathy provoked by stress in women from the United States. Circulation 2005; 111:472–9.
2. Bybee KA, Prasad A. Stress-related cardiomyopathy syndromes. Circulation 2008;118:397–409.
3. Bybee KA, Kara T, Prasad A, et al. Systematic review: transient left ventricular apical ballooning: a syndrome that mimics ST-segment elevation myocardial infarction. Ann Intern Med 2004;141:858–65.
4. Wittstein IS, Thiemann DR, Lima JA, et al. Neurohumoral features of myocardial stunning due to sudden emotional stress. N Engl J Med 2005;352: 539–48.
5. Akashi YJ, Goldstein DS, Barbaro G, et al. Takotsubo cardiomyopathy: a new form of acute, reversible heart failure. Circulation 2008;118:2754–62.
6. Tsuchihashi K, Ueshima K, Uchida T, et al. Transient left ventricular apical ballooning without coronary artery stenosis: a novel heart syndrome mimicking acute myocardial infarction. Angina Pectoris-Myocardial Infarction Investigations in Japan [see comment]. J Am Coll Cardiol 2001;38:11–8.
7. Kurowski V, Kaiser A, von Hof K, et al. Apical and midventricular transient left ventricular dysfunction

syndrome (tako-tsubo cardiomyopathy): frequency, mechanisms, and prognosis. Chest 2007;132:809–16.

8. Eitel I, von Knobelsdorff-Brenkenhoff F, Bernhardt P, et al. Clinical characteristics and cardiovascular magnetic resonance findings in stress (takotsubo) cardiomyopathy. JAMA 2011;306:277–86.

9. Anderson JL, Adams CD, Antman EM, et al. ACC/AHA 2007 guidelines for the management of patients with unstable angina/non-ST-elevation myocardial infarction: a report of the American College of Cardiology/American Heart Association Task Force on Practice Guidelines (Writing Committee to Revise the 2002 Guidelines for the Management of Patients With Unstable Angina/Non-ST-Elevation Myocardial Infarction) developed in collaboration with the American College of Emergency Physicians, the Society for Cardiovascular Angiography and Interventions, and the Society of Thoracic Surgeons endorsed by the American Association of Cardiovascular and Pulmonary Rehabilitation and the Society for Academic Emergency Medicine. J Am Coll Cardiol 2007;50:e1–157.

10. Prasad A, Lerman A, Rihal CS. Apical ballooning syndrome (Tako-Tsubo or stress cardiomyopathy): a mimic of acute myocardial infarction. Am Heart J 2008;155:408–17.

11. Dote K, Sato H, Tateishi H, et al. Myocardial stunning due to simultaneous multivessel coronary spasms: a review of 5 cases. J Cardiol 1991;21:203–14 [in Japanese].

12. Sato H, Taiteishi H, Uchida T. Takotsubo-type cardiomyopathy due to multivessel spasm. In: Kodama K, Haze K, Hon M, editors. Clinical aspect of myocardial injury: from ischemia to heart failure. Tokyo: Kagakuhyouronsha; 1990. p. 56–64.

13. Kurisu S, Sato H, Kawagoe T, et al. Tako-tsubo-like left ventricular dysfunction with ST-segment elevation: a novel cardiac syndrome mimicking acute myocardial infarction. Am Heart J 2002;143:448–55.

14. Sharkey SW, Shear W, Hodges M, et al. Reversible myocardial contraction abnormalities in patients with an acute noncardiac illness. Chest 1998;114:98–105.

15. Pavin D, Le Breton H, Daubert C. Human stress cardiomyopathy mimicking acute myocardial syndrome [see comment]. Heart 1997;78:509–11.

16. Sharkey SW, Lesser JR, Maron MS, et al. Why not just call it tako-tsubo cardiomyopathy: a discussion of nomenclature. J Am Coll Cardiol 2011;57:1496–7.

17. Sharkey SW, Windenburg DC, Lesser JR, et al. Natural history and expansive clinical profile of stress (tako-tsubo) cardiomyopathy. J Am Coll Cardiol 2010;55:333–41.

18. Park JH, Kang SJ, Song JK, et al. Left ventricular apical ballooning due to severe physical stress in patients admitted to the medical ICU. Chest 2005;128:296–302.

19. Nef HM, Mollmann H, Elsasser A. Tako-tsubo cardiomyopathy (apical ballooning). Heart 2007;93:1309–15.

20. Elesber AA, Prasad A, Lennon RJ, et al. Four-year recurrence rate and prognosis of the apical ballooning syndrome. J Am Coll Cardiol 2007;50:448–52.

21. Thygesen K, Alpert JS, Jaffe AS, et al. Third universal definition of myocardial infarction. Circulation 2012;126:2020–35.

22. Schoof S, Bertram H, Hohmann D, et al. Takotsubo cardiomyopathy in a 2-year-old girl: 3-dimensional visualization of reversible left ventricular dysfunction. J Am Coll Cardiol 2010;55:e5.

23. Sharkey SW, Lesser JR, Menon M, et al. Spectrum and significance of electrocardiographic patterns, troponin levels, and thrombolysis in myocardial infarction frame count in patients with stress (tako-tsubo) cardiomyopathy and comparison to those in patients with ST-elevation anterior wall myocardial infarction. Am J Cardiol 2008;101:1723–8.

24. Bybee KA, Prasad A, Barsness GW, et al. Clinical characteristics and thrombolysis in myocardial infarction frame counts in women with transient left ventricular apical ballooning syndrome. Am J Cardiol 2004;94:343–6.

25. Elesber A, Lerman A, Bybee KA, et al. Myocardial perfusion in apical ballooning syndrome correlate of myocardial injury. Am Heart J 2006;152:469.e9–469.e13.

26. Hurst RT, Askew JW, Reuss CS, et al. Transient mid-ventricular ballooning syndrome: a new variant. J Am Coll Cardiol 2006;48:579–83.

27. Kim S, Yu A, Filippone LA, et al. Inverted-Takotsubo pattern cardiomyopathy secondary to pheochromocytoma: a clinical case and literature review. Clin Cardiol 2010;33:200–5.

28. Elesber AA, Prasad A, Bybee KA, et al. Transient cardiac apical ballooning syndrome: prevalence and clinical implications of right ventricular involvement. J Am Coll Cardiol 2006;47:1082–3.

29. Ito K, Sugihara H, Katoh S, et al. Assessment of Takotsubo (ampulla) cardiomyopathy using 99mTc-tetrofosmin myocardial SPECT–comparison with acute coronary syndrome. Ann Nucl Med 2003;17:115–22.

30. Kurisu S, Inoue I, Kawagoe T, et al. Myocardial perfusion and fatty acid metabolism in patients with tako-tsubo-like left ventricular dysfunction. J Am Coll Cardiol 2003;41:743–8.

31. Bybee KA, Murphy J, Prasad A, et al. Acute impairment of regional myocardial glucose uptake in the apical ballooning (takotsubo) syndrome. J Nucl Cardiol 2006;13:244–50.

32. Yoshida T, Hibino T, Kako N, et al. A pathophysiologic study of tako-tsubo cardiomyopathy with F-18 fluorodeoxyglucose positron emission tomography. Eur Heart J 2007;28:2598–604.

33. Akashi YJ, Nakazawa K, Sakakibara M, et al. 123I-MIBG myocardial scintigraphy in patients with "takotsubo" cardiomyopathy. J Nucl Med 2004;45:1121–7.

34. Pessoa PM, Xavier SS, Lima SL, et al. Assessment of takotsubo (ampulla) cardiomyopathy using iodine-123 metaiodobenzylguanidine scintigraphy. Acta Radiol 2006;47:1029–35.

35. Braunwald E, Kloner RA. The stunned myocardium: prolonged, postischemic ventricular dysfunction. Circulation 1982;66:1146–9.

36. Bybee KA, Motiei A, Syed IS, et al. Electrocardiography cannot reliably differentiate transient left ventricular apical ballooning syndrome from anterior ST-segment elevation myocardial infarction. J Electrocardiol 2007;40:38.e1–6.

37. Ogura R, Hiasa Y, Takahashi T, et al. Specific findings of the standard 12-lead ECG in patients with 'Takotsubo' cardiomyopathy: comparison with the findings of acute anterior myocardial infarction. Circ J 2003;67:687–90.

38. Sharkey SW. Electrocardiogram mimics of acute ST-segment elevation myocardial infarction: insights from cardiac magnetic resonance imaging in patients with tako-tsubo (stress) cardiomyopathy. J Electrocardiol 2008;41:621–5.

39. Kosuge M, Ebina T, Hibi K, et al. Simple and accurate electrocardiographic criteria to differentiate takotsubo cardiomyopathy from anterior acute myocardial infarction. J Am Coll Cardiol 2010;55:2514–6.

40. Barker S, Solomon H, Bergin JD, et al. Electrocardiographic ST-segment elevation: takotsubo cardiomyopathy versus ST-segment elevation myocardial infarction–a case series. Am J Emerg Med 2009;27:220–6.

41. Kurisu S, Inoue I, Kawagoe T, et al. Time course of electrocardiographic changes in patients with tako-tsubo syndrome: comparison with acute myocardial infarction with minimal enzymatic release. Circ J 2004;68:77–81.

42. Hirota Y, Kita Y, Tsuji R, et al. Prominent negative T waves with QT prolongation indicate reperfusion injury and myocardial stunning. J Cardiol 1992;22:325–40.

43. Kloner RA. Inverted T waves. An electrocardiographic marker of stunned or hibernating myocardium in man? [comment]. Circulation 1990;82:1060–1.

44. Madhavan M, Borlaug BA, Lerman A, et al. Stress hormone and circulating biomarker profile of apical ballooning syndrome (Takotsubo cardiomyopathy): insights into the clinical significance of B-type natriuretic peptide and troponin levels. Heart 2009;95:1436–41.

45. Madhavan M, Rihal CS, Lerman A, et al. Acute heart failure in apical ballooning syndrome (TakoTsubo/stress cardiomyopathy): clinical correlates and Mayo Clinic risk score. J Am Coll Cardiol 2011;57:1400–1.

46. Brunetti ND, Ieva R, Rossi G, et al. Ventricular outflow tract obstruction, systolic anterior motion and acute mitral regurgitation in Tako-Tsubo syndrome. Int J Cardiol 2008;127:e152–7.

47. El Mahmoud R, Mansencal N, Pilliere R, et al. Prevalence and characteristics of left ventricular outflow tract obstruction in Tako-Tsubo syndrome. Am Heart J 2008;156:543–8.

48. Ionescu A. Subaortic dynamic obstruction: a contributing factor to haemodynamic instability in tako-tsubo syndrome? Eur J Echocardiogr 2008;9:384–5.

49. Good CW, Hubbard CR, Harrison TA, et al. Echocardiographic guidance in treatment of cardiogenic shock complicating transient left ventricular apical ballooning syndrome. JACC Cardiovasc Imaging 2009;2:372–4.

50. Syed FF, Asirvatham SJ, Francis J. Arrhythmia occurrence with takotsubo cardiomyopathy: a literature review. Europace 2011;13:780–8.

51. Samuelov-Kinori L, Kinori M, Kogan Y, et al. Takotsubo cardiomyopathy and QT interval prolongation: who are the patients at risk for torsades de pointes? J Electrocardiol 2009;42:353–357.e1.

52. Akashi YJ, Tejima T, Sakurada H, et al. Left ventricular rupture associated with Takotsubo cardiomyopathy. Mayo Clin Proc 2004;79:821–4.

53. Blessing E, Steen H, Rosenberg M, et al. Recurrence of takotsubo cardiomyopathy with variant forms of left ventricular dysfunction. J Am Soc Echocardiogr 2007;20:439.e11–2.

54. Kaushik M, Alla VM, Madan R, et al. Recurrent stress cardiomyopathy with variable regional involvement: insights into etiopathogenetic mechanisms. Circulation 2011;124:e556–7.

55. Ibanez B, Navarro F, Cordoba M, et al. Tako-tsubo transient left ventricular apical ballooning: is intravascular ultrasound the key to resolve the enigma? Heart 2005;91:102–4.

56. Citro R, Previtali M, Bovelli D, et al. Chronobiological patterns of onset of Tako-Tsubo cardiomyopathy: a multicenter Italian study. J Am Coll Cardiol 2009;54:180–1.

57. Abraham J, Mudd JO, Kapur N, et al. Stress cardiomyopathy after intravenous administration of catecholamines and beta-receptor agonists. J Am Coll Cardiol 2009;53:1320–5.

58. Nef HM, Mollmann H, Kostin S, et al. Tako-Tsubo cardiomyopathy: intraindividual structural analysis in the acute phase and after functional recovery. Eur Heart J 2007;28:2456–64.

59. Ueyama T, Kasamatsu K, Hano T, et al. Emotional stress induces transient left ventricular hypocontraction in the rat via activation of cardiac adrenoceptors: a possible animal model of 'tako-tsubo' cardiomyopathy. Circ J 2002;66:712–3.

60. Mori H, Ishikawa S, Kojima S, et al. Increased responsiveness of left ventricular apical myocardium to adrenergic stimuli. Cardiovasc Res 1993;27:192–8.

61. Sharkey SW, Maron BJ, Nelson P, et al. Adrenergic receptor polymorphisms in patients with stress

(tako-tsubo) cardiomyopathy. J Cardiol 2009;53: 53–7.

62. Miyazaki S, Fujiwara H, Onodera T, et al. Quantitative analysis of contraction band and coagulation necrosis after ischemia and reperfusion in the porcine heart. Circulation 1987;75:1074–82.

63. Sclarovsky S, Nikus KC. The role of oestrogen in the pathophysiologic process of the Tako-Tsubo cardiomyopathy. Eur Heart J 2010;31:377.

64. Maron BJ, Towbin JA, Thiene G, et al. Contemporary definitions and classification of the cardiomyopathies: an American Heart Association Scientific Statement from the Council on Clinical Cardiology, Heart Failure and Transplantation Committee; Quality of Care and Outcomes Research and Functional Genomics and Translational Biology Interdisciplinary Working Groups; and Council on Epidemiology and Prevention. Circulation 2006;113:1807–16.

65. Kono T, Morita H, Kuroiwa T, et al. Left ventricular wall motion abnormalities in patients with subarachnoid hemorrhage: neurogenic stunned myocardium. J Am Coll Cardiol 1994;24:636–40.

66. Ziegelstein RC. Acute emotional stress and cardiac arrhythmias. JAMA 2007;298:324–9.

Gender-Related Differences in Takotsubo Cardiomyopathy

Birke Schneider, MD[a],*, Anastasios Athanasiadis, MD[b],
Udo Sechtem, MD[b]

KEYWORDS

- Takotsubo cardiomyopathy • Gender-related difference • Emotional stress • Physical stress
- Cardiogenic shock • Resuscitation • Electrocardiogram • Apical ballooning syndrome

KEY POINTS

- In all studies reported so far, there is a marked gender preference in takotsubo cardiomyopathy (TTC), in which 90% of those affected are women, with a mean age of 62 to 76 years.
- Between 1% and 3% of patients presenting with a suspected acute coronary syndrome (ACS) eventually are diagnosed as having TTC. There is a gender-specific prevalence, which is higher in women (6%–9%) than in men (<0.5%).
- In contrast to studies of true ACS, mean age, prehospital delay, and clinical symptoms, such as angina, are similar in male and female patients with TTC.
- Physical stress as a triggering event is more frequent in male patients with TTC, whereas emotional stress or no identifiable trigger is more prevalent in women.
- More male patients than female patients with TTC present with cardiogenic shock and/or out-of-hospital cardiac arrest; TTC, therefore, has to be considered as another important cause of sudden cardiac death, especially in men.
- There seems to be a disproportionate corrected QT (QTc) prolongation in male patients during the acute course of TTC predisposing men to malignant ventricular arrhythmias.
- The elevation of cardiac markers is higher in men. This may in part be related to physical stress as a trigger directly before the onset of TTC in men.
- The obvious female predominance of TTC is still not well understood. Further studies are necessary to clarify the pathogenetic background and develop strategies against this potentially life-threatening disease.

INTRODUCTION

TTC, first described in Japan in 1990, has increasingly been recognized in Western countries over the past years.[1–14] This cardiac syndrome mimics acute myocardial infarction (AMI) and is characterized by transient left ventricular regional dysfunction, ischemic ECG changes, and elevation of cardiac markers in the absence of significant coronary artery disease. Frequently, this reversible form of acute heart failure is precipitated by a stressful event. In all studies reported so far, there is a marked gender discrepancy in TTC, which affects predominantly elderly women.

Men and women with AMI are known to have a different clinical presentation and outcome[15–20] but currently there is little information about gender-related differences in the clinical profile of TTC.[21,22]

PATHOPHYSIOLOGIC BACKGROUND

The precise pathophysiology of TTC is still not well understood. As possible underlying mechanisms,

a Medizinische Klinik II, Sana Kliniken Lübeck, Kronsforder Allee 71 – 73, D-23562 Lübeck, Germany;
b Abteilung für Kardiologie, Robert-Bosch-Krankenhaus, Auerbachstrasse 110, D-70376 Stuttgart, Germany
* Corresponding author.
E-mail address: b.schneider@sana-luebeck.de

Heart Failure Clin 9 (2013) 137–146
http://dx.doi.org/10.1016/j.hfc.2012.12.005
1551-7136/13/$ – see front matter © 2013 Elsevier Inc. All rights reserved.

transient multivessel coronary artery spasm,[1,23,24] coronary microvascular dysfunction,[25–29] and obstruction of the left ventricular outflow tract[5,8,9,30,31] due to a septal bulge have been proposed, all of which are more prevalent in women. The most widely accepted hypothesis suggests that TTC is caused by an excessive release of catecholamines after exposure to emotional or physical stress,[10,30,32] resulting in catecholamine-induced myocardial stunning.[33] Similar regional wall motion abnormalities have been observed in patients with high catecholamine levels due to pheochromocytoma[34,35] and subarachnoid hemorrhage.[36,37] Moreover, in a rat model of TTC, ST segment elevation and regional left ventricular dysfunction due to immobilization stress could be prevented by α-adrenoreceptor and β-adrenoreceptor antagonists.[38,39] Estrogen has a protective role on the cardiovascular system of postmenopausal women by attenuating catecholamine and glucocorticoid response to mental stress and by improving norepinephrine-induced vasoconstriction.[40,41] Thus, the reduction of estrogen levels after menopause may predispose elderly women to develop TTC[42–44] and can in part explain the striking female predominance of this syndrome.

EPIDEMIOLOGY

The exact incidence of TTC is unknown. Among patients presenting with a suspected ACS in Japan, the reported prevalence of TTC ranges from 1.2% to 2.2%.[2,45,46] In prospective studies from Western countries, between 2% and 3% of the patients undergoing coronary angiography because of suspected ACS eventually are diagnosed as having TTC.[47–51] There is a gender-specific prevalence that is higher in women, ranging from 6% to 9.8%, whereas the prevalence of TTC among male patients with an ACS is below 0.5%.[48–51]

DEMOGRAPHICS

Overall, 90% (range 65%–100%) of the patients with TTC are women.[52] In case series from Western countries, less than 11% are men.[8–14,22,25,27–29,31,47–51,53] The number of men seems higher in prospective studies from Asia, ranging from 13% to 35%.[5,7,21,30,32,45,54,55] This obvious female predominance of TTC is in contrast to patients with ACS.[15,16,18–20]

In several studies reported so far, the mean age has ranged from 62 to 76 years.[52] TTC is most frequently diagnosed in postmenopausal women over age 50 although premenopausal women and even children of both genders may

be affected.[5,53,56–59] The mean age is similar in male patients and in female patients with TTC.[14,21,22,53] This finding is in contrast to studies of true ACS, where women are consistently 7 to 9 years older than men.[15,16,18,20]

TRIGGERING EVENTS

In the majority of patients (70%–80%), the onset of TTC is preceded by a triggering event, with a similar distribution of emotional and physical stress in 30% to 40% of the patients, respectively.[52] In the largest study of gender differences reported so far,[22] physical stress (most commonly, acute noncardiac illness or surgical/diagnostic procedure) was significantly more frequent in male patients with TTC (57% vs 30%, $P = .005$) whereas emotional stress or no identifiable trigger were more prevalent in women (**Table 1**). These findings are in accordance with 2 smaller studies,[21,53] where physical stress was also found the predominant stressor in men.

PREHOSPITAL DELAY

The time interval from symptom onset to hospital admission reported in TTC patients ranges from median 2 (interquartile range 1–5) up to 10 ± 16 hours.[9,10,13,60] In a study evaluating gender differences in TTC,[22] prehospital delay was 7.5 ± 6.9 hours and comparable in women and men (see **Table 1**). In contrast, patients with an ACS enrolled in a similar hospital setting had a shorter prehospital delay, which was significantly longer in female patients than in male patients (median 6.2 vs 5.1 hours for non–ST elevation myocardial infarction and median 3.3 vs 2.5 hours for ST elevation myocardial infarction; both $P<.001$).[16,18] These data imply that in patients with TTC symptoms may be less severe than in ACS, have a more insidious onset, and often are attributed by both male and female patients to the triggering event preceding TTC onset.

SYMPTOMS

The most common presenting symptoms in TTC are chest pain and dyspnea, which have been reported in 70% and 20% of the patients, respectively.[52] Initial presentation with syncope, nausea and vomiting, cardiogenic shock, and ventricular fibrillation, however, has also been observed.[4–6,8–10,13,27,45,46,53–57,60]

When comparing female patients and male patients with TTC,[22] chest pain was reported more frequently in women (73% vs 57%, $P = .08$) whereas dyspnea, syncope, and no or other diverse symptoms occurred with similar frequency

Table 1
Clinical characteristics of 324 female patients and male patients with takotsubo cardiomyopathy

Characteristics	Female		Male		P Value
Patients	296	(91%)	28	(9%)	
Age (y)	68 ± 12	(27–90)	66 ± 12	(37–84)	0.31
Symptoms					
Chest pain	217	(73%)	16	(57%)	0.08
Dyspnea	45	(15%)	5	(18%)	0.78
Syncope	9	(3%)	1	(4%)	0.60
Shock/resuscitation	2	(1%)	4	(14%)	<0.001
Other	16	(5%)	1	(4%)	1.00
None	7	(2%)	1	(4%)	0.52
Triggering event	226	(76%)	24	(86%)	0.35
Emotional stress	111	(38%)	6	(21%)	0.10
Physical stress	88	(30%)	16	(57%)	0.005
Both	27	(9%)	2	(7%)	1.00
None	70	(24%)	4	(14%)	0.93
Time from symptom onset to hospital admission					
Hours	7.6 ± 6.8	(0–23.8)	7.2 ± 7.1	(0–23.0)	0.57
Cardiac markers					
CK median × ULN	1.17	(0.72–1.80)	1.55	(1.10–2.11)	0.05
CK-MB median × ULN	1.34	(0.85–2.20)	1.28	(0.75–1.77)	0.76
Troponin median × ULN	7.2	(2.9–17.9)	10.7	(7.6–29.0)	0.03
Angiography					
Symptom onset to angiography (days)	1	(0–2)	1	(0–2.75)	0.48
Coronary plaque (<50% stenosis)	133	(45%)	23	(82%)	<0.001
LV ejection fraction	49 ± 14	(18–81)	46 ± 15	(23–80)	0.23
Apical ballooning	189	(64%)	18	(64%)	1.00
Midventricular ballooning	107	(36%)	10	(36%)	
Intraaortic balloon pump	2	(1%)	1	(4%)	0.24

Abbreviations: CK, creatine kinase; CK-MB, creatine kinase MB fraction; LV, left ventricular; ULN, upper limit of normal.
  Data from Schneider B, Athanasiadis A, Stöllberger C, et al. Gender differences in the manifestation of takotsubo cardiomyopathy. Int J Cardiol 2011. http://dx.doi.org/10.1016/j.ijcard.2011.11.027.

in male patients and in female patients (see **Table 1**). Significantly more male patients were admitted after out-of-hospital cardiac arrest and/or in cardiogenic shock (14% vs 1%, P<.001) unable to report specific cardiac symptoms. It is known that sudden cardiac death from AMI and various other diagnoses is more frequent in men than in women.[61–64] TTC may be another important cause of cardiac arrest, especially in men, and must be added to the list of diseases potentially leading to sudden cardiac death. This is substantiated by a study including 91 Japanese patients (85% male) who underwent autopsy after sudden cardiac death. In that study, acute cardiac dysfunction related to stress was found the most likely cause of death in 19.8%.[64]

ELECTROCARDIOGRAM

The most frequently encountered finding on the admission ECG is ST segment elevation in the precordial leads, which has been documented in 60% to 90% of the patients.[5,6,9,13,25,45,52,53] Over the next days, ST segment elevation resolves and widespread deep T-wave inversion develops. The QTc interval is prolonged, and transient Q waves are present in 26% to 45% on admission.[5,9,10,13,25,52,53,60]

In a Japanese study directly comparing ECG changes in male and female patients with TTC,[21] ST segment elevation on the admission ECG was found less frequently in men (62% vs 81%) and was explained by a presumably later diagnosis of

TTC in men. This is in contrast to a large European registry,[22] where there was a trend toward a higher number of male patients with ST segment elevation (96% vs 85%, $P = .09$) despite a similar prehospital delay. Other ECG parameters in this study (heart rate, proportion of patients with ST segment elevation, T-wave inversion, or Q wave) evaluated during the first 3 days after symptom onset were not different between women and men (**Table 2**). Overall, there was a prolongation of the QTc interval (**Fig. 1**), with a maximum on the second day after symptom onset (503 ± 62 milliseconds). The QTc interval was found significantly longer in women than in men only on the day of symptom onset; however, during the following 2 days there was no significant difference between both genders (see **Table 2**). Because women normally have a longer QTc interval than men,[65] there may be a disproportionate QTc prolongation in male patients during the acute course of TTC, which may predispose them to ventricular arrhythmias. Accordingly, in a meta-analysis of QT interval prolongation in TTC patients, a higher prevalence of male gender with torsades de pointes tachycardia was reported.[66] Because especially men with a prolonged QTc

interval are at risk for malignant ventricular arrhythmias, monitoring for at least 3 days after symptom onset has been suggested.

LABORATORY FINDINGS

Elevation of creatine kinase has been reported in 50% to 60% of the patients and creatine kinase MB fraction in 40% to 70%. Cardiac troponin was found elevated in 70% to 100% of TTC patients.[5,8–10,13,22,27,45,49,52,53] In general, the increase of cardiac markers is less than in patients with AMI[10,67] and seems disproportionate to the extent of left ventricular dysfunction.

Gender-related differences in cardiac markers have been evaluated in only 1 TTC study.[22] There was a trend toward a higher level of creatine kinase in men (2.7 ± 3.6 vs 1.8 ± 3.3 times the upper limit of normal for gender, $P = .05$). Elevation of cardiac troponin was significantly higher in male patients than in female patients (see **Table 1**). The higher level of cardiac markers in male patients with TTC may in part be related to physical stress directly before the onset of TTC.

Plasma brain natriuretic peptide is invariably elevated in patients with TTC,[10,67,68] and elevation

Table 2
ECG findings in female patients and male patients with takotsubo cardiomyopathy

ECG Parameters	Female		Male		P Value
ECG day 1 (n = 312)					
Heart rate/min (range)	87 ± 22	(44–165)	96 ± 31	(40–180)	0.14
ST segment elevation	240	(85%)	27	(96%)	0.09
T-wave inversion	192	(68%)	19	(68%)	1.00
Q wave	72	(25%)	8	(29%)	0.66
ECG day 2 (n = 272)					
Heart rate/min (range)	78 ± 17	(11–159)	81 ± 22	(46–118)	0.93
ST segment elevation	154	(62%)	15	(68%)	0.65
T-wave inversion	222	(89%)	18	(82%)	0.29
Q wave	55	(22%)	4	(14%)	0.79
ECG day 3 (n = 257)					
Heart rate/min (range)	75 ± 18	(38–150)	74 ± 18	(49–123)	0.53
ST segment elevation	117	(50%)	10	(34%)	0.66
T-wave inversion	225	(97%)	21	(95%)	0.56
Q wave	38	(16%)	4	(17%)	1.00
QTc (ms)					
Day 1 (range)	468 ± 52	(354–685)	441 ± 51	(294–507)	0.047
Day 2 (range)	504 ± 61	(350–714)	488 ± 63	(403–648)	0.18
Day 3 (range)	503 ± 65	(354–745)	494 ± 53	(405–593)	0.78

Abbreviations: QTc, corrected QT interval (Bazett formula).
   Data from Schneider B, Athanasiadis A, Stöllberger C, et al. Gender differences in the manifestation of takotsubo cardiomyopathy. Int J Cardiol 2011. http://dx.doi.org/10.1016/j.ijcard.2011.11.027.

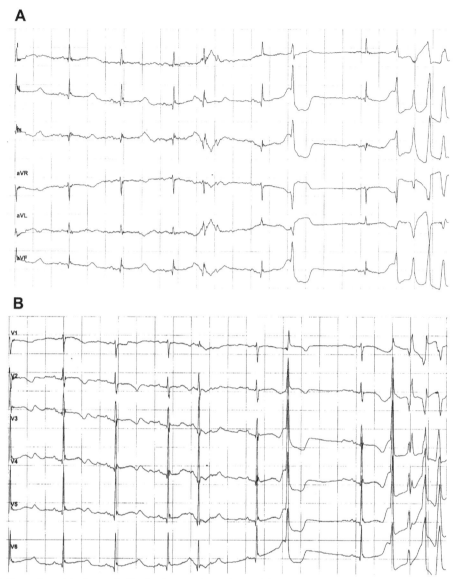

Fig. 1. Malignant ventricular arrhythmias in a male patient with TTC on day 2 after symptom onset. There is marked prolongation of the QTc interval (640 milliseconds), resulting in torsades de pointes tachycardia. (*A*) Limb leads. (*B*) Precordial leads.

of catecholamines has been observed in a subset of patients[6,10,26,67]; however, gender-related differences have not been reported so far.

ANGIOGRAPHIC FINDINGS

Despite clinically presenting as an ACS, left heart catheterization in patients with TTC typically shows normal coronary arteries or minimal coronary artery disease (lumen diameter <50%). Spontaneous coronary artery spasm is rare. Left ventriculography most commonly discloses an apical ballooning pattern in 60% and a midventricular ballooning pattern with apical sparing in 40%.[13,22,54,69] Rarely, an inverted type with basal hypokinesia can be observed. The left ventricular ejection fraction assessed by angiography, echocardiography, or cardiac MRI has ranged from 20% to 49%.[52]

In a study of gender differences in TTC,[22] time from symptom onset to angiography, left ventricular ejection fraction, and the frequency of contraction abnormalities (apical vs midventricular ballooning pattern) were not different between female patients and male patients (see **Table 1**). More men than women, however, showed minor plaque on coronary angiography.

COMPLICATIONS

A variety of complications have been reported in the course of the disease, such as malignant arrhythmias, cardiogenic shock, pulmonary edema, intraventricular pressure gradients sometimes associated with acute mitral regurgitation,[5,8–13,30,53,56,57,69] right ventricular involvement with pleural effusions,[47,70] and intraventricular thrombi resulting in acute stroke or arterial embolism.[71–74] Rarely, perforation of the left ventricle or the interventricular septum has been described.[75–78] In large studies, in-hospital mortality was observed in 1% to 2% of TTC patients but death may occur in up to 16% of the patients due to severe underlying diseases triggering TTC.[5,8,30,48,53,55,69]

Evaluating gender differences in TTC,[22] complications during hospitalization (**Table 3**) were observed in a high proportion of both women and men (53% vs 40%, respectively; P = .35). Left ventricular thrombi were diagnosed only in women (3% vs 0%) and pulmonary edema occurred more frequently in women than in men (14% vs 5%); however, this did not reach statistical significance. Regarding right ventricular involvement, occurrence of intraventricular pressure gradients, arrhythmias, need for resuscitation, or development of cardiogenic shock after hospital admission, there was no significant difference between both genders. Despite the high number of complications, mortality in the whole population was low (2%) and comparable in male patients and female patients.

RECURRENCE

A recurrence of TTC has been observed in up to 10% of the patients, the majority being women.[5,8,9,11,25,48,53,69] Because of the low numbers reported, no significant difference in the recurrence rate among men and women has been described (see **Table 3**).

GENDER DIFFERENCES IN TAKOTSUBO CARDIOMYOPATHY

TTC has a clinical presentation that is indistinguishable from myocardial infarction. This entity has, therefore, emerged as an important differential diagnosis of an ACS. One poorly understood aspect of TTC is the marked gender discrepancy. Besides pathophysiologic differences in the cardiovascular system predisposing women to develop TTC, it is currently unclear whether underdiagnosis or misdiagnosis may contribute to the apparent lower prevalence of TTC in men. The diagnosis of TTC depends to some degree on clinically considering the syndrome as a differential diagnosis if coronary angiography and left ventricular angiography in men show diffuse coronary artery disease and regional left ventricular

Table 3
Complications in female patients and male patients with takotsubo cardiomyopathy

Complications	Female		Male		P Value
All complications (n = 209)	100/189	(53%)	8/20	(40%)	0.35
Atrial fibrillation (n = 209)	29/189	(15%)	3/20	(15%)	1.00
Ventricular tachycardia (n = 209)	15/189	(8%)	2/20	(10%)	0.67
LV thrombi (echo + CMRI, n = 301)	8/274	(3%)	0/27		1.00
Intraventricular gradient (n = 276)	11/253	(4%)	1/23	(4%)	1.00
RV involvement (echo + CMRI, n = 290)	46/264	(17%)	5/26	(19%)	0.79
Pulmonary edema (n = 209)	27/189	(14%)	1/20	(5%)	0.48
Respirator therapy (n = 209)	13/189	(7%)	1/20	(5%)	1.00
CP resuscitation (n = 209)	7/189	(4%)	1/20	(5%)	0.56
Cardiogenic shock (n = 209)	13/189	(7%)	1/20	(5%)	1.00
Myocardial rupture (n = 209)	1/189	(1%)	0/20		1.00
Death (n = 324)	6/296	(2%)	1/28	(4%)	0.47
Recurrence	7/296	(2%)	0/28		1.00

Abbreviations: CMRI, cardiac MRI; CP, cardiopulmonary; echo, echocardiography; LV, left ventricular; RV, right ventricular.
Data from Schneider B, Athanasiadis A, Stöllberger C, et al. Gender differences in the manifestation of takotsubo cardiomyopathy. Int J Cardiol 2011. http://dx.doi.org/10.1016/j.ijcard.2011.11.027.

dysfunction, this is usually interpreted as the result of plaque rupture or coronary embolization. Searching for details in the history and studying serial ECGs, however, could potentially reveal more cases of TTC in male patients.

Another reason for underestimating the prevalence of TTC in men could be that men die more often suddenly in the early phase of TTC and the diagnosis cannot be established because the typical course of this syndrome, with rapid resolution of the wall abnormality, cannot be documented. The fact that men arrived at a hospital more often after resuscitation[22] indicates a greater electrical vulnerability in the early phase of TTC.[57,66]

Surprisingly, animal experiments for TTC were performed either with male animals or with female animals, and gender differences were not studied.[38,39,42,43,79,80] To the authors' knowledge, no comparison of gender-specific reactions to various types of physical or emotional stress in animal models has been reported.

SUMMARY

TTC predominantly occurs in elderly women. Men are affected in 10% of the patients with a similar clinical profile. In contrast to myocardial infarction, age distribution; symptoms, such as angina; and prehospital delay in TTC are not different between genders. In men, physical stress as a triggering event and shock or cardiac arrest on presentation are more frequent. A disproportionate QTc prolongation in male patients during the acute course of TTC has been observed, which may predispose them to malignant ventricular arrhythmias. The higher level of cardiac markers found in male patients with TTC may in part be related to the greater frequency of physical stress directly before the onset of TTC in men. Gender-related differences in TTC need to be carefully investigated at the clinical and experimental levels to explain the evident gender discrepancy in the prevalence of TTC, to clarify the pathogenetic background, and to develop preventive and therapeutic means against this life-threatening disease.

REFERENCES

1. Sato H, Tateishi H, Uchida T, et al. Takotsubo like left ventricular dysfunction due to multivessel coronary spasm. In: Kodama K, Haze K, Hon M, editors. Clinical aspect of myocardial injury: from ischemia to heart failure (in Japanese). Tokyo: Kagakuhyouronsya Publishing Co; 1990. p. 56–64.

2. Dote K, Sato H, Tateishi H, et al. Myocardial stunning due to simultaneous multivessel coronary spasms: a review of 5 cases. J Cardiol 1991;21:203–14.

3. Pavin D, Le Breton H, Daubert C. Human stress cardiomyopathy mimicking acute myocardial syndrome. Heart 1997;78:509–11.

4. Kawai S, Suzuki H, Yamaguchi H, et al. Ampulla cardiomyopathy ("Takotusbo" Cardiomyopathy). Reversible left ventricular dysfunction with ST segment elevation. Jpn Circ J 2000;64:156–9.

5. Tsuchihashi K, Ueshima K, Uchida T, et al. Transient left ventricular apical ballooning without coronary artery stenosis: a novel heart syndrome mimicking acute myocardial infarction. J Am Coll Cardiol 2001;38:11–8.

6. Kurisu S, Sato H, Kawagoe T, et al. Tako-tsubo like left ventricular dysfunction with ST-segment elevation: a novel cardiac syndrome mimicking acute myocardial infarction. Am Heart J 2002;143:448–55.

7. Abe Y, Kondo M, Matsuoka R, et al. Assessment of clinical features in transient left ventricular apical ballooning. J Am Coll Cardiol 2003;41:737–42.

8. Desmet WJ, Adriaenssens BF, Dens JA. Apical ballooning of the left ventricle: first series in white patients. Heart 2003;89:1027–31.

9. Sharkey SW, Lesser JR, Zenovich AG, et al. Acute and reversible cardiomyopathy provoked by stress in women from the United States. Circulation 2005; 111:472–9.

10. Wittstein IS, Thiemann DR, Lima JA, et al. Neurohumoral features of myocardial stunning due to sudden emotional stress. N Engl J Med 2005;352: 539–48.

11. Elesber AA, Prasad A, Lennon RJ, et al. Four-year recurrence rate and prognosis of the apical ballooning syndrome. J Am Coll Cardiol 2007;50: 448–52.

12. Parodi G, Del Pace S, Salvadori C, et al. Tuscany Registry of Tako-Tsubo Cardiomyopathy. Left ventricular apical ballooning syndrome as a novel cause of acute mitral regurgitation. J Am Coll Cardiol 2007;50:647–9.

13. Schneider B, Athanasiadis A, Schwab J, et al. Clinical spectrum of tako-tsubo cardiomyopathy in Germany: results of the tako-tsubo registry of the Arbeitsgemeinschaft Leitende Kardiologische Krankenhausärzte (ALKK). Dtsch Med Wochenschr 2010;135:1908–13 [in German].

14. Eitel I, von Knobelsdorff-Brenkenhoff F, Bernhardt P, et al. Clinical characteristics and cardiovascular magnetic resonance findings in stress (takotsubo) cardiomyopathy. JAMA 2011;306:277–86.

15. Hochman JS, Tamis JE, Thompson TD, et al. Sex, clinical presentation, and outcome in patients with acute coronary syndromes. N Engl J Med 1999; 341:226–32.

16. Heer T, Schiele R, Schneider S, et al. Gender differences in acute myocardial infarction in the era of reperfusion (the MITRA registry). Am J Cardiol 2002; 89:511–7.

17. Patel H, Rosengren A, Ekman I. Symptoms in acute coronary syndromes: does sex make a difference? Am Heart J 2004;148:27–33.

18. Heer T, Gitt AK, Juenger C, et al. ACOS Investigators. Gender differences in acute non-ST-segment elevation myocardial infarction. Am J Cardiol 2006; 98:160–6.

19. Koeth O, Zahn R, Heer T, et al. Gender differences in patients with acute ST-elevation myocardial infarction complicated by cardiogenic shock. Clin Res Cardiol 2009;98:781–6.

20. Dey S, Flather MD, Devlin G, et al. for the GRACE investigators. Sex related differences in the presentation, treatment and outcomes among patients with acute coronary syndromes: the Global Registry of Acute Coronary Events. Heart 2009;95:20–6.

21. Kurisu S, Inoue I, Kawagoe T, et al. Presentation of tako-tsubo cardiomyopathy in men and women. Clin Cardiol 2010;33:42–5.

22. Schneider B, Athanasiadis A, Stöllberger C, et al. Gender differences in the manifestation of tako-tsubo cardiomyopathy. Int J Cardiol 2011. http://dx.doi.org/10.1016/j.ijcard.2011.11.027.

23. Angelini P. Transient left ventricular apical ballooning: a unifying pathophysiologic theory at the edge of Prinzmetal angina. Catheter Cardiovasc Interv 2008;71:342–52.

24. Nojima Y, Kotani J. Global coronary artery spasm caused takotsubo cardiomyopathy. J Am Coll Cardiol 2010;55:e17.

25. Bybee KA, Prasad A, Barsness GW, et al. Clinical characteristics and thrombolysis in myocardial infarction frame counts in women with transient left ventricular apical ballooning syndrome. Am J Cardiol 2004;94:343–6.

26. Kume T, Akasaka T, Kawamoto T, et al. Assessment of coronary microcirculation in patients with takotsubo-like left ventricular dysfunction. Circ J 2005;69:934–9.

27. Elesber A, Lerman A, Bybee KA, et al. Myocardial perfusion in apical ballooning syndrome: correlate of myocardial injury. Am Heart J 2006;152:469.e9–e13.

28. Rigo F, Sicari R, Citro R, et al. Diffuse, marked, reversibile impairment in coronary microcirculation in stress cardiomyopathy: a Doppler transthoracic echo study. Ann Med 2009;41:462–70.

29. Galiuto L, De Caterina AR, Porfidia A, et al. Reversible coronary microvascular dysfunction: a common pathogenetic mechanism in apical ballooning or takotsubo syndrome. Eur Heart J 2010;31:1319–27.

30. Yoshioka T, Hashimoto A, Tsuchihashi K, et al. Clinical implications of midventricular obstruction and intravenous propranolol use in transient left ventricular apical ballooning (tako-tsubo cardiomyopathy). Am Heart J 2008;155:526.e1–7.

31. Mahmoud RE, Mansencal N, Pilliere R, et al. Prevalence and characteristics of left ventricular outflow tract obstruction in tako-tsubo syndrome. Am Heart J 2008;156:543–8.

32. Yoshida T, Hibino T, Kako N, et al. A pathophysiologic study of tako-tsubo cardiomyopathy with F-18 fluorodeoxyglucose positron emission tomography. Eur Heart J 2007;28:2598–604.

33. Nef HM, Möllmann H, Kostin S, et al. Tako-tsubo cardiomyopathy: intraindividual structural analysis in the acute phase and after functional recovery. Eur Heart J 2007;28:2456–64.

34. Spes C, Knape A, Mudra H. Recurrent tako-tsubo like left ventricular dysfunction (apical ballooning) in a patient with pheochromocytoma—a case report. Clin Res Cardiol 2006;95:307–11.

35. Ueda H, Hosokawa Y, Tsujii U, et al. An autopsy case of left ventricular apical ballooning probably caused by pheochromocytoma with persistent ST-segment elevation. Int J Cardiol 2011;149: e50–2.

36. Kono T, Morita H, Kuroiwa T, et al. Left ventricular wall motion abnormalities in patients with subarachnoid hemorrhage: neurogenic stunned myocardium. J Am Coll Cardiol 1994;24:636–40.

37. Naredi S, Lambert G, Eden E, et al. Increased sympathetic nervous activity in patients with non-traumatic subarachnoid hemorrhage. Stroke 2000; 31:901–6.

38. Ueyama T, Yoshida K, Senba E. Stress-induced elevation of the ST segment in the rat electrocardiogram is normalized by an adrenoreceptor blocker. Clin Exp Pharmacol Physiol 2000;27:384–6.

39. Ueyama T, Kasamatsu K, Hano T, et al. Emotional stress induces left ventricular hypocontraction in the rat via activation of cardiac adrenoreceptors— a possible animal model of tako-tsubo cardiomyopathy. Circ J 2002;66:712–3.

40. Komesaroff PA, Esler MD, Sudhir K. Estrogen supplementation attenuates glucocorticoid and catecholamine responses to mental stress in perimenopausal women. J Clin Endocrinol Metab 1999;84:606–10.

41. Sung BH, Ching M, Izzo JL, et al. Estrogen improves abnormal norepinephrine-induced vasoconstriction in postmenopausal women. J Hypertens 1999;17: 523–8.

42. Ueyama T, Hano T, Kasamatsu K, et al. Estrogen attenuates the emotional stress-induced cardiac responses in the animal model of tako-tsubo (ampulla) cardiomyopathy. J Cardiovasc Pharmacol 2003;42(Suppl 1):S117–9.

43. Ueyama T, Kasamatsu K, Hano T, et al. Catecholamines and estrogen are involved in the pathogenesis of emotional stress-induced acute heart attack. Ann N Y Acad Sci 2008;1148:479–85.

44. Kuo BT, Choubey R, Novaro GM. Reduced estrogen in menopause may predispose women to takotsubo cardiomyopathy. Gend Med 2010;7:71–7.

45. Akashi YJ, Nakazawa K, Sakakibara M, et al. 123I-MIBG myocardial scintigraphy in patients with takotsubo cardiomyopathy. J Nucl Med 2004;45:1121–7.

46. Matsuoka K, Okubo S, Fujii E, et al. Evaluation of the arrhythmogenecity of stress-induced takotsubo cardiomyopathy from the time course of the 12-lead surface electrocardiogram. Am J Cardiol 2003;92:230–3.

47. Haghi D, Athanasiadis A, Papavassiliu T, et al. Right ventricular involvement in tako tsubo cardiomyopathy. Eur Heart J 2006;27:2433–9.

48. Elian D, Osherov A, Matetyky S, et al. Left ventricular apical ballooning: not an uncommon variant of acute myocardial infarction in women. Clin Cardiol 2006;29:9–12.

49. Wedekind H, Möller K, Scholz KH. Tako-tsubo cardiomyopathy. Incidence in patients with acute coronary syndrome. Herz 2006;31:339–46.

50. Schneider B, Koch S, Stein J. Transient left ventricular dysfunction: differences between apical and mid-ventricular involvement. Circulation 2005;112(Suppl II):II-692.

51. Parodi G, Bellandi B, Del Pace S, et al. Natural history of tako-tsubo cardiomyopathy. Chest 2011;139:887–92.

52. Pilgrim TM, Wyss TR. Takotsubo cardiomyopathy or transient left ventricular apical ballooning syndrome: a systematic review. Int J Cardiol 2008;124:283–92.

53. Sharkey SW, Windenburg DC, Lesser JR, et al. Natural history and expansive clinical profile of stress (tako-tsubo) cardiomyopathy. J Am Coll Cardiol 2010;55:333–41.

54. Hahn JY, Gwon HC, Park SW, et al. The clinical features of transient left ventricular nonapical ballooning syndrome: comparison with apical ballooning syndrome. Am Heart J 2007;154:1166–73.

55. Lee PH, Song JC, Sun BJ, et al. Outcome of patients with stress-induced cardiomyopathy diagnosed by echocardiography in a tertiary referral hospital. J Am Soc Echocardiogr 2010;23:766–71.

56. Freitas HF, Renault R, Ribeiro ES, et al. Sudden cardiac death due to puerperal transient left ventricular apical ballooning syndrome. Int J Cardiol 2011;149:e12–3.

57. Olivotti L, Moshiri S, Nicolino A, et al. Stress cardiomyopathy and arrhythmic storm in a 14-year old boy. J Cardiovasc Med (Hagerstown) 2010;11:517–21.

58. Bajolle F, Basquin A, Lucron H, et al. Acute ischemic cardiomyopathy after extreme emotional stress in a child. Congenit Heart Dis 2009;4:387–90.

59. Schoof S, Bertram H, Hohmann D, et al. Takotsubo cardiomyopathy in a 2-year old girl. J Am Coll Cardiol 2010;55:e5.

60. Dib C, Asirvatham S, Elesber A, et al. Clinical correlates and prognostic significance of electrocardiographic abnormalities in apical ballooning syndrome (takotsubo/stress-induced cardiomyopathy). Am Heart J 2009;157:933–8.

61. Bowker TJ, Wood DA, Davies MJ. Sudden unexpected cardiac death: methods and results of a national pilot survey. Int J Cardiol 1995;52:241–50.

62. Thomas AC, Knapman PA, Krikler DM, et al. Community study of the causes of "natural" sudden death. BMJ 1988;297:1453–6.

63. Chugh SS, Jui J, Gunson K, et al. Current burden of sudden cardiac death: multiple source surveillance versus retrospective death certificate-based review in a large U.S. community. J Am Coll Cardiol 2004;44:1268–75.

64. Owada M, Aizawa Y, Kurihara K, et al. Risk factors and triggers of sudden death in the working generation: an autopsy proven case-control study. Tohoku J Exp Med 1999;189:245–58.

65. Larsen JA, Kadish AH. Effects of gender on cardiac arrhythmias. J Cardiovasc Electrophysiol 1998;9:655–64.

66. Samuelov-Kinori L, Kinori M, Kogan Y, et al. Takotsubo cardiomyopathy and QT interval prolongation: who are the patients at risk for torsades de pointes? J Electrocardiol 2009;42:353–7.

67. Madhavan M, Borlaug BA, Lerman A, et al. stress hormone and circulating biomarker profile of apical ballooning syndrome (takotsubo cardiomyopathy): insights into the clinical significance of B-type natriuretic peptide and Troponin levels. Heart 2009;95:1436–41.

68. Akashi YJ, Musha H, Nakazawa K, et al. Plasma brain natriuretic peptide in takotsubo cardiomyopathy. QJM 2004;97:599–607.

69. Kurowski V, Kaiser A, von Hof K, et al. Apical and midventricular transient left ventricular dysfunction syndrome (tako-tsubo cardiomyopathy). Frequency, mechanisms and prognosis. Chest 2007;132:809–16.

70. Elesber AA, Prasad A, Bybee KA, et al. Transient cardiac apical ballooning syndrome: prevalence and clinical implications of right ventricular involvement. J Am Coll Cardiol 2006;47:1082–3.

71. Haghi D, Papavassiliu T, Heggemann F, et al. Incidence and clinical significance of left ventricular thrombus in tako-tsubo cardiomyopathy assessed with echocardiography. QJM 2008;101:381–6.

72. de Gregorio C, Grimaldi P, Lentini C. Left ventricular thrombus formation and cardioembolic complications in patients with Takotsubo-like syndrome: a systematic review. Int J Cardiol 2008;131:18–24.

73. Andò G, Saporito F, Trio O, et al. Systemic embolism in takotsubo syndrome. Int J Cardiol 2009;134:e42–3.

74. Mitsuma W, Kodama M, Ito M, et al. Thromboembolism in takotsubo cardiomyopathy. Int J Cardiol 2010;139:98–100.

75. Akashi YJ, Tejima T, Sakurada H, et al. Left ventricular rupture associated with takotsubo cardiomyopathy. Mayo Clin Proc 2004;79:821–4.

76. Ohara Y, Hiasa Y, Hosokwa S, et al. Left ventricular free wall rupture in transient left ventricular apical ballooning. Circ J 2005;69:621–3.

77. Shinozaki K, Tamura A, Abe Y, et al. Left ventricular free wall rupture in takotsubo cardiomyopathy. Int J Cardiol 2007;115:e3–4.

78. Sacha J, Maselko J, Wester A, et al. Left ventricular apical rupture caused by takotsubo cardiomyopathy – comprehensive pathological heart investigation. Circ J 2007;71:982–5.

79. Ellison GM, Torella D, Karakikes I, et al. Acute beta-adrenergic overload produces myocyte damage through calcium leakage from the ryanodine receptor 2 but spares cardiac stem cells. J Biol Chem 2007;282:11397–409.

80. Lathers CM, Levin RM, Spivey WH. Regional distribution of myocardial beta-adrenoceptors in the cat. Eur J Pharmacol 1986;130:111–7.

Breaking Heart
Chronobiologic Insights into Takotsubo Cardiomyopathy

Roberto Manfredini, MD[a],*, Raffaella Salmi, MD[b],
Fabio Fabbian, MD[a], Fabio Manfredini, MD[c],
Massimo Gallerani, MD[d], Eduardo Bossone, MD, PhD, FESC[e,f]

KEYWORDS

- Chronobiology phenomena • Circadian rhythm • Seasons • Takotsubo cardiomyopathy
- Acute myocardial infarction • Stroke • Aortic aneurysm • Pulmonary embolism

KEY POINTS

- In a clinical emergency setting, when a prompt differential diagnosis between acute myocardial infarction and takotsubo cardiomyopathy (TTC) is needed, clinical factors (typical chest pain, female gender, postmenopausal age, recent stressful events) and instrumental examinations (electrocardiogram, echocardiography) are the first diagnostic tools.
- Although there is no consensus on the treatment of TTC, β-blockade has been suggested as a rational therapy.
- The possible identification of times of highest risk for TTC could help for tailoring appropriate use of drugs, such as β-blockers, to try to extend maximal benefit during the particularly vulnerable periods.

CHRONOBIOLOGY AND BIOLOGIC RHYTHMS

Chronobiology is a branch of biomedical sciences devoted to the study of biologic rhythms. It is known that biologic rhythms exist at any level of living organisms and, according to their cycle length, may be divided into three main types: (1) circadian rhythms (characterized by a period of approximately 24 hours); (2) ultradian rhythms (period shorter than 24 hours [eg, hours, minutes, or even seconds]); and (3) infradian rhythms (period longer than 24 hours [eg, days, weeks, months]).

Circadian rhythms are the most commonly and widely studied biologic rhythms, and are driven by circadian clocks. Circadian clocks can be defined as a transcriptionally based molecular mechanism, composed of positive and negative feedback loops, with a free-running period of approximately 24 hours.[1] The principal circadian clock or "master clock," located in the suprachiasmatic nucleus, is entrained by light and is supposed

This work was supported, in part, by a scientific grant (FAR – Fondo Ateneo Ricerca) from the University of Ferrara, Italy.

The authors have nothing to disclose.

[a] Clinica Medica, Department of Medicine, General and University Hospital of Ferrara, Via Aldo Moro, 44124 Cona, Ferrara, Italy; [b] 2nd Internal Unit of Internal Medicine, Department of Medicine, General and University Hospital of Ferrara, Via Aldo Moro, 44124 Cona, Ferrara, Italy; [c] Vascular Diseases Center, University of Ferrara, Via Gramicia 35, Ferrara 44123, Italy; [d] 1st Internal Unit of Internal Medicine, Department of Medicine, General and University Hospital of Ferrara, Via Aldo Moro, 44124 Cona, Ferrara, Italy; [e] Cardiac Surgery Department, IRCCS Policlinico San Donato, Piazza Edmondo Malan 1, 20097 San Donato Milanese, Italy; [f] Cardiology Division, "Cava de' Tirreni and Amalfi Coast" Hospital, Heart Department, University of Salerno, Via De Marinis, 84013 Cava de' Tirreni (SA), Italy

* Corresponding author.

E-mail address: roberto.manfredini@unife.it

to entrain peripheral clocks by neurohumoral modulation.[1] Circadian clocks have been identified within almost all mammalian cell types, including cardiomyocytes,[2] vascular smooth muscle cells, and endothelial cells,[3] and circadian clock genes are essential for cardiovascular health. Anticipation is the principal role of cellular biologic clocks, because the capacity to know the time of day represents critical information and selective advantage.

The cardiovascular system is organized according to a specific temporal order that is oscillatory in nature, and most cardiovascular functions exhibit circadian changes. Such predictable-in-time differences in the physiologic status of the cardiovascular system give rise to rhythmic variations in the susceptibility of human beings to morbid and mortal events. However, the pathologic mechanisms of cardiovascular disease themselves exhibit temporal changes in their manifestation and severity, leading to predictable-in-time differences in their ability to precipitate and graduate the overt expression of disease.[4] A growing body of evidence suggests that the occurrence of cardiovascular events is not evenly distributed in time, but shows peculiar temporal patterns that vary with time of the day, day of the week, and month of the year. These patterns coincide with the temporal variation in the pathophysiologic mechanisms that trigger cardiovascular events and physiologic changes in the body rhythms. These contribute to the definition of the new concept of "chronorisk," where the constellation of several factors, not harmful if taken alone, are capable to trigger unfavorable events when presenting all together within the same temporal window.

BIOLOGIC RHYTHMS AND PATTERNS OF ONSET OF ACUTE CARDIOVASCULAR DISEASES

A considerable amount of evidence shows that the major leading acute cardiovascular diseases underlying cardiac death (ie, acute myocardial infarction [AMI], stroke, pulmonary embolism, and rupture or dissection of aortic aneurysms[5]) do not randomly occur along time, but seem to exhibit specific temporal patterns in their onset, according to time of day, month, or season, and day of week, independent of gender.[6]

Acute Myocardial Infarction

Circadian (time of day)
Several decades ago, Muller and colleagues[7] first observed a circadian variation for onset of AMI, characterized by increased morning frequency

between 6 and 12 AM. Some years later, a comprehensive meta-analysis[8] considering 30 studies on nonfatal AMI (more than 66,000 cases) and 19 studies on sudden cardiac death (near 6000 cases), reported that 27.7% of morning AMIs and 22.5% of sudden cardiac death, accounting for approximately 9% and 7% of all AMIs and sudden cardiac death, respectively, were attributable to a morning excess of risk. It is possible that time of day may have an impact on clinical outcome: an excess of fatal infarctions have been reported between 6 and 12 AM, independent of patients' age and AMI site or extension.[9]

Seasonal
Data from the US Second National Registry of Myocardial Infarction reported 53% more cases in the winter than in the summer, and winter was characterized by the highest frequency of fatal cases.[10] With some exceptions, most studies have reported the lowest frequency of AMI onset in the summer and the highest frequency during winter.[11] Our group has recently confirmed this temporal pattern in more than 64,000 consecutive cases of AMI hospitalized between 1998 and 2006 in the Emilia-Romagna region of Italy.[12]

Circaseptan (weekly)
More than a decade ago, Willich and colleagues[13] in Germany, and Gnecchi-Ruscone and colleagues[14] in Italy, reported an increased risk of AMI on Monday. In particular, Willich and colleagues[13] found that this weekly variation with a Monday peak was present only in the working but not in nonworking population. A couple of years after, Spielberg and colleagues,[15] in Germany, confirmed the higher frequency of events on Monday, but with no differences between working or retired patients. A meta-analysis study aimed to quantify the excess risk associated with the Monday peak in cardiovascular mortality[16] found an increased pooled odds ratio of 1.19, without significant differences between subgroups by gender and age. Our group recently confirmed the Monday excess (16.1%) with a lower rate on Sunday (11.8%).[12]

A recent meta-analysis of 28 community-based studies[17] confirmed a statistically significant excess in coronary events on Mondays in 20 out of 28 studies. The Monday excess in events was observed in fatal and nonfatal events in both sexes, and was greater in younger compared with older subjects. However, this meta-analysis showed that, even if greater than zero, the Monday excess in coronary event was small (being calculated as less than 1 event in 100, with a relative increase of 1%), compared with the estimated excess in morning (+40%) and in winter (+45%).

Stroke

Circadian (time of day)

Since the late 1980s, several studies have indicated that the incidence of stroke shows a significant circadian rhythm, characterized by a higher frequency during morning hours.[18–21] A comprehensive meta-analysis of 31 separate studies found that approximately 55% of ischemic strokes, 34% of hemorrhagic strokes, and 50% of transient ischemic attacks occurred between 6 and 12 AM.[22] As for ischemic stroke, it has been found that the morning preference is independent of patients' age; gender; common risk factors (ie, smoke, hypertension, diabetes, dyslipidemia); and type of stroke.[23] The interesting analogy of the temporal window of occurrence of either ischemic or hemorrhagic strokes[21,23–25] seems to suggest that probably a series of common risk factors are shared by the two entities.[26]

Seasonal

Several studies have reported seasonality in the occurrence of stroke, characterized by a winter and autumn peak for its occurrence.[27–33] The complications of acute carotid surgery also exhibit a similar pattern.[34]

Circaseptan (weekly)

Several studies have indicated that Monday represents a critical day for onset of stroke,[35,36] and this seems to be independent of the presence or not of most common risk factors.[37] A recent study by our group on more than 56,000 patients with ischemic stroke admitted to the hospitals of the Emilia-Romagna region of Italy confirmed that admissions were most frequent on Monday (16.6%) and least frequent on Sunday (12.9%), also with no significant differences between fatal or nonfatal cases.[38] Such a pattern was found to be exactly the same for transient ischemic attacks (16.1% vs 11.6%).[39]

Rupture or Dissection of Aortic Aneurysms

Circadian (time of day)

Also for abdominal or thoracic aortic aneurysms, several studies have found a circadian variation, characterized by an increased risk of rupture or dissection during early morning hours.[40–42] Analysis of the IRAD registry showed that this morning peak (around 8–9 AM) was independent of gender, type A or B dissection, age less than or greater than or equal to 70 years, and presence or absence of hypertension.[43] Such pattern coincides with the temporal variation in the pathophysiology

mechanisms that trigger cardiovascular events and the physiologic changes in body rhythms.[44]

Seasonal

Most available studies indicate a greater occurrence of aortic rupture or dissection during the fall and winter months,[45–49] although temporal pattern seems to be independent of climatic variables.[50] Moreover, mortality does not seem to be affected by seasonal (or circadian) patterns.[51]

Circaseptan (weekly)

A few studies have investigated this temporal aspect. Sumiyoshi and coworkers[42] found a small peak on Monday and a trough on Thursday and Friday, but the distribution was homogenous as a whole. The IRAD Registry study[43] did not find any significant weekly variation. A weekly pattern, characterized by a decreasing frequency from Monday to Sunday, was shown in more than 4500 cases in the Emilia-Romagna region of Italy.[52] Fatal cases showed an opposite trend with a peak on Sunday. Moreover, mortality is higher in cases admitted on weekends compared with weekdays.[53]

Pulmonary Embolism

Circadian (time of day)

Previous studies reported the existence of a circadian variation also in the occurrence of acute pulmonary embolism[54,55] characterized by the same main morning peak observed also for arterial embolism.[56]

Seasonal

A seasonal pattern, characterized by an autumnal but especially a winter peak, has been reported for venous thromboembolism (deep vein thrombosis and pulmonary embolism[57–64]), although some studies did not confirm this pattern.[65] A recent meta-analysis of the available literature (about 35,000 cases) confirmed the increased incidence of venous thromboembolism in winter, with a relative risk of 1.14 (1.19 in the month of January).[66] Such a pattern seems to be independent of risk factors and patients' comorbid conditions.[67]

Circaseptan (weekly)

No reports are available dealing with weekly variation of pulmonary embolism, although a higher mortality has been found in patients hospitalized during weekends compared with weekdays.[68]

TAKOTSUBO CARDIOMYOPATHY

A novel cardiac syndrome, characterized by transient left ventricular and dysfunction, has been recently described in Japanese patients. It has been named "tako-tsubo," from the Japanese terms indicating the particular shape of the end-systolic left ventricle in ventriculography resembling that of the round-bottom and narrow-neck pot used for trapping octopuses.[69] Other terms, in addition to takotsubo cardiomyopathy (TTC), have been used to define this cardiac entity (ie, "apical ballooning," "acute stress cardiomyopathy," or "broken heart"). The diagnostic criteria[69] include transient hypokinesis, akinesis, or dyskinesis in the left ventricular mid segments with or without apical involvement; regional wall motion abnormalities that extend beyond a single epicardial vascular distribution; frequently but not always, a stressful trigger[2]; absence of obstructive coronary disease or angiographic evidence of acute plaque rupture[3]; new electrocardiogram abnormalities (ST-segment elevation or T-wave inversion) or modest elevation in cardiac troponin; and absence of myocarditis or pheochromocytoma.[4]

Recent data on a large population of more than 6800 cases of TTC in the United States, referring to the National Inpatient Sample database,[70] reported an overall frequency of 5.2 per 100,000 for women and 0.6 per 100,000 for men, with a preferite age between 66 and 80 years, a uniform distribution in the different regions, and a higher frequency in whites compared with African Americans and Hispanics.

TTC has gained growing interest among cardiologists and emergency doctors, because it is usually triggered by severe emotional or physical stress, and generally mimics the clinical scenario of AMI.[71,72] The prevalence among patients with symptoms suggestive of AMI is 0.7% to 2.5%,[73] and approximately 2% of ST-elevation acute coronary syndromes referring to the hospital are consistent with TTC.[74]

This clinical similarity with AMI suggested investigating whether a temporal pattern of onset could be demonstrated for TTC. Our group performed a computer-assisted MEDLINE search of the literature, years 2000 to 2010,[75] with the following search terms: transient left ventricular apical ballooning syndrome, takotsubo-like left ventricular dysfunction, ampulla cardiomyopathy, takotsubo or takotsubo cardiomyopathy, tako-tsubo, and apical ballooning. Criteria for inclusion in the study were set a priori[76] and included (1) reporting of original data, (2) inclusion of at least 30 or more cases, and (3) adherence to the requested diagnostic criteria for TTC. **Table 1** reports the results of the original study updated with three further studies.

Table 1
Time of onset of takotsubo cardiomyopathy: analysis of 2000–2012 studies

Author (Year)	Country	Cases (N)	Peak
Deshmukh et al,[70] 2012	United States	6837	July (and through January) (P = not given)
Sharkey et al,[80] 2012	United States	186	Afternoon (noon–4 PM) (P<.001) December (P = ns) Tuesday (P = ns)
Parodi et al,[88,89] 2011	Italy	116	Spring and Summer (P = ns) No weekend/weekday variation
Summers et al,[87] 2010	United States	186	January and August (P = ns) No seasonal peak
Mansecal et al,[86] 2010	France	51	April (P = not given)
Regnante et al,[83] 2009	United States	70	Summer (P<.001)
Manfredini et al,[12,37,38,64,84] 2009[a]	Italy	112	July (P = .006)
Citro et al,[78] 2009	Italy	88	July (P = .016) Morning (P = .021)
Eshtehardi et al,[85] 2009	Switzerland	41	Winter (P = .003)
Kurisu et al,[77] 2007	Japan	50	Morning-afternoon (P = ns) Daytime vs nighttime (P = .004)
Abdulla et al,[79] 2007	Australia	35	Morning-afternoon-night (P = ns) Summer (P = ns)
Hertting et al,[81] 2006	Germany	32	Summer July (P = .026)

[a] The data by Manfredini et al represent a further update of those by Citro et al.

Circadian (Time of Day)

Two studies reported a morning preference for TTC onset[77,78] but another did not find significant variations.[79] Kurisu and colleagues,[77] in a study on 50 subjects in Japan, found a nonsignificant trend for TTC occurrence during the morning and afternoon 6-hour periods (6 AM to noon and 12 PM to 6 PM, respectively). However, when comparing daytime (6 AM TO 6 PM) with nighttime (6 PM to 6 AM), the distribution was statistically different (73% vs 27%; $P = .004$). Citro and colleagues,[78] in a series of 79 patients in Italy, confirmed a higher frequency of events in the morning and fewest at night (40.5% vs 10.2%; $P = .021$). Abdulla and colleagues[79] did not find significant differences in the timing of onset of symptom in 35 subjects in Australia by splitting the day into three 8-hour periods (morning, 6 AM to 2 PM; afternoon, 2 PM to 10 PM; night, 10 PM to 6 AM). Recently, Sharkey and colleagues[80] reported for TTC a nonuniform distribution with a distinctive afternoon peak from 12 noon to 4 PM, and a nadir at 12 to 4 AM ($P<.001$).

Seasonal

More studies reported this information. Abdulla and colleagues[79] found a slight, statistically not significant, summer preference. Hertting and colleagues[81] found that one-half of their 32 German patients had an event during summer months. When reanalyzing the raw monthly data by means of a chronobiologic software Chronolab,[82] a significant peak was found in July. A significant summer preference was confirmed also from studies in the United States, Rhode Island Registry[83] and in a multicenter series in Italy.[78,84] Different results were reported by Eshtehardi and colleagues[85] in Switzerland (peak in winter; $P = .03$); Sharkey and colleagues[80] in the United States (peak in December, but uniform distribution; $P = .77$); and Mansecal and colleagues[86] in France (peak in April; P value not given). Further studies conducted in the United States on 186 consecutive patients[87] and in Italy (116 subjects)[88,89] did not confirm the preference of a chronobiologic pattern (not significant peaks in August and January, and spring and summer, respectively). Very recently, data on 6837 patients from the US Nationwide Inpatients Sample database confirmed a peak in July (and a trough in January).[70]

Circaseptan (Weekly)

Only one positive study is available, and it refers to the Italian collaborative study.[90] The highest number of cases was found on Monday and the lowest on Saturday, with a significant rhythmic reproducible pattern. Parodi and colleagues[88,89] analyzed their cohort of patients according to weekend or weekdays, but there was no significant difference. Again, Sharkey and colleagues[80] found highest frequency of events on Tuesday and lowest on Sunday, but events were uniformly distributed throughout the week ($P = .18$).

PATHOPHYSIOLOGIC FACTORS AND TIME: IS THERE A POSSIBLE LINK?

The overt and underlying causes of TTC remain unclear. Several possible pathologic mechanisms[73] have been put forward: vasospasm of coronary arteries; disturbance of the microcirculation; obstruction of the left ventricular outflow tract; and catecholamine-mediated effect, secondary to exposure to either endogenous or exogenous stress, and increased sympathetic activity. Other supported hypotheses[91] include estrogen deficiency theory, genetic predisposition, and ruptured plaque theory.

A series of factors, some of them leading to an increase of oxygen demand and others reducing oxygen supply, potentially related with vasospasm of coronary arteries, disturbance of the microcirculation, and obstruction of the left ventricular outflow tract, may be temporally related to the morning hours. A first group of causes includes activation of sympathetic nervous system during the rapid eye movement phase of sleep, the rise of heart rate and blood pressure (BP) (morning BP surge) on awakening and commencing daily activities, the morning rise in plasma cortisol levels, contributing to the sensitivity of vessels to vasoconstrictor stimuli. However, morning reduction in myocardial oxygen supply may derive from the enhanced vascular tone (with consequently reduced flow), mediated by an increased α-sympathetic vasoconstrictor activity, the imbalance between hypercoagulation (increased levels of fibrinogen, plasma viscosity, hematocrit, platelet aggregability), and reduced endogenous fibrinolysis.[92,93]

The hypothesis of catecholamine (CA)-mediated effect, secondary to exposure to either endogenous or exogenous stress, and increased sympathetic activity, is based on the possible relationship between increased sympathetic activity, stress and stressful events, and TTC. Wittstein and colleagues[94] found significantly higher plasma CAs levels in a group of patients with stress-induced cardiomyopathy compared with patients with MI. Moreover, most TTC patients have experienced a prior stressful event, emotional or physical. As for possible time-related circadian aspects, catecholamines show a circadian periodicity, with a urinary peak in late morning.[95] Moreover, in healthy women under routine lifestyle, the excretion of norepinephrine (NE) was higher during the working hours (9 AM to 3 PM).[96] Also, the stress hormone cortisol in healthy individuals exhibits a diurnal pattern with an early morning peak, then a decline throughout the day, and a nadir around 2 or 3 AM.[97]

Stress, both chronic and acute, is a potential trigger for cardiovascular disease. Acute stressful events (in the recent 48 hours), independent of traditional risk factors, may play a triggering role on the occurrence of acute coronary syndrome, and chronic stress also may play a role.[98] The circadian system and the stress response system together play a crucial role in the adaptation of the organism to environmental challenges. The central master clock uses light as its primary synchronizer, whereas peripheral clocks are influenced by neurohumoral factors (ie, angiotensin for the circadian clock within vascular smooth muscle cells[99] and NE within the cardiomyocyte[100]). Acute exposure of cardiomyocytes to NE, mimicking a burst of sympathetic activity, induced oscillations in three circadian clock components (bmal1, rev-erbα, and per2) and the circadian clock–regulated gene dbp. A tight link between catecholamines and molecular clock exists[101]: (1) the molecular clock influences sympathoadrenal function, and NE and epinephrine (Epi) exhibit a diurnal variation, with higher levels during the active phase; (2) genes relevant to CAs synthesis and disposition are under the control of the molecular clock; (3) BMAL1 and CLOCK are indispensable for the circadian rhythm of BP; and (4) the circadian clock modulates selective stress response. In humans, stress is capable of exerting major effects on the circulatory system, particularly in the morning, by multiple mechanisms, including catecholamine activation, and changes in heart rate, systemic and diastolic BP, blood viscosity, and coagulation.[102]

Very little is known regarding seasonal aspects of catecholamines, although several studies have reported a summer peak for NE and Epi.[95,96] Some authors have described a summer frequency of onset of TTC, and this pattern is opposite to that reported for MI. Changes in ambient temperature, with consequences on coagulation, BP, and endothelial function, have been called as potential favoring factors for the winter peak of MI.[103]

Finally, only one study has shown a day-of-week variation in the onset of TTC.[90] Monday is a critical day for onset of other unfavorable cardiac events (eg, MI and sudden death).[13,14,104,105] The stress of commencing the weekly activities has been proposed as a potential triggering factor. In fact, a Monday morning surge in BP has been demonstrated,[106] and the average BP on a workday was higher than on a nonworkday.[107] However, Parodi and colleagues[88,89] did not find differences in the occurrence of TTC between weekend and weekdays. Other confirmation studies on larger sample populations and in different countries are needed.

SUMMARY

Although the onset of TTC seems to be more frequent during morning hours and summer months, it is not possible to draw definite conclusions. Thus, time of onset may not represent a useful tool in diagnosing TTC.[108] However, the morning frequency of TTC is similar to that of acute MI. It is possible that these two clinical entities share several concurrent underlying risk factors, and circadian rhythms and stress play a pivotal role in the diurnal regulation of multiple cardiovascular parameters. However, the seasonal summer preference is quite different, compared with the well-known winter peak of MI. In a clinical emergency setting, when a prompt differential diagnosis between AMI and TTC is needed, clinical factors (typical chest pain, female gender, postmenopausal age, recent stressful events) and instrumental examinations (electrocardiogram, echocardiography) are the first diagnostic tools. However, it has been shown that emergency department arrivals respect a different temporal pattern depending on the type of acute disease,[109] and also the clinical severity of certain diseases (ie, acute coronary syndrome), could be different at different times.[110] The possibility of a chronotherapeutic approach to cardiovascular diseases was hypothesized as far back as a few decades ago.[111] Although there is no consensus on the treatment of TTC, β-blockade has been suggested as a rational therapy.[91] The possible identification of times of highest risk for TTC could help for tailoring appropriate use of drugs, such as β-blockers, to try to extend maximal benefit during the particularly vulnerable periods.

REFERENCES

1. Edery I. Circadian rhythms in a nutshell. Physiol Genomics 2000;3:59–74.
2. Durgan DJ, Young ME. The cardiomyocyte circadian clock. Emerging roles in health and disease. Circ Res 2010;106:647–58.
3. Takeda N, Maemura K, Horie S, et al. Thrombomodulin is a clock-controlled gene in vascular endothelial cells. J Biol Chem 2007;282:32561–7.

4. Portaluppi F, Manfredini R, Fersini C. From a static to a dynamic concept of risk: the circadian epidemiology of cardiovascular events. Chronobiol Int 1999;16:33–49.

5. Manfredini R, Portaluppi F, Grandi E, et al. Out of hospital sudden death referring to an emergency department. J Clin Epidemiol 1996;49:865–8.

6. Manfredini R, Fabbian F, Pala M, et al. Seasonal and weekly patterns of occurrence of acute cardiovascular diseases: does a gender difference exist? J Womens Health 2011;20:1663–8.

7. Muller JE, Stone PH, Turi ZG, et al. Circadian variation in the frequency of onset of acute myocardial infarction. N Engl J Med 1985;313:1315–22.

8. Cohen MC, Rohtla KM, Lavery CE, et al. Meta-analysis of the morning excess of acute myocardial infarction and sudden cardiac death. Am J Cardiol 1997;79:1512–5.

9. Manfredini R, Boari B, Bressan S, et al. Influence of circadian rhythm on mortality after myocardial infarction: data from a prospective cohort of emergency calls. Am J Emerg Med 2004;22:555–9.

10. Ornato JP, Peberdy MA, Chandra NC, et al. Seasonal pattern of acute myocardial infarction in the National Registry of Myocardial Infarction. J Am Coll Cardiol 1996;28:1684–8.

11. Manfredini R, Boari B, Smolensky MH, et al. Seasonal variation in onset of myocardial infarction-a 7-year single-center study in Italy. Chronobiol Int 2005;22:1121–35.

12. Manfredini R, Manfredini F, Boari B, et al. Seasonal and weekly patterns of hospital admissions for nonfatal and fatal myocardial infarction. Am J Emerg Med 2009;27:1096–102.

13. Willich SN, Lowel H, Lewis M, et al. Weekly variation of acute myocardial infarction: increased Monday risk in the working population. Circulation 1994;90:87–93.

14. Gnecchi-Ruscone T, Piccaluga E, Guzzetti S, et al. Mornings and Monday: critical periods for the onset of acute myocardial infarction. Eur Heart J 1994;15:882–7.

15. Spielberg C, Falkenhahm D, Willich SH, et al. Circadian, day of week and seasonal variability in myocardial infarction: comparison between working and retired patients. Am Heart J 1996;132:579–84.

16. Witte DR, Grobbee DE, Bots ML, et al. Meta-analysis of excess cardiac mortality on Monday. Eur J Epidemiol 2005;20:401–6.

17. Barnett AG, Dobson AJ. Excess in cardiovascular events on Mondays: a meta-analysis and perspective study. J Epidemiol Community Health 2005;59:109–14.

18. Marler JR, Price RT, Clark GL, et al. Morning increase in onset of ischemic stroke. Stroke 1989;20:473–6.

19. Marsh EE, Biller J, Adams HP Jr, et al. Circadian variation in onset of acute ischemic stroke. Arch Neurol 1990;47:1178–80.

20. Kelly-Hayes M, Wolf PA, Kase CS, et al. Temporal patterns of stroke onset. The Framingham Study. Stroke 1995;26:1343–7.

21. Gallerani M, Portaluppi F, Maida G, et al. Circadian and circannual rhythmicity in the occurrence of subarachnoid hemorrhage. Stroke 1996;27:1793–7.

22. Elliott WJ. Circadian variation in the time of stroke onset: a meta-analysis. Stroke 1998;29:992–6.

23. Casetta I, Granieri E, Fallica E, et al. Patient demographic and clinical features and circadian variation in onset of ischemic stroke. Arch Neurol 2002;59:48–53.

24. Gallerani M, Trappella G, Manfredini R, et al. Acute intracerebral haemorrhage: circadian and circannual patterns of onset. Acta Neurol Scand 1994;89:280–6.

25. Casetta I, Granieri E, Portaluppi F, et al. Circadian variability in hemorrhagic stroke. JAMA 2002;287:1266–7.

26. Manfredini R, Boari B, Smolensky MH, et al. Circadian variation in stroke onset: identical temporal pattern in ischemic and hemorrhagic events. Chronobiol Int 2005;22:417–53.

27. Alter M, Christoferson L, Resch J, et al. Cerebrovascular disease: frequency and population selectivity in an upper Midwestern community. Stroke 1970;1:454–65.

28. Haberman S, Capildeo R, Rose FC. The seasonal variation in mortality from cerebrovascular disease. J Neurol Sci 1981;52:25–36.

29. Suzuki K, Kutzusawa T, Takita K, et al. Clinico-epidemiologic study of stroke in Japan. Stroke 1987;18:402–6.

30. Giroud M, Beuriat P, Vion P, et al. Stroke in a French prospective population study. Neuroepidemiology 1989;8:97–104.

31. Ricci S, Celani MG, Vitali R, et al. Diurnal and seasonal variations in the occurrence of stroke: a community-based study. Neuroepidemiology 1992;11:59–64.

32. Gallerani M, Manfredini R, Ricci L, et al. Chronobiological aspects of acute cerebrovascular diseases. Acta Neurol Scand 1993;87:482–7.

33. Manfredini R, Gallerani M, Portaluppi F, et al. Chronobiological patterns of onset of acute cerebrovascular diseases. Thromb Res 1997;88:451–63.

34. Coen M, Manfredini F, Agnati M, et al. Seasonal variation of acute carotid surgery: does it exist? J Vasc Surg 2010;51:285–6.

35. Manfredini R, Casetta I, Paolino E, et al. Monday preference in onset of ischemic stroke. Am J Med 2001;111:401–3.

36. Jakovljevic D. Day of the week and ischemic stroke: is it Monday high or Sunday low? Stroke 2004;35:2089–93.

37. Manfredini R, Manfredini F, Boari B, et al. The Monday peak in the onset of ischemic stroke is independent of major risk factors. Am J Emerg Med 2009;27:244–6.

38. Manfredini R, Manfredini F, Malagoni AM, et al. Day-of-week distribution of fatal and nonfatal stroke in elderly subjects. J Am Geriatr Soc 2009;57: 1511–3.

39. Manfredini R, Manfredini F, Boari B, et al. Temporal patterns of hospital admissions for transient ischemic attack. A retrospective population-based study in the Emilia-Romagna region of Italy. Clin Appl Thromb Hemost 2010;16:153–60.

40. Manfredini R, Portaluppi F, Zamboni P, et al. Circadian variation in spontaneous rupture of abdominal aorta. Lancet 1999;353:643–4.

41. Gallerani M, Portaluppi F, Grandi E, et al. Circadian rhythmicity in the occurrence of spontaneous acute dissection and rupture of thoracic aorta. J Thorac Cardiovasc Surg 1997;113:603–4.

42. Sumiyoshi M, Kojima S, Arima M, et al. Circadian, weekly, and seasonal variation at the onset of acute aortic dissection. Am J Cardiol 2002;89:619–23.

43. Mehta RH, Manfredini R, Hassan F, et al. Chronobiological patterns of acute aortic dissection. Circulation 2002;106:1110–5.

44. Manfredini R, Boari B, Gallerani M, et al. Chronobiology of rupture and dissection of aortic aneurysms. J Vasc Surg 2004;40:382–8.

45. Liapis C, Sechas M, Iliopoulos D, et al. Seasonal variation in the incidence of ruptured abdominal aortic aneurysms. Eur J Vasc Surg 1992;6:416–8.

46. Manfredini R, Portaluppi F, Gallerani M, et al. Seasonal variation in the rupture of abdominal aortic aneurysms. Jpn Heart J 1997;38:67–72.

47. Manfredini R, Portaluppi F, Salmi R, et al. Seasonal variation in the occurrence of non traumatic rupture of thoracic aorta. Am J Emerg Med 1999;17:672–4.

48. Kobza R, Ritter M, Seifert B, et al. Variable seasonal peaks for different types of aortic dissection? Heart 2002;88:640.

49. Manfredini R, Boari B, Manfredini F, et al. Seasonal variation in occurrence of aortic diseases: the database of hospital discharge data of the Emilia-Romagna region, Italy. J Thorac Cardiovasc Surg 2008;135:442–4.

50. Mehta RH, Manfredini R, Bossone E, et al. The winter peak in the occurrence of acute aortic dissection is independent of the climate. Chronobiol Int 2005;22:723–9.

51. Mehta RH, Manfredini R, Bossone E, et al. Does circadian and seasonal variation in the occurrence of acute aortic dissection influence in-hospital mortality outcomes? Chronobiol Int 2005;22:343–51.

52. Manfredini R, Boari B, Salmi R, et al. Day-of-week variability in the occurrence and outcome of aortic diseases: does it exist? Am J Emerg Med 2008;26: 363–6.

53. Gallerani M, Imberti D, Bossone E, et al. Higher mortality in patients hospitalized for acute aortic rupture or dissection during weekends. J Vasc Surg 2012;55:1247–54.

54. Gallerani M, Manfredini R, Ricci L, et al. Sudden death from pulmonary thromboembolism: chronobiological aspects. Eur Heart J 1992;13:661–5.

55. Sharma GV, Frisbie JH, Tow DE, et al. Circadian and circannual rhythm of nonfatal pulmonary embolism. Am J Cardiol 2001;87:922–4.

56. Manfredini R, Gallerani M, Portaluppi F, et al. Circadian variation in the onset of acute critical limb ischemia. Thromb Res 1998;92:163–9.

57. Colantonio D, Casale R, Natali G, et al. Seasonal periodicity in fatal pulmonary thromboembolism. Lancet 1990;335:56–7.

58. Manfredini R, Gallerani M, Salmi R, et al. Fatal pulmonary embolism in hospitalized subjects: evidence for a winter peak. J Int Med Res 1994; 22:85–9.

59. Chau KY, Yuen ST, Wong MP. Seasonal variation in the necropsy incidence of pulmonary thromboembolism in Hong Kong. J Clin Pathol 1995;48:578–9.

60. Boulay F, Berthier F, Schoukroun G, et al. Seasonal variations in hospital admissions for deep vein thrombosis and pulmonary embolism: analysis of discharge data. BMJ 2001;323:601–2.

61. Bilora F, Boccioletti V, Manfredini R, et al. Seasonal variation in the incidence of deep vein thrombosis in patients with deficiency of protein C or protein S. Clin Appl Thromb Hemost 2002;8:231–7.

62. Gallerani M, Boari B, De Toma D, et al. Seasonal variation in the occurrence of deep vein thrombosis. Med Sci Monit 2004;10:191–6.

63. Gallerani M, Boari B, Smolensky MH, et al. Seasonal variation in occurrence of pulmonary embolism: analysis of the database of the Emilia-Romagna region, Italy. Chronobiol Int 2007;24: 143–60.

64. Manfredini R, Imberti D, Gallerani M, et al. Seasonal variation in the occurrence of venous thromboembolism: data from the MASTER registry. Clin Appl Thromb Hemost 2009;15:309–15.

65. Stein PD, Kayali F, Olson RE. Analysis of occurrence of venous thromboembolic disease in the four seasons. Am J Cardiol 2004;93:511–3.

66. Dentali F, Ageno W, Rancan E, et al. Seasonal and monthly variability in the incidence of venous thromboembolism: a systematic review and a meta-analysis of the literature. Thromb Haemost 2011; 106:439–47.

67. Manfredini R, Gallerani M, Boari B, et al. The seasonal variation in the onset of pulmonary

embolism is independent of patients' underlying risk comorbid conditions. Clin Appl Thromb Hemost 2004;10:39–43.

68. Gallerani M, Imberti D, Ageno W, et al. Higher mortality rate in patients hospitalised for acute pulmonary embolism during weekend. Thromb Haemost 2011;106:83–9.

69. Prasad A, Lerman A, Rihal CS. Apical ballooning syndrome (tako-tsubo or stress cardiomyopathy): a mimic of acute myocardial infarction. Am Heart J 2008;155:408–17.

70. Deshmukh A, Kumar G, Pant S, et al. Prevalence of takotsubo cardiomyopathy in the United States. Am Heart J 2012;164:66–71.e1.

71. Kurisu S, Sato H, Kawagoe T, et al. Tako-tsubo-like left ventricular dysfunction with ST-segment elevation: a novel cardiac syndrome mimicking acute myocardial infarction. Am Heart J 2002; 143:448–55.

72. Kolkebeck TE, Cotant CL, Krasuski RA. Takotsubo cardiomyopathy: an unusual syndrome mimicking an ST-elevation myocardial infarction. Am J Emerg Med 2007;25:92–5.

73. Nef HM, Mollmann H, Akashi YI, et al. Mechanisms of stress (takotsubo) cardiomyopathy. Nat Rev Cardiol 2010;7:187–93.

74. Bybee KA. Clinical characteristics and thrombolysis in myocardial infarction frame counts in women with transient left ventricular apical ballooning syndrome. Am J Cardiol 2004;94:343–6.

75. Gianni M, Dentali F, Grandi AM, et al. Apical ballooning syndrome or takotsubo cardiomyopathy: a systematic review. Eur Heart J 2006;27:1523–9.

76. Bossone E, Citro R, Eagle KA, et al. Tako-tsubo cardiomyopathy: is there a preferred time of onset? Intern Emerg Med 2011;6:221–6.

77. Kurisu S, Inoue I, Kawagoe T, et al. Circadian variation in the occurrence of tako-tsubo cardiomyopathy: comparison with acute myocardial infarction. Int J Cardiol 2007;115:270–1.

78. Citro R, Previtali M, Bovelli D, et al. Chronobiological patterns of onset of tako-tsubo cardiomyopathy. J Am Coll Cardiol 2009;54:180–1.

79. Abdulla I, Kay S, Mussap C, et al. Apical sparing in tako-tsubo cardiomyopathy. Intern Med J 2007;36: 414–8.

80. Sharkey SW, Lesser JR, Garberich RF, et al. Comparison of circadian rhythm patterns in takotsubo cardiomyopathy versus ST- segment elevation myocardial infarction. Am J Cardiol 2012;110: 795–9. http://dx.doi.org/10.1016/j.amjcard.2012. 04.060.

81. Hertting K, Krause K, Harle T, et al. Transient left ventricular apical ballooning in a community hospital in Germany. Int J Cardiol 2006;112:282–8.

82. Mojòn A, Fernàndez JR, Hermida RC. Chronolab: an interactive software package for chronobiologic time series analysis written for the Macintosh computer. Chronobiol Int 1992;9:403–12.

83. Regnante R, Zuzek RW, Weinsier SB, et al. Clinical characteristics and four-year outcomes of patients in the Rhode Island Takotsubo Cardiomyopathy Registry. Am J Cardiol 2010;103:1015–9.

84. Manfredini R, Citro R, Previtali M, et al. Summer preference in the occurrence of takotsubo cardiomyopathy is independent of age. J Am Geriatr Soc 2009;57:1509–11.

85. Eshtehardi P, Koestner SC, Adorjan P, et al. Transient apical ballooning syndrome: clinical characteristics, ballooning pattern, and long-term follow-up in a Swiss population. Int J Cardiol 2009;135:370–5.

86. Mansecal N, El Mahmoud R, Dubourg O. Occurrence of tako-tsubo cardiomyopathy and chronobiological variation. J Am Coll Cardiol 2010;55: 500–1.

87. Summers MR, Dib C, Prasad A. Chronobiology of tako-tsubo cardiomyopathy (apical ballooning syndrome). J Am Geriatr Soc 2010;58:805–6.

88. Parodi G, Bellandi B, Del Pace S, et al. Natural history of tako-tsubo cardiomyopathy. Chest 2011;139:887–92.

89. Parodi G, Bellandi B, Antonucci D. Tako-tsubo cardiomyopathy: is a temporal pattern of onset confirmed? [reply]. Chest 2011;140:1101–2.

90. Manfredini R, Citro R, Previtali M, et al. Monday preference in onset of takotsubo cardiomyopathy. Am J Emerg Med 2010;28:715–9.

91. Milinis K, Fisher M. Takotsubo cardiomyopathy: pathophysiology and treatment. Postgrad Med J 2012; 88:530–8. http://dx.doi.org/10.1136/postgradmedj-2012-130761.

92. Manfredini R, Gallerani M, Portaluppi F, et al. Relationships of the circadian rhythms of thrombotic, ischemic, hemorrhagic, and arrhythmic events to blood pressure rhythms. Ann N Y Acad Sci 1996; 783:141–58.

93. Manfredini R, Boari B, Salmi R, et al. Circadian variation of cardiovascular events and morning blood pressure surge. Vasc Dis Prev 2008;5: 246–51.

94. Wittstein IS, Thiemann DR, Lima JA, et al. Neurohumoral features of myocardial stunning due to sudden emotional stress. N Engl J Med 2005;352: 539–48.

95. Descovich GC, Montalbetti N, Kiahl JF, et al. Age and catecholamine rhythms. Chronobiologia 1974;1:163–71.

96. Hansen AM, Garde AH, Skovgaard LT, et al. Seasonal and biological variation of urinary epinephrine, norepinephrine, and cortisol in healthy women. Clin Chim Acta 2001;309:25–35.

97. Van Cauter E, Leproult R, Kupfer DJ. Effects of gender and age on the levels and circadian

rhythmicity of plasma cortisol. J Clin Endocrinol Metab 1996;81:2468–73.

98. Roohafza H, Talaei M, Sadeghi M, et al. Association between acute and chronic life events on acute coronary syndrome: a case-control study. J Cardiovasc Nurs 2010;25:E1–7.

99. Nonaka H, Emoto N, Ikeda K, et al. Angiotensin II induces circadian genes expression of clock genes in cultured vascular smooth muscle cells. Circulation 2001;104:1746–8.

100. Durgan JD, Hotze MA, Tomlin TM, et al. The intrinsic circadian clock within the cardiomyocyte. Am J Physiol Heart Circ Physiol 2005;289: H1530–41.

101. Curtis AM, Cheng Y, Kapoor S, et al. Circadian variation of blood pressure and the vascular response to asynchronous stress. Proc Natl Acad Sci U S A 2007;104:3450–5.

102. Manfredini R, Boari B, Salmi R, et al. Circadian rhythm effects on cardiovascular and other stress-related events. In: Fink G, editor. Encyclopedia of stress, vol. 1, 2nd edition. Oxford: Academic Press; 2007. p. 500–5.

103. Manfredini R, Manfredini F, Malagoni AM, et al. Chronobiology of vascular disorders: a "seasonal" link between arterial and venous thrombotic diseases? J Coagul Disord 2010;2:61–7.

104. Arntz HR, Willich SN, Schreiber C, et al. Diurnal, weekly, and seasonal variation of sudden death. Population-based analysis of 24,061 consecutive cases. Eur Heart J 2000;21:315–20.

105. Gruska M, Gaul GB, Winkler M, et al. Increased occurrence of out-of-hospital cardiac arrest on Mondays in a community-based study. Chronobiol Int 2005;20:401–6.

106. Murakami S, Otsuka K, Kubo Y, et al. Repeated ambulatory monitoring reveals a Monday morning surge in blood pressure in a community-dwelling population. Am J Hypertens 2004;17(12 Pt 1): 1179–83.

107. Pieper C, Warren K, Pickering TC. A comparison of ambulatory blood pressure and heart rate at home on work and nonwork days. J Hypertens 1993;11: 177–83.

108. Manfredini R, Eagle KA, Bossone E. Acute myocardial infarction and tako-tsubo cardiomyopathy: could time of onset help to diagnose? Expert Rev Cardiovasc Ther 2011;9:123–6.

109. Manfredini R, la Cecilia O, Boari B, et al. Circadian pattern of emergency calls: implications for ED organization. Am J Emerg Med 2002;20:282–6.

110. LaBounty T, Eagle KA, Manfredini R, et al. The impact of time and day on the presentation of acute coronary syndromes. Clin Cardiol 2006;29:542–6.

111. Manfredini R, Gallerani M, Salmi R, et al. Circadian rhythms and the heart: implications for chronotherapy of cardiovascular diseases. Clin Pharmacol Ther 1994;56:244–7.

Role of Echocardiography in Takotsubo Cardiomyopathy

Rodolfo Citro, MD, FESC[a,b,*], Federico Piscione, MD[c],
Guido Parodi, MD[d], Jorge Salerno-Uriarte, MD[e],
Eduardo Bossone, MD, PhD, FESC[f,g]

KEYWORDS

- Takotsubo cardiomyopathy • Echocardiography • Left ventricular systolic dysfunction
- Noninvasive assessment

KEY POINTS

- Diagnosis of takotsubo cardiomyopathy (TTC) and the early identification of possible precipitating factors have important implications for clinical management.
- Despite a good long-term prognosis, approximately one-third of patients with TTC experience life-threatening complications during the acute phase.
- Echocardiography is a safe and easy to perform imaging modality; its widespread availability probably accounts for the increase in the prevalence of clinically recognized TTC.
- Echocardiography can provide useful information about LV morphology, and regional and global systolic or diastolic function.
- Specific findings that have been associated with TTC, such as LV outflow tract obstruction, mitral regurgitation, and right ventricular involvement, can also be detected by echocardiography, which also allows noninvasive assessment of coronary microcirculation impairment during the acute phase of TTC.

INTRODUCTION

Takotsubo cardiomyopathy (TTC) is characterized by transient and reversible left ventricular (LV) systolic dysfunction in the absence of significant atherosclerotic narrowing of epicardial coronary arteries.[1–4] Typically, LV apical ballooning can be appreciated during the acute phase using common diagnostic imaging methods, such as echocardiography, cardiac magnetic resonance, and left ventriculography. Variant forms, such as midventricular ballooning or basal ballooning, have also been described.[5] TTC usually occurs in postmenopausal women and is often triggered by severe emotional or physical stress.[6,7] Although the pathophysiologic mechanisms remain unclear, catecholamine excess seems to play a central role. Diagnosis of TTC and the early identification of possible precipitating factors have important implications for clinical management. Despite a good long-term prognosis, approximately one-third of patients with TTC experience life-threatening complications during the acute phase.

[a] Department of Heart Sciences, Circolo Hospital and Macchi Foundation, University of Insubria, Varese, Italy; [b] Heart Department, University Hospital "San Giovanni di Dio e Ruggi d'Aragona," Heart Tower, Room 810, Largo Città di Ippocrate, 84131 Salerno, Italy; [c] Department of Medicine and Surgery, San Giovanni di Dio and Ruggi D'Aragona Academic Hospital, University of Salerno, Cardiology Tower - Room S1, Largo Città d'Ippocrate, 84131 Salerno, Italy; [d] Division of Cardiology, Careggi Hospital, Florence, Italy; [e] Cardiology Clinics, Circolo University Hospital and Macchi Foundation, University of Insubria, 21100 Varese, Italy; [f] Cardiology Division, "Cava de' Tirreni and Amalfi Coast" Hospital, Heart Department, University of Salerno, Via De Marinis, 84013 Cava de' Tirreni (SA), Italy; [g] Cardiac Surgery Department, IRCCS Policlinico San Donato, Piazza Edmondo Malan 1, 20097 San Donato Milanese, Italy
* Corresponding author. University Hospital "San Giovanni di Dio e Ruggi d'Aragona," Heart Tower Room 810, Largo Città di Ippocrate, Salerno 84131, Italy.
E-mail address: rodolfocitro@gmail.com

Heart Failure Clin 9 (2013) 157–166
http://dx.doi.org/10.1016/j.hfc.2012.12.014
1551-7136/13/$ – see front matter © 2013 Elsevier Inc. All rights reserved.

Echocardiography is a safe and easy-to-perform imaging modality also in emergency settings, and its widespread availability probably accounts for the increase in the prevalence of clinically recognized TTC. It can provide useful information about LV morphology and regional and global systolic or diastolic function. In addition, specific findings that have been associated with TTC, such as LV outflow tract obstruction (LVOTO), mitral regurgitation (MR), and right ventricular (RV) involvement, can also be detected.[8] Moreover, echocardiography allows noninvasive assessment of coronary microcirculation impairment during the acute phase of TTC. Each of these topics is discussed in the following sections.

LV MORPHOLOGY

In the acute phase echocardiography and ventriculography are useful to identify peculiar LV morphology associated with TTC (**Fig. 1**). The typical form characterized by LV apical ballooning with hypercontractility of the basal segments can be detected in most cases. However variant forms, such as midventricular ballooning, apical sparing, and basal ballooning, have been described (**Fig. 2**).[3,5,9] Furthermore, seriated echocardiographic controls are a useful noninvasive technique to monitor the recovery of myocardial contractile function and the silhouette of the left ventricle.

LV SYSTOLIC FUNCTION

We previously compared LV regional wall motion abnormalities (RWMA) in 37 patients with TTC and in 37 patients with anterior ST-elevation myocardial infarction (STEMI) who underwent standard two-dimensional echocardiography.[10] The TTC cohort showed higher LV diastolic and systolic volumes (55.5 ± 17 vs 44.7 ± 10.1 mL/m^2 and 34.5 ± 10.8 vs 26.5 ± 6.9 mL/m^2; $P = .001$ and $P<.001$, respectively), lower LV ejection fraction (EF) (37.6 ± 5.1 vs and 40.9 ± 3.7%; $P = .002$), and higher WMSI (1.98 ± 0.2 vs 1.51 ± 0.14; $P<.001$) than patients with anterior STEMI. RWMA involving the apex with sparing of the base were detected in 29% and 2% of patients with TTC and anterior STEMI, respectively ($P = .002$). Considering LV segmentation, according to the American Society of Echocardiography/European Association of Echocardiography classification,[11] apical segments were similarly involved in both groups, with the exception of the apical inferior and lateral segments (34 vs 13 and 37 vs 31; $P<.001$ and $P = .011$, respectively), which were more often involved in patients with TTC. Patients with TTC showed more frequent involvement of the midposteroseptal (31 vs 6; $P<.001$), inferior (31 vs 0; $P<.001$), inferolateral (33 vs 5; $P<.001$), and lateral walls (34 vs 7; $P<.001$). Finally, only a few patients with TTC showed hypokinesis in the basal segments of the anteroseptal (2 vs 11; $P = .006$), posteroseptal

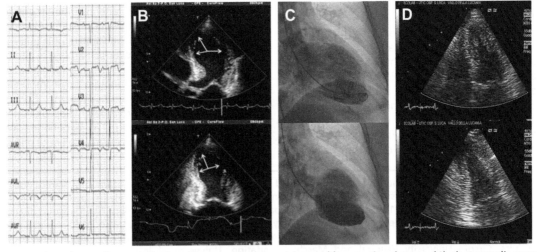

Fig. 1. Takotsubo cardiomyopathy in a 69-year-old woman triggered by emotional stress. (*A*) electrocardiogram on admission; note the slight ST-segment elevation in the anterior precordial leads. (*B*) Transthoracic echocardiography on admission: apical four-chamber view (*top*) and two-chamber view (*bottom*). Involvement of the apex and mid segments of the opposite left ventricular wall (*arrows*) can be appreciated (ejection fraction, 38%). (*C*) Left ventriculography: diastolic frame (*top*) and systolic frame (*bottom*). Note the typical morphology of left ventricular apical ballooning that in systole resembles the shape of a Japanese pot (tako-tsubo) with a narrow neck and wide base. (*D*) Transthoracic echocardiography at 1-month follow-up: same views as *B* showing recovery of left ventricular contractility and global systolic function (ejection fraction, 65%).

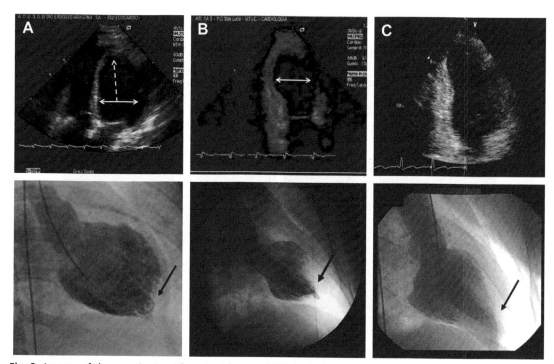

Fig. 2. Images of three patients with variant forms of TTC (apical sparing, midventricular, and basal ballooning, respectively). (*A*) Transthoracic echocardiography, apical four-chamber view (*top*). Note the involvement of the basal and mid segments (*solid arrow*) of the left ventricle, despite normal contractility of the apex (*dotted arrow*). Systolic frame from left ventriculography confirming an apical-sparing variant of TTC (*black arrow*). (*B*) Transthoracic echocardiography, apical two-chamber view (*top*). Note the involvement of the midsegments only (*solid arrow*). Systolic frame from left ventriculography showing ballooning confined to the midsegments (midventricular ballooning). (*C*) Transthoracic echocardiography, apical two-chamber view (*top*). Note the involvement of the basal segments only (*solid arrow*). Systolic frame from left ventriculography showing ballooning confined to the basal segments (basal ballooning) with normal contraction of the remaining walls (*black arrow*). (*Modified from* Reuss CS, Lester SJ, Hurst RT, et al. Isolated left ventricular basal ballooning phenotype of transient cardiomyopathy in young women. Am J Cardiol 2007;99:1451–3; with permission.)

(1 vs 1; $P = 1$), and inferior walls (4 vs 1; $P = .165$). No significant differences were observed between groups with regard to RWMA in the territory supplied by the left anterior descending coronary artery (LAD) (37 vs 37; $P = 1$). Conversely, the territories supplied by the LAD/left circumflex coronary artery (37 vs 31; $P = .011$), LAD/right coronary artery (RCA) (34 vs 13; $P<.001$), RCA (33 vs 5; $P<.001$), and RCA/left circumflex coronary artery (31 vs 2; $P<.001$) were more frequently involved in patients with TTC. Topography of LV segmental myocardial dysfunction was characterized by symmetric RWMA extending equally into the anterior, inferior, and lateral walls, supporting the hypothesis of extensive myocardial stunning in the pathogenesis of TTC (**Fig. 3**).

Using two-dimensional speckle tracking echocardiography, Mansencal and colleagues[12] compared patients with TTC with patients affected by coronary artery disease caused by LAD occlusion. At speckle tracking analysis, patients with TTC showed a peculiar pattern of contraction, characterized by similarly reduced peak systolic velocities between opposite LV walls (eg, interventricular septum and lateral walls, or inferior and anterior walls), different from those observed in patients with LAD occlusion. In patients with TTC, LV dysfunction extended beyond the territory of LAD distribution with a circular pattern.

Heggemann and colleagues[13] compared global and regional myocardial function in 12 patients with TTC and 12 patients with anterior STEMI using two-dimensional strain imaging to measure longitudinal and radial strain of the left ventricle. In the midsegments, radial strain was reduced along the entire LV circumference in patients with TTC, whereas it was predominantly reduced in the anterior and anteroseptal walls in patients with STEMI. In patients with TTC, LVEF and global strain were significantly lower compared with patients with STEMI. Moreover, in midventricular and apical segments, longitudinal strain was reduced with lower strain values in inferior, posterior, and lateral segments. The findings of Heggemann

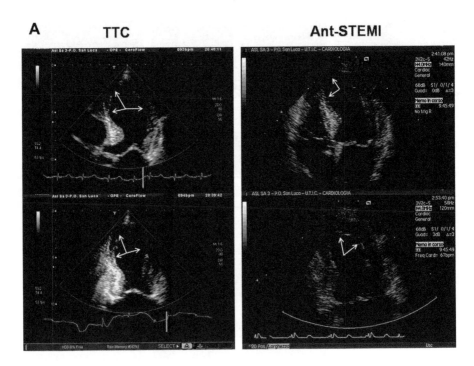

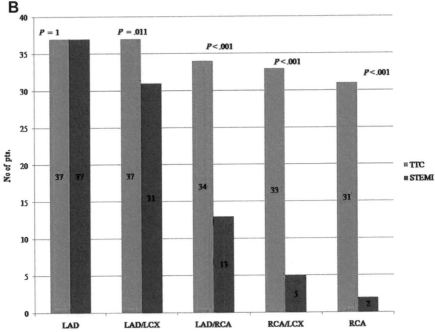

Fig. 3. (A) Apical four-chamber view (top) and two-chamber view (bottom) in TTC (left) and anterior STEMI (right). In patients with TTC, akinesis of apical and mid segments of the opposite walls (interventricular septum and lateral wall in four-chamber view; inferior and anterior walls in two-chamber view) can be appreciated. Conversely, in patients with anterior STEMI only the mid and apical segments of the interventricular septum and anterior wall (supplied only by the LAD) are involved (arrows). (B) Left ventricular segmental systolic dysfunction according to coronary artery distribution in TTC versus patients with STEMI. In patients with TTC, the territories not exclusively supplied by the LAD are more significantly involved. Ant-STEMI, anterior ST-elevation myocardial infarction; LCX, left circumflex coronary artery. (Modified from Citro R, Rigo F, Ciampi Q, et al. Echocardiographic assessment of regional left ventricular wall motion abnormalities in patients with tako-tsubo cardiomyopathy: comparison with anterior myocardial infarction. Eur J Echocardiogr 2011;12:542–9; with permission.)

and colleagues are consistent with our results, confirming a peculiar pattern of RWMA that can be considered a hallmark for the early suspicion of TTC. In addition, the severity of global systolic dysfunction seems to have prognostic implications, in particular in the elderly. Reduced LVEF on admission has been associated with an increased risk of in-hospital hard events in patients with TTC older than 75 years old.[14]

LV DIASTOLIC FUNCTION

Several studies suggested that TTC may also cause LV diastolic dysfunction.[15–17] Madhavan and colleagues[16] compared the neurohormonal and cardiac biomarker profile of 15 patients with TTC with that of 10 patients with STEMI. Patients with TTC showed lower troponin and higher B-type natriuretic peptide levels, indicating elevated LV filling pressures despite less extensive myocardial damage. The disproportionate increase in B-type natriuretic peptide levels compared with the slight troponin rise should be considered suggestive of TTC. Basal hyperkinesis and apical LV wall stress induce intraventricular diastolic and systolic pressure gradients and are believed to be the predominant mechanisms responsible for increased LV end-diastolic pressure. In addition, E/e' ratio, a simple, reproducible and easy to measure echocardiographic index considered a good predictor of LV filling pressure, was higher in TTC compared with patients with STEMI.

Meimoun and colleagues[17] evaluated LV twist mechanics in 17 patients with TTC and 17 patients with anterior STEMI using two-dimensional speckle tracking echocardiography. Patients with TTC showed a transient impairment of systolic and diastolic function. In some cases, an inverted pattern of apical rotation with abnormal LV twist was observed. In addition, diastolic function was found to be altered even in the early phase of TTC, as evidenced by impaired LV untwisting rate (a regional diastolic index) and increased E/e' ratio (a global diastolic index). Using standard echocardiography, we evaluated LV diastolic function in a large cohort of patients with TTC enrolled in the Takotsubo Italian Network.[18] E/e' ratio was significantly increased in patients with hard events compared with those without. In addition, in the overall population, E/e' ratio was the strongest predictor of adverse short-term outcome. This finding is not surprising because patients with TTC may show volume and pressure overload related to acute systolic and diastolic dysfunction, or to other cardiac diseases. In 156 patients with heart failure undergoing conventional echocardiography and pulsed-wave tissue Doppler imaging, Olson and colleagues[19] demonstrated that E/e' ratio is a strong prognostic predictor of long-term cardiovascular mortality in patients with heart failure and systolic dysfunction. E/e' ratio is less affected by loading conditions, age, and heart rate compared with other conventional echocardiographic parameters of diastolic function. Early and systematic assessment of E/e' ratio in patients with TTC is therefore advisable to identify those at higher risk of acute hard events.

LEFT VENTRICULAR OUTFLOW TRACT OBSTRUCTION

LVOTO is a dynamic phenomenon that depends on loading conditions, and may be associated with systolic anterior motion of the mitral valve (SAM) with subsequent MR (**Fig. 4**).[20] In a study

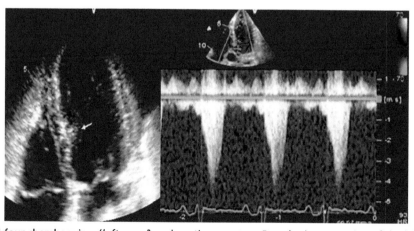

Fig. 4. Apical four-chamber view (*left panel*) and continuous-wave Doppler interrogation of the left ventricular outflow tract showing significant intraventricular gradient in a patient with TTC. Note the small left ventricular cavity with bulging of the basal interventricular septum (*arrow*). (*Modified from* Merli E, Sutcliffe S, Gori M, et al. Tako-tsubo cardiomyopathy: new insights into the possible underlying pathophysiology. Eur J Echocardiogr 2006;7:53–61; with permission.)

of El Mahmoud and colleagues,[21] LVOTO, defined as an intraventricular gradient greater than or equal to 25 mm Hg by standard transthoracic echocardiography (TTE), was detected in 8 (25%) of 32 patients with TTC. All patients with LVOTO had SAM and localized hypertrophy of the proximal interventricular septum (septal bulge). Prevalence of septal bulge was 100% in patients with TTC and LVOTO versus 29% in patients without LVOTO ($P = .002$). Moderate MR was significantly prevalent in patients with TTC and LVOTO (2.1 $\pm$ 0.7 vs 0.9 $\pm$ 0.7), although recovery of systolic function at follow-up was similar in both groups. Echocardiographic detection of LVOTO in patients with TTC has important therapeutic implications, in particular for patients with advanced systolic heart failure.

In older postmenopausal women with small left ventricles and septal bulge, LVOTO may be induced by basal hypercontractility, as occurs in the typical forms of TTC, and may be precipitated by inappropriate administration of catecholamines.[22] In this clinical scenario, inotropic agents causing enhanced contractility of the basal segments and diuretics causing volume depletion may increase the intraventricular pressure gradient and induce hemodynamic instability, ultimately leading to cardiogenic shock. In clinical conditions, the use of intra-aortic counterpulsation should be preferred, and inotropic agents and excessive dehydration should be avoided.

The onset of LVOTO is accompanied by an increase in LV afterload and systolic wall stress leading to subendocardial ischemia and acute myocardial stunning. Initially, it was thought that LVOTO was the unique pathogenetic mechanism of TTC characterized by apical ballooning, but this hypothesis was later disproved in large series of patients with TTC demonstrating a low prevalence of LVOTO. More attention should be paid in patients with TTC and severe LVOTO because of the occurrence of life-threatening arrhythmias and fatal LV wall rupture.

TTE should be performed as early as possible in patients with TTC, especially when a new murmur is heard. If TTE is not feasible, such as in critically ill patients, transesophageal echocardiography is indicated to detect LVOTO and MR.

MITRAL REGURGITATION

Significant (moderate-to-severe, or severe) MR was detected in 19% to 25.5% of patients affected by TTC (**Fig. 5**).[23–25] Parodi and colleagues[23] were the first to study MR secondary to TTC. They collected data from 68 patients with TTC, and significant acute MR was observed in 21% of the

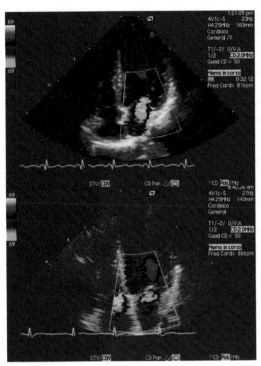

Fig. 5. Apical four-chamber view showing color flow mapping of the mitral valve in a patient with TTC. A significant reduction in mitral regurgitation from moderate-severe on admission (*top*) to mild at 1-month follow-up (*bottom*) can be appreciated.

study population. Echocardiographic MR grade was the only predictor of Killip class III to IV on admission (hazard ratio, 2.24; 95% confidence interval, 1.11–4.50; $P = .024$). Moreover, LVEF on admission (hazard ratio, 0.85; 95% confidence interval, 0.75–0.96; $P = .009$) and SAM (hazard ratio, 18.00; 95% confidence interval, 1.63–98.51; $P = .018$) were the only independent predictors of acute MR. Patients with significant MR required more frequently treatment with an intra-aortic balloon pump (36% vs 7%; $P = .006$). In the MR group, predischarge LVEF was lower and overall mortality rates were higher (14% vs 2%; $P = .044$) than in patients with TTC without MR.

In contrast to these results, Haghi and colleagues[24] did not find clear evidence that significant MR can be considered a predictor of acute adverse events and worse outcome. These authors prospectively evaluated 60 patients with TTC, and significant acute MR was detected in 19% of them (95% confidence interval, 10%–34%). No significant statistical differences in LVEF were reported between patients with and without MR (45 $\pm$ 12 vs 48 $\pm$ 12%; $P = .51$). However, LVEF was significantly lower in patients with classical apical ballooning syndrome than in patients affected by the apical-sparing variant of

TTC ($44 \pm 12\%$ vs $52 \pm 11\%$; $P = .006$). At follow-up, echocardiography performed 47 ± 56 days (range, 2–156 days) after TTC onset, MR resolution was documented in all patients.

The discrepancies between the two aforementioned studies are most likely caused by differences in patient profiles (classical TTC in the study of Parodi and colleagues vs classical and variant TTC in the study of Haghi and colleagues) and in diagnostic methods used to assess LV function (echocardiography vs ventriculography), MR grade (echocardiography vs ventriculography), and pulmonary edema (auscultation vs chest radiograph).

The mechanisms underlying MR in TTC seem to be multiple. SAM has been reported in 33% to 50% of patients with TTC with significant MR.[23,25] In the study of Izumo and colleagues,[25] patients without SAM showed lower LVEF and higher wall motion score (WMS) index and end-systolic volume than those with MR caused by SAM. These findings led the authors to hypothesize that mitral tenting area (leaflet tethering by papillary muscle displacement caused by regional or global LV dysfunction) plays a role in the genesis of MR without SAM. Patients with TTC with MR also had a significantly higher pulmonary artery systolic pressure than patients without MR.

RIGHT VENTRICULAR INVOLVEMENT

Elesber and colleagues[26] first described RV involvement in 8 (27%) of 27 patients by visual assessment with standard TTE. RV dysfunction was identified as uniform involvement of the RV apex (dyskinesis, akinesis, or severe hypokinesis) and sparing of the RV base. RV involvement was associated with lower LVEF; longer hospital stay; and higher complication rates, such as severe congestive heart failure, use of intra-aortic counterpulsation, and cardiopulmonary resuscitation. In TTC variants with biventricular involvement, RV involvement has a similar pattern of LV apical ballooning, with transient and reversible wall motion abnormalities (**Fig. 6**).[27] Its real incidence is probably underestimated because of the intrinsic limitations of conventional echocardiography in assessing the complex RV anatomy. Notwithstanding, in a study conducted with cardiac magnetic resonance imaging, the prevalence of RV involvement was similar to that reported using TTE.[28] RV dysfunction associated with LV apical ballooning represents an additional finding of TTC that can help early recognition of this peculiar syndrome. Its detection increases the suspicion of TTC and should be taken into consideration in the differential diagnosis with anterior STEMI.

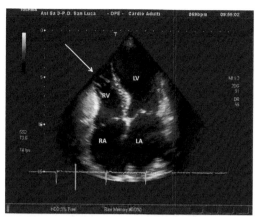

Fig. 6. Transthoracic echocardiography, apical four-chamber view. Right (*arrow*) and left ventricular apical ballooning (biventricular ballooning) in an elderly woman with TTC. LA, left atrium; LV, left ventricle; RA, right atrium; RV, right ventricle. (*Modified from* Citro R, Caso I, Provenza G, et al. Right ventricular involvement and pulmonary hypertension in an elderly woman with tako-tsubo cardiomyopathy. Chest 2010;137:973–5; with permission.)

Isolated RV ballooning without simultaneous involvement of the left ventricle has also been reported.[29] Intracavity thrombi can be detected also in dilated right ventricles, as occurs in LV apical ballooning. RV involvement should be ruled out in patients with TTC, because of its negative impact on hemodynamics, cardiac morbidity, and length of hospitalization.

CORONARY MICROCIRCULATION IMPAIRMENT

In patients with TTC, Kume and colleagues[30] found a significant reduction in coronary flow reserve (CFR) of the three coronary arteries recorded by invasive Doppler flow wire, but in all cases it improved during follow-up.

We reported a case of a 70-year-old woman with TTC triggered by emotional stress, presenting with chest pain and electrocardiogram (ECG) changes in the anterior precordial leads. Coronary angiography showed normal coronary arteries, and echocardiography and left ventriculography revealed typical apical ballooning. For the first time, CFR was measured noninvasively using TTE after adenosine infusion in the distal part of the LAD during the acute phase and at the time of LV myocardial function recovery and ECG normalization. CFR showed a reduction in the acute phase (1.54) and improvement (2.68) at predischarge, suggesting that coronary microvascular dysfunction may be a causative mechanism of TTC, which reverses on recovery of LV systolic function (**Fig. 7**).[31]

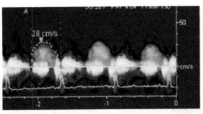 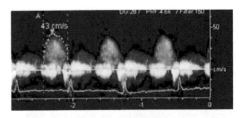

CFR= 1.54

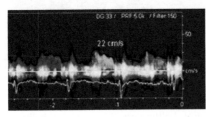 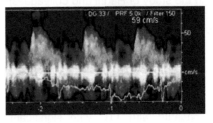

CFR= 2.68

Fig. 7. Transthoracic pulsed-wave Doppler of coronary flow in the distal tract of the LAD before (*left panels*) and after (*right panels*) adenosine infusion. Note the increase in coronary flow reserve (CFR) from 1.54 on Day 1 to 2.68 on Day 8, demonstrating microvascular dysfunction in the acute phase that reverses with recovery. (*From Citro R, Galderisi M, Maione A, et al. Sequential transthoracic ultrasound assessment of coronary flow reserve in a patient with tako-tsubo syndrome. J Am Soc Echocardiogr 2006;19:1402.e5–8; with permission.*)

Our findings were subsequently conformed by Meimoun and colleagues[32] in 12 consecutive patients with TTC undergoing serial CFR measurements using the same methodology. CFR significantly increased from the acute phase to recovery (ΔCFR = 0.73 ± 0.39), whereas WMS decreased (ΔWMS = −14.6 ± 6), and a significant correlation was observed between ΔCFR and ΔWMS. In a larger series, the same authors demonstrated that the improvement of CFR was closely correlated not only with the decrease in WMS, but also with the reduction in LV systolic volume. They concluded that the acute phase of TTC is characterized by reduced vasodilating capacity of the coronary microcirculation, which correlates with LV systolic parameters.[33]

Rigo and colleagues[34] evaluated 30 consecutive patients with TTC using dual imaging with dipyridamole (0.84 mg/kg over 6 minutes), which allows CFR and WMS to be measured simultaneously. All examinations were performed on Day 1, Day 7 (±2 days), and at 6 months after TTC onset. CFR was assessed on the middistal LAD and posterior descending branch of the RCA. In the acute phase, CFR was reduced in both the LAD and posterior descending branch of the RCA, suggesting diffuse and marked coronary microvascular impairment. This study also showed the parallel recovery of CFR and myocardial contraction, confirming that coronary microvascular dysfunction is reversible.

Galiuto and colleagues[35] compared coronary microcirculation in patients with TTC and anterior STEMI undergoing myocardial contrast echocardiography at baseline during adenosine infusion and at 1-month follow-up. In patients with TTC, clear perfusion defects as assessed by quantitative analysis were detected within the dysfunctional myocardium. The extent of perfusion defects was transiently reduced by adenosine infusion and recovered at 1-month follow-up. Microvascular dysfunction was closely related to microvascular perfusion defects, and adenosine-induced recovery of microcirculatory perfusion was associated with a significant improvement in regional myocardial contraction at 1-month follow-up. Conversely, in patients with STEMI neither change in perfusion defect area nor wall motion recovery were observed at follow-up. This study confirms that multiterritorial reversible coronary microvascular vasoconstriction leading to extensive myocardial dysfunction is the pathogenetic mechanism of TTC.

POTENTIAL COMPLICATIONS

The extensive ventricular asynergy that characterizes apical ballooning involves a decrease in intraventricular systolic flow velocity and represents a major predisposing condition for thrombus formation. Mural or pedunculated thrombi, usually localized at the apex, may occur especially in the acute phase during the first 2 days after TTC onset, albeit only rarely (1%–2%).[36] The diagnosis is usually made during an echocardiographic examination performed early. The ultrasound detection of intraventricular thrombosis has important therapeutic (use of heparin or oral anticoagulants) and prognostic implications. De Gregorio and colleagues[36] reported stroke or systemic embolization (renal or lower limb embolism) in 21% and 33% of patients with TTC, respectively, complicated by LV thrombus formation. Thrombus resolution was documented in approximately one-third of patients within 14 days. However, in some cases, thrombi were observed even up to 30 days. Serial echocardiographic studies should be performed to monitor the efficacy of anticoagulation therapy and thrombus evolution. In doubtful cases, use of contrast agents may be helpful in detecting formation of small size thrombi.

LV free wall rupture is another extremely rare but life-threatening complication. It can occur especially in elderly patients with high systolic blood pressure and marked hyperkinesis of the basal segments, and can be favored by high intraventricular pressure fluctuations.[37] Although cardiac rupture is usually fatal, early diagnosis and prompt cardiac surgery may increase the chance of survival. Cardiac wall rupture should therefore be ruled out by echocardiography if sudden hemodynamic deterioration occurs.

SUMMARY

Echocardiography can identify important distinctive features of TTC. The discrepancy between extension of myocardial dysfunction and ECG changes or troponin levels, the detection of wall motion abnormalities in the apical or midventricular segments, which typically extend beyond the distribution of a single coronary artery, and CFR measurement in the distal tract of the LAD provide useful information for the early recognition of TTC. In addition, assessment of LV systolic and diastolic function and the early identification of any potential complications (ie, LVOTO, significant MR, RV involvement, thrombus formation, and cardiac rupture) are crucial for the management, risk stratification, and follow-up of patients with this peculiar syndrome.

REFERENCES

1. Tsuchihashi K, Ueshima K, Uchida T, et al. Transient left ventricular apical ballooning without coronary artery stenosis: a novel heart syndrome mimicking acute myocardial infarction. J Am Coll Cardiol 2001;8:11–8.
2. Abe Y, Kondo M, Matsuoka R, et al. Assessment of clinical features in transient left ventricular apical ballooning. J Am Coll Cardiol 2003;41:737–42.
3. Bybee KA, Kara T, Prasad A, et al. Systematic review: transient left ventricular apical ballooning: a syndrome that mimics ST-segment elevation myocardial infarction. Ann Intern Med 2004;141:858–65.
4. Kurisu S, Sato H, Kawagoe T, et al. Tako-tsubo-like left ventricular dysfunction with ST-segment elevation: a novel cardiac syndrome mimicking acute myocardial infarction. Am Heart J 2002;143:448–55.
5. Hurst RT, Prasad A, Askew JW III, et al. Takotsubo cardiomyopathy: a unique cardiomyopathy with variable ventricular morphology. JACC Cardiovasc Imaging 2010;3:641–9.
6. Sharkey SW, Lesser JR, Zenovich AG, et al. Acute and reversible cardiomyopathy provoked by stress in women from the United States. Circulation 2005;111:472–9.
7. Parodi G, Del Pace S, Carrabba N, et al. Incidence, clinical findings, and outcome of women with left ventricular apical ballooning syndrome. Am J Cardiol 2007;99:182–5.
8. van der Wall EE, Holman ER, Scholte AJ, et al. Echocardiography in takotsubo cardiomyopathy; a useful approach? Int J Cardiovasc Imaging 2010;26:537–40.
9. Reuss CS, Lester SJ, Hurst RT, et al. Isolated left ventricular basal ballooning phenotype of transient cardiomyopathy in young women. Am J Cardiol 2007;99:1451–3.
10. Citro R, Rigo F, Ciampi Q, et al. Echocardiographic assessment of regional left ventricular wall motion abnormalities in patients with tako-tsubo cardiomyopathy: comparison with anterior myocardial infarction. Eur J Echocardiogr 2011;12:542–9.
11. Lang RM, Bierig M, Devereux RB, et al. Recommendations for chamber quantification: a report from the American Society of Echocardiography's Guidelines and Standards Committee and the Chamber Quantification Writing Group, developed in conjunction with the European Association of Echocardiography, a branch of the European Society of Cardiology. J Am Soc Echocardiogr 2005;18:1440–63.
12. Mansencal N, Abbou N, Pillière R, et al. Usefulness of two-dimensional speckle tracking echocardiography for assessment of tako-tsubo cardiomyopathy. Am J Cardiol 2009;103:1020–4.
13. Heggemann F, Hamm K, Kaelsch T, et al. Global and regional myocardial function quantification in takotsubo cardiomyopathy in comparison to acute anterior myocardial infarction using two-dimensional (2D) strain echocardiography. Echocardiography 2011;28:715–9.
14. Citro R, Rigo F, Previtali M, et al. Differences in clinical features and in-hospital outcomes of older adults with tako-tsubo cardiomyopathy. J Am Geriatr Soc 2012;60:93–8.
15. Akashi YJ, Goldstein DS, Barbaro G, et al. Takotsubo cardiomyopathy: a new form of acute, reversible heart failure. Circulation 2008;118:2754–62.
16. Madhavan M, Borlaug BA, Lerman A, et al. Stress hormone and circulating biomarker profile of apical

ballooning syndrome (takotsubo cardiomyopathy): insights into the clinical significance of B-type natriuretic peptide and troponin levels. Heart 2009;95: 1436–41.

17. Meimoun P, Passos P, Benali T, et al. Assessment of left ventricular twist mechanics in tako-tsubo cardiomyopathy by two-dimensional speckle-tracking echocardiography. Eur J Echocardiogr 2011;12:931–9.

18. Citro R, Rigo F, Provenza G, et al. Echocardiographic predictors of hard events in patient with tako-tsubo cardiomyopathy [abstract 1294]. Eur Heart J 2012; 33:Suppl 1.

19. Olson JM, Samad BA, Alam M. Prognostic value of pulse-wave tissue Doppler parameters in patients with systolic heart failure. Am J Cardiol 2008;102: 722–5.

20. Merli E, Sutcliffe S, Gori M, et al. Tako-tsubo cardiomyopathy: new insights into the possible underlying pathophysiology. Eur J Echocardiogr 2006;7: 53–61.

21. El Mahmoud R, Mansencal N, Pillière R, et al. Prevalence and characteristics of left ventricular outflow tract obstruction in tako-tsubo syndrome. Am Heart J 2008;156:543–8.

22. Chockalingan A, Xie GY, Dellsperger KC. Echocardiography in stress cardiomyopathy and acute LVOT obstruction. Int J Cardiovasc Imaging 2010;26: 527–35.

23. Parodi G, Del Pace S, Salvadori C, et al. Left ventricular apical ballooning syndrome as a novel cause of acute mitral regurgitation. J Am Coll Cardiol 2007; 50:647–9.

24. Haghi D, Rohm S, Suselbeck T, et al. Incidence and clinical significance of mitral regurgitation in takotsubo cardiomyopathy. Clin Res Cardiol 2010;99:93–8.

25. Izumo M, Nalawadi S, Shiota M, et al. Mechanisms of acute mitral regurgitation in patients with takotsubo cardiomyopathy. Circ Cardiovasc Imaging 2011;4:392–8.

26. Elesber AA, Prasad A, Bybee KA, et al. Transient cardiac apical ballooning syndrome: prevalence and clinical implications of right ventricular involvement. J Am Coll Cardiol 2006;47:1082–3.

27. Citro R, Caso I, Provenza G, et al. Right ventricular involvement and pulmonary hypertension in an elderly woman with tako-tsubo cardiomyopathy. Chest 2010;137:973–5.

28. Haghi D, Athanasiadis A, Papavassiliu T, et al. Right ventricular involvement in takotsubo cardiomyopathy. Eur Heart J 2006;27:2433–9.

29. Mrdovic I, Kostic J, Perunicic J, et al. Right ventricular takotsubo cardiomyopathy. J Am Coll Cardiol 2010;55:1751.

30. Kume T, Akasaka T, Kawamoto T, et al. Assessment of coronary microcirculation in patients with takotsubo-like left ventricular dysfunction. Circ J 2005;69:934–9.

31. Citro R, Galderisi M, Maione AG, et al. Sequential transthoracic ultrasound assessment of coronary flow reserve in a patient with tako-tsubo syndrome. J Am Soc Echocardiogr 2006;19:1402.e5–8.

32. Meimoun P, Malaquin D, Sayah S, et al. The coronary flow reserve is transiently impaired in takotsubo cardiomyopathy: a prospective study using serial Doppler transthoracic echocardiography. J Am Soc Echocardiogr 2008;21:72–7.

33. Meimoun P, Malaquin D, Benali T, et al. Transient impairment of coronary flow reserve in tako-tsubo cardiomyopathy is related to left ventricular systolic parameters. Eur J Echocardiogr 2009;10: 265–70.

34. Rigo F, Sicari R, Citro R, et al. Diffuse, marked, reversible impairment in coronary microcirculation in stress cardiomyopathy: a Doppler transthoracic echo study. Ann Med 2009;41:462–70.

35. Galiuto L, De Caterina AR, Porfidia A, et al. Reversible coronary microvascular dysfunction: a common pathogenetic mechanism in apical ballooning or tako-tsubo syndrome. Eur Heart J 2010;31:1319–27.

36. de Gregorio C, Grimaldi P, Lentini C. Left ventricular thrombus formation and cardioembolic complications in patients with takotsubo-like syndrome: a systematic review. Int J Cardiol 2008;131:18–24.

37. Kumar S, Kaushik S, Nautiyal A, et al. Cardiac rupture in takotsubo cardiomyopathy: a systematic review. Clin Cardiol 2011;34:672–6.

Role of Cardiovascular Magnetic Resonance in Takotsubo Cardiomyopathy

Anastasios Athanasiadis, MD[a],*, Birke Schneider, MD[b],
Udo Sechtem, MD[a]

KEYWORDS

- CMR • Takotsubo cardiomyopathy • Apical ballooning syndrome

KEY POINTS

- Cardiac MRI (CMR) has become an important tool in the diagnosis of cardiomyopathies.
- CMR is a unique tool for further evaluating and characterizing patients with takotsubo cardiomyopathy (TTC) and studying the underlying causes and pathophysiologic mechanisms of TTC.
- Using CMR, regional wall motion abnormalities, right ventricular (RV) involvement, intraventricular thrombi, and reversible myocardial injury (inflammation or ischemic edema) or irreversible myocardial injury (necrosis or fibrosis) can be detected in patients presenting with TTC.
- CMR imaging can distinguish between acute myocardial infarction (AMI) and TTC.

INTRODUCTION

CMR has become an important tool for the evaluation of cardiac diseases. In the clinical setting, CMR is frequently used in the diagnosis of ischemic heart disease and, increasingly in the recent years, in the diagnosis of congestive heart failure/cardiomyopathies.[1] Advances in scanner hardware and novel pulse sequences continue to improve and to expand the diagnostic utility and capability of CMR. The advantages of CMR include the lack of radiation, the variety of tissue contrast mechanisms, and the ability to image the heart in any arbitrary direction. A comprehensive CMR study enables evaluating cardiac structure, function, tissue characteristics, perfusion, and scarring or fibrosis.

Because the underlying pathophysiology of TTC is not yet elucidated, CMR is a unique tool for further evaluating and characterizing patients with TTC, obtaining possible explanations of the underlying cause and pathophysiologic mechanisms, and distinguishing TTC from other cardiac diseases. CMR can accurately visualize regional wall motion abnormalities and allows precise quantification of RV and left ventricular (LV) function. Furthermore, during a CMR study, additional abnormalities can be observed (pericardial and pleural effusion, thrombi, and so forth). CMR is also helpful for distinguishing between reversible injury (inflammation or ischemic edema) and irreversible injury (necrosis or fibrosis). This distinction may be important for verifying TTC and excluding similar acute cardiac diseases, such as myocardial infarction or myocarditis.[2–4]

This article reviews advances in the diagnostic abilities of CMR for evaluating TTC.

LEFT VENTRICULAR FUNCTION AND BALLOONING PATTERN

Functional images of heart contraction throughout the cardiac cycle are obtained in multiple orientations using cine–steady-state free precession (SSFP) pulse sequences. SSFP has become the reference standard for functional cine CMR imaging because of its superior contrast between myocardium and the blood pool.[5] Conventional

---

[a] Department of Cardiology, Robert-Bosch-Krankenhaus, Auerbachstrasse 110, Stuttgart 70376, Germany;
[b] Department of Cardiology, Sana Kliniken Lübeck GmbH, Kronsdorfer Allee 71-73, Lübeck 23560, Germany
* Corresponding author.
E-mail address: anastasios.athanasiadis@rbk.de

Heart Failure Clin 9 (2013) 167–176
http://dx.doi.org/10.1016/j.hfc.2012.12.011

cine gradient-echo pulse sequences have poorer contrast between the blood pool and myocardium but remain useful for evaluating valvular disease due to their inherent dephasing of the regurgitant blood signal. Quantitative evaluation of cine-images provides accurate and reproducible measures of ejection fraction and cardiac chamber dimensions.[6,7] The application of parallel imaging techniques, which reduce the amount of data that need to be collected, has improved the temporal and spatial resolution of single breath-hold cine-SSFP imaging.[8] Techniques for real-time cine imaging, which enable imaging of myocardial function without ECG gating or breath-holds, have extended the usefulness of CMR to patients with cardiac arrhythmias or those who are unable to hold their breath.[9] Thus, CMR has advantages for identification of the peculiar LV form of the TTC. High precision and reproducibility have been reported for the evaluation of the form and function of the LV by CMR, and this imaging modality thus has become the reference standard.[10]

In a large TTC population of 207 patients examined with CMR, within a median of 3 days after presentation, 3 different patterns of LV wall motion abnormalities could be identified.[11] In this CMR study, the majority of the patients (82%) showed apical ballooning with apical akinesia and basal hyperkinesia (**Fig. 1**), whereas 17% of the patients presented with midventricular ballooning and mid-ventricular akinesia, normal motion of the apex, and basal hyperkinesia (**Fig. 2**) and 2 patients (1%) showed an isolated basal ballooning with normokinesia or hyperkinesia of the other LV segments (**Fig. 3**). The frequencies of these wall motion abnormality patterns vary from study to study and it is not clear whether this is related to different patient populations or an effect of the different imaging modalities. In the German Tako-Tsubo Registry, which included 324 patients, the distribution was 64% apical ballooning and 36% midventricular ballooning. No patient with basal ballooning was included in this German registry.[12]

Many recent studies have in common that the number of patients with midventricular ballooning is increasing compared with the initial description of TTC.[13–15] It is still unclear why there are different patterns of regional wall abnormalities. No investigation could identify significant clinical differences between these different manifestations.

RIGHT VENTRICULAR INVOLVEMENT

The RV has long been the forgotten ventricle because it is difficult to assess RV function, especially by standard echocardiography owing to its

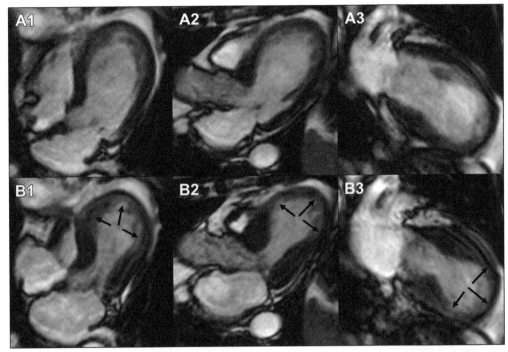

Fig. 1. Representative example of a patient with an apical ballooning. (*A*) Images of end diastole in a 4-chamber view (*A1*), 3-chamber view (*A2*), and 2-chamber view (*A3*). (*B*) Images of end systole in a 4-chamber view (*B1*), 3-chamber view (*B2*), and 2-chamber view (*B3*). *Black arrows* highlight the area of apical akinesia in the different views.

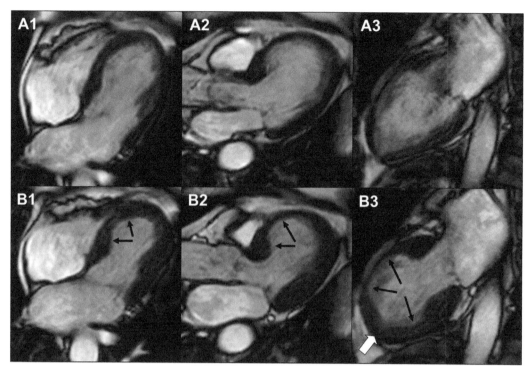

Fig. 2. Representative example of a patient with a midventricular ballooning. (*A*) Images of end diastole in a 4-chamber view (*A1*), 3-chamber view (*A2*), and 2-chamber view (*A3*). (*B*) Images of end systole in a 4-chamber view (*B1*), 3-chamber view (*B2*), and 2-chamber view (*B3*). *Black arrows* (*B1, B2, B3*) highlight the area of mid-LV akinesia in the different views. White arrow (*B3*) indicates the apex with normal wall motion.

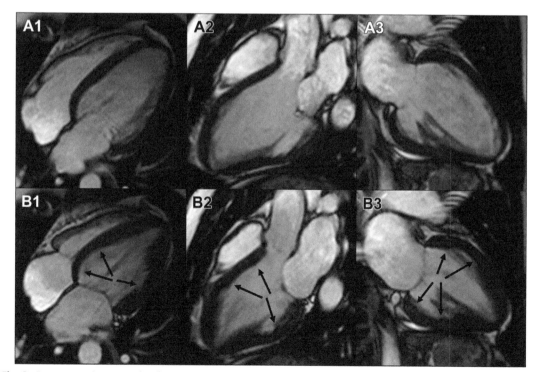

Fig. 3. Representative example of a patient with a basal ballooning. (*A*) Images of end diastole in a 4-chamber view (*A1*), 3-chamber view (*A2*), and 2-chamber view (*A3*). (*B*) Images of end systole in a 4-chamber view (*B1*), 3-chamber view (*B2*), and 2-chamber view (*B3*). *Black arrows* (*B1, B2, B3*) highlight the area of basal akinesia in the different views.

complex morphology, structure, and function. Developments in CMR imaging and echocardiography have provided new insights into RV structure and function.[16] The evaluation of the RV is largely performed by echocardiography in daily clinical practice despite limitations, such as limited echo windows and difficulties in viewing all parts of the RV in many patients. CMR imaging provides a unique opportunity to image the RV in motion and in 3-D without view-limiting echocardiographic windows. Therefore, CMR imaging is increasingly used for the assessment of the RV in a wide variety of cardiopulmonary diseases, including TTC.[17,18]

Using CMR evaluation at a median of 3 days, Haghi and colleagues[19] first described RV involvement in 9 of 34 patients (26%) with TTC. In their study, pleural effusion was significantly more common in patients with RV involvement than in those without (67% vs 8%, $P<.01$). Eitel and colleagues[11] observed in their larger population a similar rate of 34% of patients with biventricular involvement. RV ballooning was associated with longer hospitalization, heart failure with a high incidence of bilateral pleural effusion, and older age. Thus, CMR may be advantageous in TTC for precisely detecting the often subtle signs of RV involvement and for predicting a longer and more severe course of the disease, which may have an effect on treatment and outcome of these patients. An example of a patient with RV involvement and bilateral effusion, which completely disappeared after 1 month, is shown in **Fig. 4**.

TTC may also appear as isolated RV TTC.[20,21] Thus, serial CMR examinations may also be indicated in patients with unexplained sudden RV failure if echocardiography is not able to fully depict RV anatomy.

INTRAVENTRICULAR THROMBI

LV apical thrombus formation is a known complication of TTC and has been reported in up to 8% of case series by echocardiography.[22] Echocardiography studies, however, have reported significant interobserver variability in diagnosing LV thrombus.[23] Up to 46% of echocardiograms may be diagnostically inconclusive for thrombus.[24] In contrast, delayed-enhancement CMR using gadolinium chelates as contrast agents is a sensitive method for detecting LV thrombus[25]; delayed-enhancement CMR differentiates thrombus from surrounding myocardium because thrombus is avascular and thus characterized by an absence of contrast uptake.[26] Hence, CMR provides improved sensitivity and specificity for the detection of LV thrombus compared with echocardiography.[26]

Despite the advantages of CMR in the detection of LV thrombus, only a few case reports of LV thrombus formation in TTC patients with CMR have been published.[27,28] In the large CMR study by Eitel and colleagues,[11] the incidence of left thrombus in TTC patients was only 2% and, hence, considerably lower than the previously reported 8%[22] by echocardiography. De Gregorio and colleagues,[28] in their review of 15 reports of patients with TTC complicated by LV thrombus, also concluded that the incidence of this complication was low, approximately 2.5%. This estimation was based on relating their 15 cases to all cases reported in the same time interval in the literature. In contrast to de Gregorio, Leurent and colleagues,[29] in a similar review of the literature, reported a higher incidence of apical LV thrombus either detected by CMR or echocardiography of 5.1% (range 3% to 9%). The lower incidence of

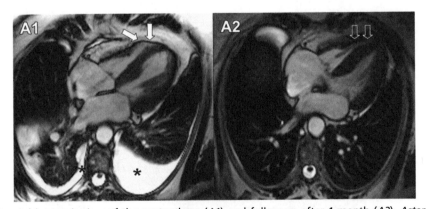

Fig. 4. Horizontal long axis view of the acute phase (*A1*) and follow-up after 1 month (*A2*). *Asterisks* indicate bilateral pleural effusion at acute presentation. *White filled arrows* indicate the RV involvement with apical akinesia in the presence of an apical ballooning. After 1 month, the RV presented with normal wall motion (*white opened arrows*).

thrombus detected by CMR compared with echocardiography may be explained by false-positive findings due to the suboptimal specificity of echo for the detection of apical thrombi.[30] Thus, sensitive and specific detection of thrombi is another advantage of using CMR in patients with suspected TTC (**Fig. 5**).

MYOCARDIAL EDEMA

Sequences in which image contrast is weighted by intrinsic magnetic relaxation times, such as T1, T2, or T2* relaxation times, may be obtained depending on the specific clinical question. Because T2 relaxation time is linearly correlated to the percentage of free water, edema is visible on T2-weighted MRI sequences. T2-weighted sequences, equipped with inversion techniques to null the signal of fat and blood, are now the most commonly used for edema imaging.[31] Eitel and colleagues,[11] for example, used in their CMR imaging protocol a triple inversion recovery fast spin-echo sequence (short TI inversion recovery) to study the presence and extent of myocardial edema in TTC patients.

The characteristic finding on such short TI inversion recovery CMR images in TTC patients is edema of the LV myocardium, showing high signal intensity with a diffuse or transmural distribution.

The edema is located in the parts of the ventricle showing the wall motion abnormality and—like the wall motion abnormality—is not related to a single coronary artery (**Fig. 6**). These features allow distinguishing between TTC and AMI, in which edema is usually located transmurally but always has a vascular distribution. In patients with acute myocarditis, however, short TI inversion recovery sequences similarly shows a high signal intensity in the ventricular wall, but the signal is more heterogeneously distributed and is frequently located in middle layer of the ventricular wall or subepicardially and often seen in the inferolateral wall of the LV.[32]

In Abdel-Aty and colleagues'[33] small series of 7 patients with TTC, all had edema in the acute setting and there was a strong and significant relation to the severity of ventricular dysfunction. Nakamori and colleagues[34] reported the presence of myocardial edema in 96% of their Japanese patients with TTC. Eitel and colleagues[11] found myocardial edema in the majority of their white patients (70%) in the region with abnormal systolic function. The time course of edema in TTC can also be studied by CMR.[35] In the first days after beginning of the symptoms, the T2 signal is very evident. After 2 weeks, however, signal intensity decreases and becomes difficult to differentiate from the signal intensity of the normal wall.[35] In

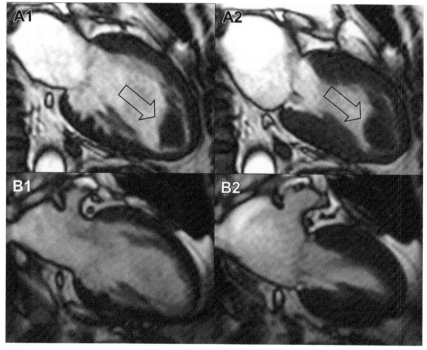

Fig. 5. Vertical long axis views at the acute presentation (*A1, A2*) and at follow-up after 3 months (*B1, B2*). *Arrows* indicate a large thrombus in the apex of the LV, which is seen in end diastole (*A1*) and end systole (*A2*). After 3 months, the thrombus completely disappeared in end diastole (*B1*) and end systole (*B2*).

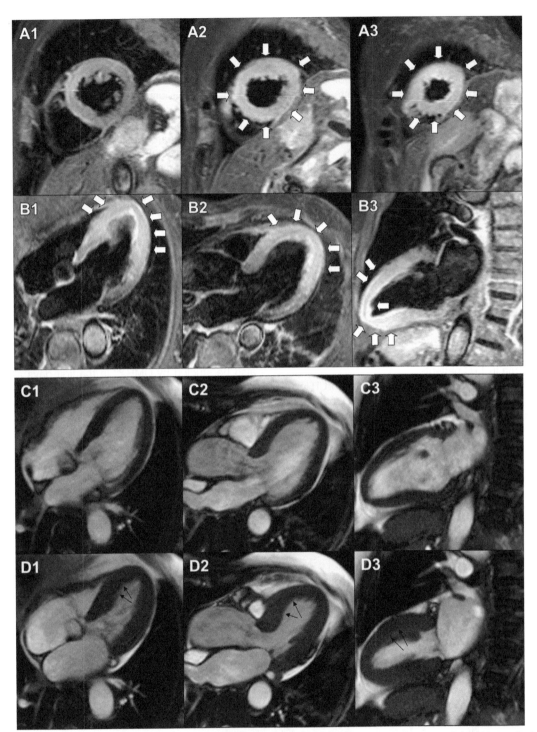

Fig. 6. T2-weighted images in short-axis views (*A*) and long-axis views (*B*), demonstrating normal signal intensity in the basal segments of the left myocardium (*A1*) and a global edema in the mid (*A2*) and apical segments (*A3*) of the left myocardium (*white arrows*). In the long-axis 4-chamber view (*B1*), the 3-chamber vies (*B2*) and 2-chamber view (*B3*) white arrows indicate the global edema in the mid and apical segments. In (*C*) (end diastolein a 4-chamber view (*C1*), 3-chamber view (*C2*), and 2-chamber view (*C3*)) and (*D*) (end systolein a 4-chamber view (*D1*), 3-chamber view (*D2*), and 2-chamber view (*D3*)) the corresponding cine images show the already diminishing wall motion abnormalities of a apical ballooning (*black arrows*) 2 days after onset of symptoms.

contrast to the situation in TTC, the T2 signal remains visible for a longer time period in patients with AMI or myocarditis.[35,36]

The pathophysiologic mechanism underlying the development of myocardial edema in TTC remains unclear. It has been suggested that inflammation, increased LV wall stress, and/or transient ischemia may contribute to this phenomenon.

LATE GADOLINIUM ENHANCEMENT

To date, the paramagnetic gadolinium-chelated contrast agents are the only licensed group of paramagnetic agents for routine cardiac imaging. Gadolinium contrast agents are not disease specific; as such, myocardial enhancement is nonspecific, whereas the location and pattern of enhancement give important information regarding the underlying cause. T1-weighted turbo spin-echo images are usually acquired approximately 10 to 15 minutes after the intravenous application of gadolinium-based contrast agents for the assessment of the late gadolinium enhancement (LGE) images.[37]

Typically, LGE is absent in TTC and the absence of LGE is an important criterion in the differential diagnosis between AMI and TTC.[38,39] It remains, however, controversial, whether minor amounts of LGE may be present in some patients with TTC and which type of LGE may be observed in patients with TTC.

Several studies have reported LGE in patients with TTC.[33,40–42] Eitel and colleagues[11] found that LGE by CMR showed minute focal or patchy nonischemic myocardial scarring in 9% of the patients. Nakamori and colleagues[34] and Rolf and colleagues[43] observed LGE in 22% and in 33% of their TTC patients whereas Naruse and colleagues[44] reported LGE even in 40% of TTC patients. A representative example is shown in **Fig. 7**.

To reliably determine the presence of LGE in TTC, it is important to define the threshold for differentiating between normal myocardium and abnormal myocardium on LGE MRI and to evaluate the signal intensity characteristics in patients with TTC in comparison to those with myocardial infarction. Only when a threshold is lower than

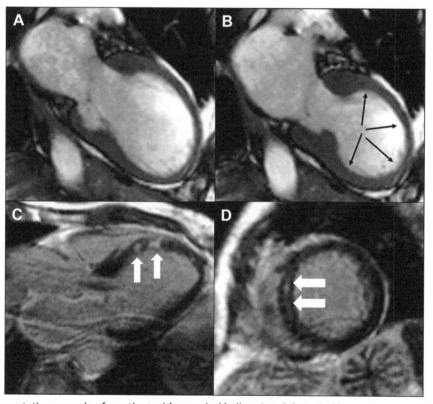

Fig. 7. Representative example of a patient with an apical ballooning. (*A*) Vertical long-axis view of the end diastole. (*B*) Vertical long-axis view of the end systole. *Black arrows* indicate the area of akinesia. (*C*) Long-axis view with a small area of LGE located in the midventricular portion of the LV (*white arrows*). (*D*) Short-axis view in the same patient. White arrows indicate an area of LGE located in the septum.

5 SD above the signal intensity of remote normally contracting myocardium (which is commonly used for defining LGE in myocardial infarction) may selected LGE become detectable in TTC. Focal and patchy LGE was seen by Eitel and colleagues[11] in 9% of their patients only when a threshold of 3 SD instead of 5 SD was used. None of their patients had evidence of LGE when using a threshold of 5 SD. Although Nakamori and colleagues[34] applied a similar threshold of 3.1 ± 0.3 SD, they found a higher rate of LGE (22%). The even higher rate of LGE in the studies of Rolf and colleagues[43] and Naruse and colleagues[44] may be explained by their using a definition of a lower threshold of 2 SD. When a threshold of 5 SD was applied to their population, no patient had LGE in either the subacute phase or the chronic phase.

The presence LGE of lower signal intensity may indicate a more severe form of TTC. Cardiogenic shock was observed more frequently in patients with LGE than in those without LGE and the patients with LGE had a longer duration to ECG normalization and recovery of wall motion than did those without LGE.[44] Similar to T2 edema, LGE disappeared over time but at later stage (within 45–180 days from onset of TTC).

The contrast-to-noise ratio may be another useful parameter for distinguishing the LGE in TTC from that in AMI. The contrast-to-noise ratio in TTC is lower than that of AMI and a contrast-to-noise ratio less than 4 may be optimal for the differentiation between LGE associated with TTC versus AMI with a sensitivity of 100% and a specificity of 94% with values greater than 4 indicating AMI.[34]

More information is necessary before the value of low threshold LGE for determining the prognosis of TTC can finally be determined.

EARLY GADOLINIUM UPTAKE

Early gadolinium uptake images are acquired prior and during the first 3 minutes after intravenous bolus of gadolinium-based contrast agent.[32] Early gadolinium uptake in TTC patients has been found in 67% of TTC patients in the large series of Eitel and colleagues.[11] They interpreted this as indicative of myocardial inflammation. Consistent with this hypothesis, they also found pericardial effusions in 70% of these patients and concluded that an inflammatory process might play a role in the acute setting of TCT. No other CMR study in TTC patients has yet reported similar findings. Thus, it remains unclear whether inflammation contributes to the LV dysfunction. Further studies are needed to investigate whether inflammation is a primary phenomenon of the syndrome or secondary due to other abnormalities.

WHEN CMR, WHEN ECHOCARDIOGRAPHY?

Echocardiography imaging can rapidly performed at the bedside and, hence, is the most commonly used imaging technique for visualizing LV function in patients with suspected cardiomyopathies. The widespread use of echocardiography in the emergency room has contributed to more frequent recognition of TTC. Meticulous evaluation by echocardiography by an experienced physician may be the only imaging procedure necessary for verifying a suspected diagnosis of TTC. The definitive diagnosis of TTC can only be confirmed, however, when echocardiography is repeated after a few days to weeks showing complete normalization of regional wall motion abnormalities and LV function.[45,46]

CMR may be helpful as a second-line technique in patients with suspected TTC but suboptimal images by echocardiography. In patients with large areas of LV akinesia, however, CMR should be used to detect thrombus and RV involvement, which may be difficult to detect by echocardiography. The tissue differentiation possible with CMR may also be helpful to distinguish TTC from other cardiac diseases. These unique features of CMR may also provide insights into possible underlying pathophysiologic mechanisms of TTC.

Using CMR, the following precise diagnostic criteria for TTC can be defined:

1. LV dysfunction in a noncoronary regional distribution pattern with or without RV involvement
2. Myocardial edema located in the segments with wall motion abnormalities (akinesia or hypokinesia)
3. Absence of high-signal areas (>5 SD above normal) in LGE images

The authors believe that a more thorough definition and understanding of TTC require the use of CMR as a routine add-on to the initially performed echocardiogram.

In summary, echocardiography and CMR have their own specific value in evaluation of patients with TTC. Echocardiography, however, remains the first imaging modality of choice in clinical routine practice due to its availability and accessibility.

REFERENCES

1. Salerno M, Kramer CM. Advances in cardiovascular MRI for diagnosis: application in coronary artery disease and cardiomyopathies. Expert Opin Med Diagn 2009;3:673–87.

2. Eitel I, Behrendt F, Schindler K, et al. Differential diagnosis of suspected apical ballooning syndrome using contrast-enhanced magnetic resonance imaging. Eur Heart J 2008;29:2651–9.

3. Eitel I, Lücke C, Grothoff M, et al. Inflammation in takotsubo cardiomyopathy: insights form cardiovascular magnetic resonance imaging. Eur Radiol 2010; 20:422–31.

4. Friedrich MG. Tissue characterization of acute myocardial infarction and myocarditis by cardiac magnetic resonance. JACC Cardiovasc Imaging 2008;1:652–62.

5. Carr JC, Simonetti O, Bundy J, et al. Cine MR angiography of the heart with segmented true fast imaging with steady-state precession. Radiology 2001;219(3):828–34.

6. Fieno DS, Jaffe WC, Simonetti OP, et al. TrueFISP: assessment of accuracy for measurement of left ventricular mass in an animal model. J Magn Reson Imaging 2002;15:526–31.

7. Lorenz CH, Walker ES, Morgan VL, et al. Normal human right and left ventricular mass, systolic function, and gender differences by cine magnetic resonance imaging. J Cardiovasc Magn Reson 1999;1: 7–21.

8. Wintersperger BJ, Nikolaou K, Dietrich O, et al. Single breath-hold real-time cine MR imaging: improved temporal resolution using generalized auto calibrating partially parallel acquisition (GRAPPA) algorithm. Eur Radiol 2003;13:1931–6.

9. Lee VS, Resnick D, Bundy JM, et al. Cardiac function: MR evaluation in one breath hold with real-time true fast imaging with steady-state precession. Radiology 2002;222:835–42.

10. Budoff MJ, Cohen MC, Garcia MJ, et al. ACCF/AHA clinical competence statement on cardiac imaging with computed tomography and magnetic resonance: a report of the American College of Cardiology Foundation/American Heart Association/American College of Physicians Task Force on Clinical Competence and Training. J Am Coll Cardiol 2005;46:383–402.

11. Eitel I, von Knobelsdorff-Brenkenhoff F, Bernhardt P, et al. Clinical characteristics and cardiovascular magnetic resonance findings in stress (takotsubo) cardiomyopathy. JAMA 2011;306:277–86.

12. Schneider B, Athanasiadis A, Schwab J, et al. Clinical spectrum of tako-tsubo cardiomyopathy in Germany: results of the tako-tsubo registry of the Arbeitsgemeinschaft Leitende Kardiologische Krankenhausärzte (ALKK). Dtsch Med Wochenschr 2010;135:1908–13 [in German].

13. Hurst RT, Askew JW, Reuss CS, et al. Transient midventricular ballooning syndrome: a new variant. J Am Coll Cardiol 2006;48:579–83.

14. Van de Walle SO, Gevaert SA, Gheeraert PJ, et al. Transient stress-induced cardiomyopathy with an inverted "takotsubo" contractile pattern. Mayo Clin Proc 2006;81:1499–502.

15. Hurst RT, Prasad A, Askew JW, et al. Takotsubo cardiomyopathy: a unique cardiomyopathy with variable ventricular morphology. JACC Cardiovasc Imaging 2010;3:641–9.

16. Valsangiacomo Buechel ER, Mertens LL. Imaging the right heart: the use of integrated multimodality imaging. Eur Heart J 2012;33:949–60.

17. Mertens LL, Friedberg MK. Imaging the right ventricle—current state of the art. Nat Rev Cardiol 2010;7:551–63.

18. Le Tourneau T, Piriou N, Donal E, et al. Imaging and modern assessment of the right ventricle. Minerva Cardioangiol 2011;59:349–73.

19. Haghi D, Athanasiadis A, Papavassiliu T, et al. Right ventricular involvement in Takotsubo cardiomyopathy. Eur Heart J 2006;27:2433–9.

20. Stähli BE, Ruschitzka F, Enseleit F. Isolated right ventricular ballooning syndrome: a new variant of transient cardiomyopathy. Eur Heart J 2011;32: 1821.

21. Burgdorf C, Hunold P, Radke PW, et al. Isolated right ventricular stress-induced ("Tako-tsubo") cardiomyopathy. Clin Res Cardiol 2011;100:617–9.

22. Haghi D, Papavassiliu T, Heggemann F, et al. Incidence and clinical significance of left ventricular thrombus in tako-tsubo cardiomyopathy assessed with echocardiography. QJM 2008;101:381–6.

23. Berger AK, Gottdiener JS, Yohe MA, et al. Epidemiological approach to quality assessment in echocardiographic diagnosis. J Am Coll Cardiol 1999;34: 1831–6.

24. Thanigaraj S, Schechtman KB, Perez JE. Improved echocardiographic delineation of left ventricular thrombus with the use of intravenous second-generation contrast image enhancement. J Am Soc Echocardiogr 1999;12:1022–6.

25. Weinsaft JW, Kim HW, Shah DJ, et al. Detection of left ventricular thrombus by delayed-enhancement cardiovascular magnetic resonance. J Am Coll Cardiol 2008;52:148–57.

26. Srichai MB, Junor C, Rodriguez LL, et al. Clinical, imaging, and pathologic characteristics of left ventricular thrombus: a comparison of contrast enhanced magnetic resonance imaging, transthoracic echocardiography and transesophageal echocardiography with surgical or pathological validation. Am Heart J 2006;152:75–84.

27. Singh V, Mayer T, Salanitri J, et al. Cardiac MRI documented left ventricular thrombus complicating acute Takotsubo syndrome: an uncommon dilemma. Int J Cardiovasc Imaging 2007;23:591–3.

28. de Gregorio C, Grimaldi P, Lentini C. Left ventricular thrombus formation and cardioembolic complications in patients with Takotsubo-like syndrome: a systematic review. Int J Cardiol 2008;131:18–24.

29. Leurent G, Larralde A, Boulmier D, et al. Cardiac MRI studies of transient left ventricular apical ballooning syndrome (takotsubo cardiomyopathy): a systematic review. Int J Cardiol 2009;135:146–9.

30. Sechtem U, Theissen P, Heindel W, et al. Diagnosis of left ventricular thrombi by magnetic resonance imaging and comparison with angiocardiography, computed tomography and echocardiography. Am J Cardiol 1989;64:1195–9.

31. Simonetti OP, Finn JP, White RV. "Black blood" T2-weighted inversion-recovery MR imaging of the heart. Radiology 1996;199:49–57.

32. Friedrich MG, Sechtem U, Schulz-Menger J, et al. Cardiovascular magnetic resonance in myocarditis: a JACC white paper. J Am Coll Cardiol 2009;53:1475–87.

33. Abdel-Aty H, Cocker M, Friedrich MG. Myocardial edema is a feature of Tako-Tsubo cardiomyopathy and is related to the severity of systolic dysfunction: insights from T2-weighted cardiovascular magnetic resonance. Int J Cardiol 2009;132:291–3.

34. Nakamori S, Matsuoka K, Onishi K, et al. Prevalence and signal characteristics of late gadolinium enhancement on contrast-enhanced magnetic resonance imaging in patients with takotsubo cardiomyopathy. Circ J 2012;76:914–21.

35. Fernández-Pérez GC, Aguilar-Arjola JA, de la Fuente GT, et al. Takotsubo cardiomyopathy: assessment with cardiac MRI. AJR Am J Roentgenol 2010;195:W139–45.

36. Assomull GR, Lyne JC, Keenan N, et al. The role of cardiovascular magnetic resonance in patients presenting with chest pain, raised troponin, and unobstructed coronary arteries. Eur Heart J 2007;28:1242–9.

37. Mahrholdt H, Wagner A, Judd RM, et al. Delayed enhancement cardiovascular magnetic resonance assessment of non-ischemic cardiomyopathies. Eur Heart J 2005;26:1461–71.

38. Wittstein IS, Thiemann DR, Lima JA, et al. Neurohumoral features of myocardial stunning due to sudden emotional stress. N Engl J Med 2005;352:539–48.

39. Gerbaud E, Montaudon M, Leroux L, et al. MRI for the diagnosis of left ventricular apical ballooning syndrome (LVABS). Eur Radiol 2008;18:947–54.

40. Sharkey SW, Lesser JR, Zenovich AG, et al. Acute and reversible cardiomyopathy provoked by stress in women from the United States. Circulation 2005;111:472–9.

41. Haghi D, Fluechter S, Suselbeck T, et al. Cardiovascular magnetic resonance findings in typical versus atypical forms of the acute apical ballooning syndrome (Takotsubo cardiomyopathy). Int J Cardiol 2007;120:205–11.

42. Balaguer JR, Estornell J, Planas AM, et al. Transient left ventricular apical ballooning and cardiac magnetic resonance. Int J Cardiol 2006;108:262–3.

43. Rolf A, Nef HM, Mollmann H, et al. Immunohistological basis of the late gadolinium enhancement phenomenon in tako-tsubo cardiomyopathy. Eur Heart J 2009;30:1635–42.

44. Naruse Y, Sato A, Kasahara K, et al. The clinical impact of late gadolinium enhancement in Takotsubo cardiomyopathy: serial analysis for cardiovascular magnetic resonance imaging. J Cardiovasc Magn Reson 2011;13:67.

45. Chockalingam A, Xie GY, Dellsperger KG. Echocardiography in stress cardiomyopathy and acute LVOT obstruction. Int J Cardiovasc Imaging 2010;26:527–35.

46. Van der Wall EE, Holman ER, Scholte AJ, et al. Echocardiography in takotsubo cardiomyopathy; a useful approach? Int J Cardiovasc Imaging 2010;26:537–40.

Clinical Management of Takotsubo Cardiomyopathy

Raymond Bietry, MD, Alex Reyentovich, MD,
Stuart D. Katz, MD, MS*

KEYWORDS

- Takotsubo cardiomyopathy • Stress-induced cardiomyopathy • Apical ballooning • Pharmacology

KEY POINTS

- The diagnosis of takotsubo cardiomyopathy must be made on clinical grounds and differentiated from a variety of alternative diagnoses with echocardiography, serum biomarkers, cardiac catheterization, and cardiac magnetic resonance imaging.
- Acute therapy includes supportive care, targeting the precipitating trigger if known, β-blockade (especially in the presence of left ventricular outflow tract obstruction), inhibitors of the renin-angiotensin system, and consideration of systemic anticoagulation in all patients, especially those with confirmed ventricular thrombus.
- Recovery of left ventricular function to normal is expected regardless of early therapy.
- Although the prognosis is generally favorable, monitoring for early dangerous complications is essential.
- There is no evidence to support use of long-term medical therapy to reduce the risk of recurrence.

INTRODUCTION

Takotsubo cardiomyopathy was first described in 1991 in Japan (**Fig. 1**).[1] The name tako-tsubo was taken from the appearance on ventriculogram of apical ballooning with a contractile ventricular base that resembles a traditional Japanese octopus trap. Although first described in Japan, it has been increasingly recognized worldwide. The syndrome has also been described as *broken heart syndrome*, *apical ballooning syndrome*, or *stress-induced cardiomyopathy*.

Takotsubo cardiomyopathy is often clinically difficult to distinguish from a broad differential of alternative diagnoses, and there remains significant uncertainty regarding its optimal management. This review summarizes current knowledge of the clinical management of takotsubo cardiomyopathy including diagnostic strategies, monitoring for potential complications, and pharmacologic therapies to consider for both short- and long-term management.

CONFIRMATION OF DIAGNOSIS

The initial step in the management of takotsubo cardiomyopathy is confirmation of the clinical diagnosis. Clinical suspicion of the diagnosis is increased in patients with known risk factors as described in **Box 1**. The prototypical description of takotsubo cardiomyopathy includes the presence of a preceding emotional stressor. However, a broad range of other types of triggers is also known to be associated with the syndrome. Case reports of physical stress triggers of takotsubo cardiomyopathy include acute stroke,[2] seizures,[3] alcohol withdrawal,[4] near drowning,[5] and noncardiac surgical procedures.[6] Furthermore, more than

Disclosures: R. Bietry and A. Reyentovich: None; S.D. Katz: None related to subject of manuscript; Other: Consulting/Advisory Committees, Bristol Meyers Squibb (modest), Amgen, Inc (modest), Terumo, Inc (modest), Speaker Bureau, Otsuka Pharmaceuticals, Inc (>modest).
Leon H. Charney Division of Cardiology, Department of Medicine, 530 First Avenue, NYU Langone Medical Center, New York, NY 10016, USA
* Corresponding author. NYU Langone Medical Center, 530 First Avenue, Skirball 9R, New York, NY 10016.
E-mail address: stuart.katz@nyumc.org

Heart Failure Clin 9 (2013) 177–186
http://dx.doi.org/10.1016/j.hfc.2012.12.003
1551-7136/13/$ – see front matter © 2013 Elsevier Inc. All rights reserved.

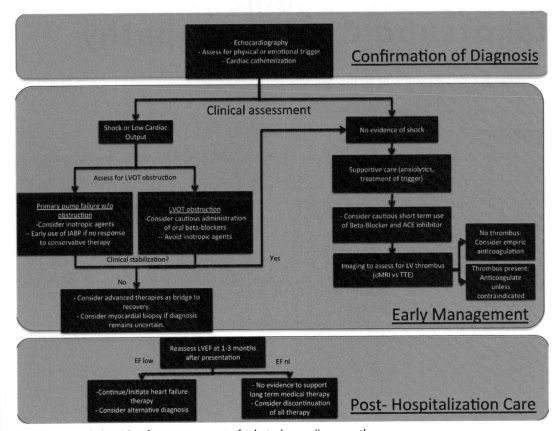

Fig. 1. Proposed algorithm for management of takotsubo cardiomyopathy.

20 drugs have been reported to be associated with takotsubo cardiomyopathy, including epinephrine, atropine, dobutamine, ergonovine, nortriptyline venlafaxine, and levothyroxine.[7]

Patients often present with chest pain, dyspnea, electrocardiogram changes including ST segment elevations in the precordial leads, positive biomarkers of cardiac injury, and left ventricular systolic dysfunction, a constellation that makes the diagnosis of takotsubo cardiomyopathy difficult to distinguish from other disorders, including acute coronary syndrome, syndrome X, coronary vasospasm (variant angina), and myocarditis.

One feature that distinguishes takotsubo cardiomyopathy from these other diseases is the relatively rapid recovery of left ventricular function. Accordingly, the Mayo Clinic proposed criteria in 2004 for the diagnosis of takotsubo cardiomyopathy (**Box 2**).[8]

Box 1
Risk factors for takotsubo cardiomyopathy

1. Postmenopause
2. Preceding emotional stressor
3. Physical stressors: surgery, seizures, stroke
4. Drugs

Data from Akashi YJ, Goldstein DS, Barbaro G, et al. Takotsubo cardiomyopathy: a new form of acute, reversible heart failure. Circulation 2008;118(25):2754–62.

Box 2
Mayo clinic criteria for diagnosis of takotsubo cardiomyopathy

1. Transient hypokinesis, akinesis, or dyskinesis of the mid left ventricle with or without apical involvement that extends beyond the distribution of a single vascular territory
2. Absence of obstructive coronary artery disease
3. New electrocardiographic abnormalities (either ST-segment elevations or t wave inversions) or modest elevation in cardiac troponin
4. Absence of pheochromocytoma, myocarditis

Data from Akashi YJ, Goldstein DS, Barbaro G, et al. Takotsubocardiomyopathy: anewformof acute, reversible heart failure. Circulation 2008;118(25):2754–62.

Echocardiography

Echocardiography is used in takotsubo cardiomyopathy to assist in the diagnosis of the disease and to evaluate for potential complications. Transthoracic echocardiography typically reveals a reduced overall left ventricular ejection fraction with hypokinesis or akinesis of the mid and apical segments and normal wall motion or hyperkinesis of the base. The Mayo Clinic Criteria require the ventricular dysfunction to extend beyond a single coronary territory; however, this is often difficult to determine in clinical practice unless coronary anatomy is already known. Without knowledge of the coronary anatomy, it is often difficult to distinguish the regional wall motion abnormality in takotsubo cardiomyopathy from an anterior wall myocardial infarction because of occlusion of a left anterior descending artery that extends around to the apex to the inferior portion of left ventricle.

Although cardiac catheterization remains necessary to distinguish anterior wall myocardial infarction from takotsubo cardiomyopathy, certain echocardiographic findings are suggestive of the takotsubo cardiomyopathy diagnosis. In a study by Citro and colleagues,[9] the echocardiographic findings of 37 patients with takotsubo cardiomyopathy were compared with those of 37 patients with an anterior wall ST-Elevation Myocardial Infarction (STEMI). In the patients with takotsubo cardiomyopathy, 29% had wall motion abnormalities involving the apex with sparing of the base compared with only 2% of patients with anterior wall STEMI. Classification according to regional wall motion abnormalities based on coronary distribution with a cutoff of ≥ 4 territories affected on echocardiography was 84% sensitive and 97% specific for the diagnosis of takotsubo cardiomyopathy. Right ventricular involvement (29% vs 2%, $P<.002$) and left ventricular outflow tract obstruction (16% vs 0%, $P<.011$) were also more frequently detected in patients with takotsubo cardiomyopathy diagnosis.

When analyzed with speckle tracking, acute takotsubo cardiomyopathy can be differentiated from left anterior descending (LAD) artery occlusion by a characteristic circular pattern of LV dysfunction.[10] In acute takotsubo cardiomyopathy, the velocities and strain of the different segments of the basal, mid, and apical regions were identical. In contrast, ventricular function after an LAD occlusion generally reveals differences in velocities within different segments of the basal, mid, and apical region. After the acute phase of the disease, the ventricular function of takotsubo detected by speckle tracking may mimic ventricular dysfunction because of LAD occlusion and become indistinguishable from an echocardiographic perspective. This information supports the use of speckle tracking and strain imaging in the assessment and differentiation of takotsubo cardiomyopathy from atherosclerosis related ventricular dysfunction, especially if the timeline of the symptoms are well-defined and the echocardiogram can be performed early in the course of symptoms.

Although traditionally described as isolated apical ballooning and hypokinesis, variants of the wall motion abnormalities in stress-induced cardiomyopathies have been described. Variants include reverse type, midventricular type, and localized type.[11] In reverse takotsubo cardiomyopathy, ventricular dysfunction extends beyond a single coronary distribution; however, the base of the heart is hypocontractile when compared with the apex. Patients with this less common pattern of left ventricular dysfunction have been reported to be younger in age (54 vs 64 years, $P<.006$) but have a similar clinical course with regard to morbidity and mortality.[12] The same study also noted that reverse takotsubo cardiomyopathy has significantly lower rates of significant mitral regurgitation and systolic anterior motion of the mitral valve, consistent with the unique hemodynamic changes that occur with apical ballooning.

Echocardiography can also be used to assess for coexisting right ventricular dysfunction. The finding of biventricular dysfunction portends a longer hospitalization and increased risk of complications, including severe heart failure and placement of an intra-aortic balloon pump.[13]

Echocardiographic evaluation for left ventricular outflow tract (LVOT) obstruction is important to guide medical management of takotsubo cardiomyopathy. Basal hypercontractility can lead to increased gradients across the LVOT and subsequently reduced cardiac output. Further, systolic anterior motion of the anterior leaflet of the mitral valve can occur because of the increased gradient of the LVOT and cause significant mitral regurgitation and therefore reduce forward flow. LVOT obstruction has been seen in 25% of patients with takotsubo cardiomyopathy and generally occurs in patients with a baseline abnormality of a septal knuckle or asymmetric septal hypertrophy.[14]

Coronary Angiography

Coronary angiography is performed to rule out significant underlying coronary artery disease in the clinical setting of chest pain, electrocardiographic changes, and elevated cardiac enzymes. The angiographic appearance of nonobstructive or normal coronaries may not be sufficient to exclude atherosclerosis as a pathologic mechanism in some patients with suspected takotsubo cardiomyopathy. A significant proportion of patients, particularly women, have no angiographic evidence of plaque rupture in the setting of myocardial infarction.[15] Multiple pathophysiologic mechanisms for this finding have been hypothesized, including plaque ulceration and thrombosis with spontaneous recanalization, vasospasm, and microvascular endothelial dysfunction. In patients with angiographically normal coronary arteries, intravascular ultrasound found nonobstructive plaque rupture in 29% of patients.[15] Therefore, the use of intravascular ultrasound in selected patients may be useful to help exclude plaque ulceration in patients, especially if the ventricular dysfunction is distributed largely within a single vascular territory.

Endomyocardial Biopsy

The typical histopathologic findings of takotsubo cardiomyopathy include mild neutrophilic infiltration, contraction band necrosis, and increased production of extracellular matrix. Although the Mayo criteria do not specifically call for routine endomyocardial biopsy, this procedure may be considered on an individual basis in cases with a strong clinical suspicion of acute myocarditis, especially if the patient is hemodynamically unstable. A published case report has shown that despite a patient satisfying all clinical criteria for takotsubo cardiomyopathy, a subsequent biopsy found underlying viral myocarditis.[16] Despite these findings, endomyocardial biopsy is seldom performed in patients with clinically suspected takotsubo cardiomyopathy. Given the risks of endomyocardial biopsy and uncertain impact in clinical decision making, endomyocardial biopsy is not recommended unless the patient does not clinically improve with conservative management or myocarditis is suspected on clinical grounds.

Biomarker and Laboratory Evaluation

Cardiac biomarkers may be useful to differentiate patients with takotsubo cardiomyopathy from acute coronary syndrome. Plasma brain natriuretic peptide (BNP), a peptide hormone released by ventricular myocytes in response to increased wall stress, was elevated in 92.9% of patients with takotsubo cardiomyopathy and was independent of the patient's measured ejection fraction.[17] Compared with a cohort of patients with ST-elevation myocardial infarction, the measured BNP level was higher in patients with takotsubo cardiomyopathy (554.5 pg/mL vs 168.5 pg/mL, $P = .005$), whereas peak troponin was only modestly elevated in takotsubo cardiomyopathy

when compared with STEMI patients (0.5 ng/mL vs 2.8 ng/mL, $P<.001$). The ratio of BNP/peak troponin was higher in patients with takotsubo cardiomyopathy when compared with that of patients with acute STEMI (1089.4 vs 97.4, $P = .042$).

Although increased release of stress hormones is suspected to be involved the pathogenesis of takotsubo cardiomyopathy, routine measurement of these hormones does not have proven clinical utility for the diagnosis of the disease. Measurement of metanephrines, catecholamines, cortisol, or C-reactive protein (CRP) is often normal or indistinguishable from patients with acute coronary syndrome.[18] This may be attributable, in part, to the short half-life of epinephrine and the presence of secondary activation of the sympathetic nervous system in the setting of ischemic cardiac injury.[19] However, given the need to exclude pheochromocytoma in the diagnosis of takotsubo cardiomyopathy, it is reasonable to measure plasma-free metanephrines or urine metanephrines after the acute phase of the disease.[20]

Cardiac Magnetic Resonance Imaging

Cardiac magnetic resonance imaging (MRI) can also be used in the diagnosis of takotsubo cardiomyopathy.[21] In one large series, myocardial edema was noted in 81% of patients. Unlike myocarditis, the distribution of edema was uniform across all layers of the heart. Myocardial inflammation (using Lake Louise consensus criteria) was detected in 67% of patients. The findings of both inflammation and edema were noted in the absence of fibrosis, as manifested by absence of late gadolinium enhancement. Late gadolinium enhancement (LGE) was present in 9% of patients with takotsubo cardiomyopathy and was generally focal or patchy, distinct from a typical postinfarction pattern. Cardiac MRI may also be useful in the detection of LV thrombus, which was incidentally found in 2% of patients with takotsubo cardiomyopathy who underwent MRI. Based on the above findings, Eitel and colleagues[21] have proposed the following diagnostic criteria for takotsubo cardiomyopathy by MRI (**Box 3**).

THERAPEUTIC STRATEGIES
General Principles of Therapy

Takotsubo cardiomyopathy has, by definition, a self-limited course with anticipation of complete recovery of ventricular function. There are no randomized trials, or even expert consensus, to guide medical therapy. Given the absence of trials to compare the efficacy of treatment strategies for takotsubo cardiomyopathy, the management recommendations are based on current

---

Box 3
MRI criteria for diagnosis of takotsubo cardiomyopathy

1. Severe left ventricular dysfunction in a non-coronary regional distribution pattern
2. Myocardial edema colocated with the regional wall motion abnormality
3. Absence of high signal areas in late gadolinium enhancement images
4. Increased early myocardial gadolinium uptake (suggestive of inflammation)

Data from Akashi YJ, Goldstein DS, Barbaro G, et al. Takotsubocardiomyopathy: anewformof acute, reversible heart failure. Circulation 2008;118(25):2754–62.

---

understanding of the pathophysiology and natural history of the disease. Although the specific pathophysiologic mechanisms are not fully characterized, several lines of evidence suggest that excessive catecholamines play a role in the pathogenesis of the disease. The theory of catecholamine-mediated myocardial injury is supported by the observation of left ventricular dysfunction in patients with pheochromocytoma,[22] cases of takotsubo cardiomyopathy after inadvertent overdose of epinephrine,[23] cases after initiation of norepinephrine reuptake inhibitors including venlafaxine,[24] and temporally associated emotional and physical stress triggers to symptoms onset.

It is established in both human and animal models that epinephrine has a cardiotoxic effect. Chronic and repeated exposure to epinephrine has been used as an animal model for heart failure.[25] In humans, chronic exposure to epinephrine via neuroendocrine tumors such as pheochromocytoma has been associated with reduced ventricular function.[22] While prolonged exposure to catecholamines is linked to the development of cardiomyopathy, the mechanism of injury from acute exposure is less certain. Proposed mechanisms of myocardial dysfunction in response to short-term exposure to catecholamines include direct myocardial injury, epicardial vasospasm, and microvascular ischemic injury.[26]

Animal models have shown that supraphysiologic concentrations of catecholamine are detrimental to myocyte function.[19] In a transgenic mouse model with overexpression of human β-2 receptors, epinephrine can both increase and decrease myocyte contractility in a concentration-dependent manner. With high concentrations of epinephrine, β-2 receptors shift from coupling with Gs protein signaling to Gi protein signaling with consequent downstream negative inotropic effect.[27] A primate model has also shown

that epinephrine-induced ventricular wall motion abnormalities are associated with increased expression of RNA involving the renin-angiotensin system and markers of heart failure, including brain natriuretic peptide at the myocardial apex.[26]

The regional wall motion abnormalities typical of takotsubo cardiomyopathy may be attributable to the regional differences in sympathetic innervation and adrenoreceptor concentration within the ventricle. In normal human hearts, the base of the heart has a higher density of sympathetic nerve innervation.[28] Perhaps as a compensatory feature, the apex has a higher density of sympathetic adrenoreceptors.[29] Thus, the apex of the heart may be more susceptible to excess systemic catecholamines exposure in response to stress.

Apart from direct myocardial injury, epicardial spasm and microvascular disease has also been implicated in the pathogenesis of takotsubo. Kurisu and colleagues[30] found ergonovine- or acetylcholine-induced coronary vasospam in 10 of 14 patients with transient apical ballooning detected by ventriculography. Microvascular disease has been implicated by both noninvasive and invasive measurements. Galiuto and colleagues[31] found that patients with acute takotsubo cardiomyopathy have a perfusion defect on myocardial contrast echocardiography that, unlike that in STEMI patients, is reduced with the administration of adenosine. Microvascular disease also has been measured invasively with calculation of microcirculatory resistance with an intracoronary pressure wire and found to be abnormal.[32] The unique geometry of the ventricular apex, with high degree of curvature and myocyte orientation, may make the apical region more susceptible to microvascular ischemic injury.[33]

Whether directly linked to catecholamine surge or not, management of the precipitating trigger is important in the acute and long-term management of takotsubo cardiomyopathy. Emotional stressors should be managed with anxiolytic agents as needed, although the potential of acute QT prolongation should be considered before the administration of any psychiatric agent. Accordingly, optimal medical management of any identified physical stressor that may have triggered the event (ie, seizure, pain, asthma) is an important consideration for therapy.

β-blocker Therapy

Based on the putative role of excessive catecholamines in the pathogenesis of takotsubo cardiomyopathy, beta-adrenergic receptor blockers have been proposed as a potential therapeutic strategy. In an animal model of takotsubo cardiomyopathy in a cynomolgus monkey induced by high-dose epinephrine, early administration of metoprolol improved the rate of left ventricular recovery and diminished severity of cardiomyocy-tolysis.[26] However, placebo-treated animals also eventually fully recovered normal ventricular function, albeit at a later timepoint.

There are no randomized, clinical trials to support the use of β-blockade as routine therapy in all patients with takotsubo cardiomyopathy. The subset of patients with left ventricular outflow (LVOT) obstruction may benefit from β-blockade. Yoshioka and colleagues[34] reported the hemody-namic and echocardiographic effects of intrave-nous propranolol (0.05 mg/kg, maximum 4 mg) in 34 patients with takotsubo cardiomyopathy. Among the 8 patients who had baseline mid-ventricular obstruction (mean pressure gradient, 90 ± 42 mm Hg), intravenous propranolol de-creased the pressure gradient to 22 ± 9 mm Hg with a subsequent increase in systolic blood pres-sure and left ventricular ejection fraction. However, in the subset of patients without LVOT obstruction, propranolol had no effect in systolic blood pressure or left ventricular ejection fraction. In patients without LVOT, recommendations for use of β-blockers are based on the general recommenda-tions by the American College of Cardiology/Amer-ican Heart Association for all patients with reduced systolic function.[35] The relevance of clinical trials results in populations with chronic left ventricular systolic dysfunction to patients with transient left ventricular systolic dysfunction caused by takot-subo cardiomyopathy is uncertain. Because takot-subo cardiomyopathy is a self-limited disease associated with anticipated recovery of left ventric-ular systolic function, the potential unproven bene-fits of β-blockers must be carefully weighed against the risk of precipitating hemodynamic compromise. Given the underlying role of cate-cholamines in the pathophysiology of takotsubo, if β-blockade is initiated, consideration should be made to use nonselective β-adrenergic receptor blocking agents such a propranolol, nadolol, or carvedilol, which act as an antagonist on both α- and β-adrenoreceptors. Blockade of α-adrenor-eceptors may acutely improve cardiovascular function by limitation of vasoconstriction in re-sponse to catecholaminergic stimuli.

Angiotensin-converting Enzyme Inhibitor Therapy

Apart from general guidelines that recommend routine use of angiotensin converting enzyme (ACE) inhibitors in all patients with reduced ven-tricular systolic function,[35] there is little evidence to support use in patients with takotsubo cardiomyop-athy. There is a known synergistic interaction between the renin-angiotensin system and the sympathetic nervous system in the mediation of vasoconstriction.[36,37] In a retrospective study, long-term use of ACE inhibitors before the onset of takotsubo cardiomyopathy was protective against cardiogenic shock, sustained ventricular arrhythmia, and death.[38] In contrast, in a retrospective non-randomized observational report of 36 patients with takotsubo cardiomyopathy, left ventricular function improved back to normal in all subjects regardless of treatment with ACE inhibitor (n = 9).[39] Thus, although ACE inhibitor therapy may modulate the pathologic sequelae of excess catecholamine signaling, the clinical benefits remain uncertain.

Anticoagulation Therapy

Intraventricular thrombus is a known complication of takotsubo cardiomyopathy, with a prevalence estimated at 2%–5% of all cases.[21] Echocardiog-raphy and cardiac MRI are useful imaging modal-ities for the detection of ventricular thrombus. Risk factors for the development of left ventricular thrombus include female gender, age greater than 65 years, electrocardiogram with deeply negative t-wave inversions, and an elevated CRP.[40] In fact, an elevated CRP level was found in one small study to be highly sensitive (100%) for the devel-opment of thrombus, although not specific (42%).[41] The estimated risk of a cardioembolic complication in patients with takotsubo cardiomy-opathy with a left ventricular thrombus is as high as 33.3%.[42] Therefore, systemic anticoagulation is recommended in all patients with a known thrombus until the thrombus and ventricular dys-function has resolved.

It is reasonable to consider systemic anticoagu-lation in all patients with takotsubo cardiomyop-athy until ventricular function returns to normal. Evidence to support the empiric use of anticoagu-lation in all patients includes relatively high incidence of thrombus in all cases, high embolic potential in those that have intracavitary thrombus, and the observation that half of patients who have ventricular thrombus have no evidence of thro-mbus on initial imaging.[42] Because a relatively short course of anticoagulation is anticipated, the potential benefits may outweigh risks in patients thought to be at low risk for bleeding.

Estrogen in the Treatment of Takotsubo Cardiomyopathy

Given the epidemiologic observation of increased risk of takotsubo cardiomyopathy in postmeno-pausal women, gonadal hormones have been theorized to contribute to the pathophysiology of the disease. In animal models, estrogen depletion predisposes the heart to a stress-induced myopathy.[43] In mammalian hearts, estrogen is involved in regulation of calcium in cardiac tissue and regulates the release of epinephrine in cardiac nerve fibers.[44]

Animal studies have shown that estrogen depletion can predispose the heart to stress-induced cardiac dysfunction. Ueyama and colleagues[43] examined the effect of estrogen supplementation in oophorectomized mice. Estrogen-depleted mice had increased cardiac dysfunction when subjected to immobilization stress (an animal model of takotsubo cardiomyopathy). This effect was mitigated by estrogen supplementation. Interestingly, estrogen supplementation seemed to confer protective effects via reduction of stress-induced c-fos mRNA expression not only in cardiac tissue but in adrenal and brain tissue as well.

There are limited data to support a link between estrogen signaling and cardiac injury in humans. Estradiol levels of 16 patients admitted with takotsubo cardiomyopathy did not differ from that of age-matched patients admitted with an acute myocardial infarction.[44] However, estradiol levels in patients were noted to decrease after the acute presentation. There are no controlled trials to support the use of estrogen supplementation in the management of takotsubo cardiomyopathy. Given the known risks of estrogen supplementation, including a possible increased risk of venous thromboembolism and coronary heart disease,[45] use of supplementation for treatment or prevention of takotsubo cardiomyopathy is not recommended.

MANAGEMENT OF COMPLICATIONS

The complications of takotsubo cardiomyopathy are summarized in **Box 4**.

Box 4
Complications of takotsubo cardiomyopathy

1. Cardiogenic shock
   a. Caused by LVOT obstruction
   b. Caused by pump failure
2. Arrhythmias: atrioventricular block, ventricular tachycardia, ventricular fibrillation
3. Systemic embolism and stroke caused by ventricular thrombus
4. Cardiac rupture

Data from Akashi YJ, Goldstein DS, Barbaro G, et al. Takotsubocardiomyopathy: anewformof acute, reversible heart failure. Circulation 2008;118(25):2754–62.

Cardiogenic Shock

Cardiogenic shock has been reported to occur in 9%–20% of patients with takotsubo cardiomyopathy.[38,46] Management of this subset of patients requires early identification and differentiation of patients with LVOT obstruction versus primary pump failure. Identification of LVOT obstruction can be diagnosed with hemodynamic measurements in the cardiac catheterization laboratory or noninvasive imaging with echocardiography.

In patients with LVOT obstruction and hypotension, β-blockers may reduce the ventricular gradient and improve blood pressure and organ perfusion. Beta-blockers have been shown to improve the hemodynamics of midventricular obstruction with takotsubo cardiomyopathy.[34] The use of inotropes may have a paradoxical effect and lead to further hemodynamic compromise in patients with LVOT obstruction. Abe and colleagues[47] reported a case of a 78-year-old woman who had hypotension with ST elevations during a surgical procedure. The patient received a continuous infusion of dopamine and was persistently hypotensive. Echocardiography found apical ballooning with an intraventricular pressure gradient of 104 mm Hg. Discontinuation of dopamine improved the patient's systolic blood pressure with reduction of the intraventricular pressure gradient.

In the absence of LVOT obstruction, patients with takotsubo cardiomyopathy with hypotension caused by primary pump failure do not seem to benefit from inotropic therapy. Fujiwara and colleagues[48] found that in 11 patients with takotsubo cardiomyopathy without LVOT obstruction, the administration of 10 μg/kg/min of dobutamine did not improve regional wall motion abnormalities in the affected regions. The use of inotropes that stimulate the β-2 and α-adrenergic receptor may have deleterious effects given the proposed pathophysiology of the disease. As an alternative, noncatecholamine inotropes such as levosimendan have been proposed for use in takotsubo cardiomyopathy.[49] Given the potentially deleterious effects of and limited clinical response to inotropic agents, early consideration of an intra-aortic balloon pump is reasonable in patients with low cardiac output syndrome or cardiogenic shock.

In rare patients with refractory shock caused by takotsubo cardiomyopathy, there have been successful reports of the use of advanced therapies. Case reports have shown the successful use of extracorporeal cardiopulmonary bypass[50] and a left ventricular assist device, which was eventually explanted after recovery of ventricular function.[51]

Arrhythmias

The electrocardiogram changes associated with takotsubo cardiomyopathy evolve during the course of the disease. Early ST elevations in the precordial leads are typically followed by marked t-wave inversions and QT prolongation.[52] Arrhythmias have been described with takotsubo cardiomyopathy, including atrioventricular block,[53] torsade de pointe,[54] and monomorphic ventricular tachycardia.[55] In most cases, the arrhythmias are transient, although permanent atrioventricular block after an episode of takotsubo cardiomyopathy has been reported.[53] Management of arrhythmias in takotsubo cardiomyopathy should be approached on an individual basis, keeping in mind the anticipated resolution of arrhythmias after recovery of left ventricular function.

Ventricular Rupture

Cardiac rupture is a rare but known complication of takotsubo cardiomyopathy.[56] A recent review found 12 cases of takotsubo cardiomyopathy complicated by cardiac rupture.[57] The demographics were notable for an entirely female cohort with a mean age of 76 years. Ten of 12 patients died. Of note, only 36% of patients with ventricular rupture were treated with β-blockers despite an average mean arterial pressure on presentation of 98 mm Hg, suggesting β-blockers may have a protective role in this unusual complication.

PROGNOSIS AND RISK OF RECURRENCE

The natural history of takotsubo cardiomyopathy is generally favorable. The acute risk of in-hospital death is low, estimated at 2% of all cases.[58] The risk of recurrence of takotsubo cardiomyopathy is rare and estimated to range from 2%–5%.[38,59,60] Little evidence supports long-term use of heart failure medications after ventricular function improves. It has been theorized that β-blockade could prevent recurrence of takotsubo cardiomyopathy; however, patients are frequently taking β-adrenergic receptor blockers before presentation of takotsubo cardiomyopathy,[38] and 3 of 7 patients with recurrence of takotsubo were taking β-blockers at the time of presentation.[59] Therefore, long-term use of β-blockers and ACE inhibitors are not routinely considered. For a patient with more than 2 recurrences, the primary intervention should be directed at control of the triggering events, with secondary consideration of chronic treatment with β-blockers or ACE inhibitors.

SUMMARY

Takotsubo cardiomyopathy is a challenging diagnosis to confirm and differentiate from diseases with overlapping presentations. Once the diagnosis is confirmed, the treatment of the patient is based primarily on the current limited knowledge of the underlying pathophysiologic mechanisms of the disease. The clinician must maintain vigilance for detection and treatment of complications that may arise because in-hospital mortality related to hemodynamic compromise or arrhythmias is not rare. Because the long-term prognosis of the disease is favorable, and the benefits of medical therapy largely unproven, routine medical therapy for this condition after recovery of LV function is not recommended. Short-term anticoagulation therapy and neurohormonal antagonists can be considered on an individualized basis.

REFERENCES

1. Dote K, Sato H, Tateishi H, et al. Myocardial stunning due to simultaneous multivessel coronary spams: a review of 5 cases. J Cardiol 1991;21(2):12.
2. Yoshimura S, Toyoda K, Ohara T, et al. Takotsubo cardiomyopathy in acute ischemic stroke. Ann Neurol 2008;64(5):547–54.
3. Stollberger C, Wegner C, Finsterer J. Seizure-associated Takotsubo cardiomyopathy. Epilepsia 2011;52(11):e160–7.
4. Alexandre J, Benouda L, Champ-Rigot L, et al. Takotsubo cardiomyopathy triggered by alcohol withdrawal. Drug Alcohol Rev 2011;30(4):434–7.
5. Citro R, Patella M, Bossone E, et al. Near-drowning syndrome: a possible trigger of tako-tsubo cardiomyopathy. J Cardiovasc Med (Hagerstown) 2008;9(5):501–5.
6. Joo I, Lee JM, Han JK, et al. Stress (tako-tsubo) cardiomyopathy following radiofrequency ablation of a liver tumor: a case report. Cardiovasc Intervent Radiol 2011;34(Suppl 2):S86–9.
7. Amariles P. A comprehensive literature search: drugs as a possible trigger of Takotsubo Cardiomyopathy. Curr Clin Pharmacol 2011;6:11.
8. Madhavan M, Rihal CS, Lerman A, et al. Acute heart failure in apical ballooning syndrome (TakoTsubo/stress cardiomyopathy): clinical correlates and Mayo Clinic risk score. J Am Coll Cardiol 2011;57(12):1400–1.
9. Citro R, Rigo F, Ciampi Q, et al. Echocardiographic assessment of regional left ventricular wall motion abnormalities in patients with tako-tsubo cardiomyopathy: comparison with anterior myocardial infarction. Eur J Echocardiogr 2011;12(7):542–9.
10. Mansencal N, Abbou N, Pilliere R, et al. Usefulness of two-dimensional speckle tracking echocardiography

for assessment of Tako-Tsubo cardiomyopathy. Am J Cardiol 2009;103(7):1020–4.

11. Ramaraj R, Movahed MR. Reverse or inverted takotsubo cardiomyopathy (reverse left ventricular apical ballooning syndrome) presents at a younger age compared with the mid or apical variant and is always associated with triggering stress. Congest Heart Fail 2010;16(6):284–6.

12. Song BG, Chun WJ, Park YH, et al. The clinical characteristics, laboratory parameters, electrocardiographic, and echocardiographic findings of reverse or inverted takotsubo cardiomyopathy: comparison with mid or apical variant. Clin Cardiol 2011;34(11): 693–9.

13. Elesber AA, Prasad A, Bybee KA, et al. Transient cardiac apical ballooning syndrome: prevalence and clinical implications of right ventricular involvement. J Am Coll Cardiol 2006;47(5):1082–3.

14. El Mahmoud R, Mansencal N, Pilliere R, et al. Prevalence and characteristics of left ventricular outflow tract obstruction in Tako-Tsubo syndrome. Am Heart J 2008;156(3):543–8.

15. Reynolds HR, Srichai MB, Iqbal SN, et al. Mechanisms of myocardial infarction in women without angiographically obstructive coronary artery disease. Circulation 2011;124(13):1414–25.

16. Caforio AL, Tona F, Vinci A, et al. Acute biopsy-proven lymphocytic myocarditis mimicking Takotsubo cardiomyopathy. Eur J Heart Fail 2009;11(4):428–31.

17. Ahmed KA, Madhavan M, Prasad A. Brain natriuretic peptide in apical ballooning syndrome (Takotsubo/stress cardiomyopathy): comparison with acute myocardial infarction. Coron Artery Dis 2012;23(4): 259–64.

18. Madhavan M, Borlaug BA, Lerman A, et al. Stress hormone and circulating biomarker profile of apical ballooning syndrome (Takotsubo cardiomyopathy): insights into the clinical significance of B-type natriuretic peptide and troponin levels. Heart 2009; 95(17):1436–41.

19. Lyon AR, Rees PS, Prasad S, et al. Stress (Takotsubo) cardiomyopathy–a novel pathophysiological hypothesis to explain catecholamine-induced acute myocardial stunning. Nat Clin Pract Cardiovasc Med 2008;5(1):22–9.

20. Lenders JW, Pacak K, Walther MM, et al. Biochemical diagnosis of pheochromocytoma: which test is best? JAMA 2002;287(11):1427–34.

21. Eitel I, von Knobelsdorff-Brenkenhoff F, Bernhardt P, et al. Clinical characteristics and cardiovascular magnetic resonance findings in stress (takotsubo) cardiomyopathy. JAMA 2011;306(3):277–86.

22. Chia PL, Foo D. Tako-tsubo cardiomyopathy precipitated by pheochromocytoma crisis. Cardiol J 2011; 18(5):564–7.

23. Volz HC, Erbel C, Berentelg J, et al. Reversible left ventricular dysfunction resembling Takotsubo syndrome after self-injection of adrenaline. Can J Cardiol 2009;25(7):e261–2.

24. Rotondi F, Manganelli F, Carbone G, et al. "Takotsubo" cardiomyopathy and duloxetine use. South Med J 2011;104(5):345–7.

25. Muders F, Friedrich E, Luchner A, et al. Hemodynamic changes and neurohumoral regulation during development of congestive heart failure in a model of epinephrine-induced cardiomyopathy in conscious rabbits. J Card Fail 1999;5(2):109–16.

26. Izumi Y, Okatani H, Shiota M, et al. Effects of metoprolol on epinephrine-induced takotsubo-like left ventricular dysfunction in non-human primates. Hypertens Res 2009;32(5):339–46.

27. Heubach JF, Ravens U, Kaumann AJ. Epinephrine activates both Gs and Gi pathways, but norepinephrine activates only the Gs pathway through human beta2-adrenoceptors overexpressed in mouse heart. Mol Pharmacol 2004;65(5):1313–22.

28. Kawano H, Okada R, Yano K. Histological study on the distribution of autonomic nerves in the human heart. Heart Vessels 2003;18(1):32–9.

29. Mori H, Ishikawa S, Kojima S, et al. Increased responsiveness of left ventricular apical myocardium to adrenergic stimuli. Cardiovasc Res 1993; 27:7.

30. Kurisu S, Sato H, Kawagoe T, et al. Tako-tsubo-like left ventricular dysfunction with ST-segment elevation: a novel cardiac syndrome mimicking acute myocardial infarction. Am Heart J 2002;143(3): 448–55.

31. Galiuto L, De Caterina AR, Porfidia A, et al. Reversible coronary microvascular dysfunction: a common pathogenetic mechanism in Apical Ballooning or Tako-Tsubo Syndrome. Eur Heart J 2010;31(11): 1319–27.

32. Daniels DV, Fearon WF. The index of microcirculatory resistance (IMR) in takotsubo cardiomyopathy. Catheter Cardiovasc Interv 2011;77(1):128–31.

33. Streeter DD, Hanna WT. Engineering mechanics for successive states in Canine left ventricular Myocardium: II. Fiber angle and sarcomere length. Circ Res 1973;33(6):656–64.

34. Yoshioka T, Hashimoto A, Tsuchihashi K, et al. Clinical implications of midventricular obstruction and intravenous propranolol use in transient left ventricular apical ballooning (Tako-tsubo cardiomyopathy). Am Heart J 2008;155(3):526.e1–7.

35. Hunt SA, Abraham WT, Chin MH, et al. 2009 focused update incorporated into the ACC/AHA 2005 Guidelines for the Diagnosis and Management of Heart Failure in Adults: a report of the American College of Cardiology Foundation/American Heart Association Task Force on Practice Guidelines: developed in collaboration with the International Society for Heart and Lung Transplantation. Circulation 2009; 119(14):e391–479.

36. Vittorio TJ. Vasopressor response to Angiotensin II infusion in patients with chronic heart failure receiving beta-blockers. Circulation 2002;107(2):290–3.

37. Hryniewicz K, Androne AS, Hudaihed A, et al. Comparative effects of carvedilol and metoprolol on regional vascular responses to adrenergic stimuli in normal subjects and patients with chronic heart failure. Circulation 2003;108(8):971–6.

38. Regnante RA, Zuzek RW, Weinsier SB, et al. Clinical characteristics and four-year outcomes of patients in the Rhode Island Takotsubo Cardiomyopathy Registry. Am J Cardiol 2009;103(7):1015–9.

39. Fazio G, Pizzuto C, Barbaro G, et al. Chronic pharmacological treatment in takotsubo cardiomyopathy. Int J Cardiol 2008;127(1):121–3.

40. de Gregorio C, Grimaldi P, Lentini C. Left ventricular thrombus formation and cardioembolic complications in patients with Takotsubo-like syndrome: a systematic review. Int J Cardiol 2008;131(1):18–24.

41. Haghi D, Papavassiliu T, Heggemann F, et al. Incidence and clinical significance of left ventricular thrombus in tako-tsubo cardiomyopathy assessed with echocardiography. QJM 2008;101(5):381–6.

42. de Gregorio C. Cardioembolic outcomes in stress-related cardiomyopathy complicated by ventricular thrombus: a systematic review of 26 clinical studies. Int J Cardiol 2010;141(1):11–7.

43. Ueyama T, Ishikura F, Matsuda A, et al. Chronic estrogen supplementation following ovariectomy improves the emotional stress-induced cardiovascular responses by indirect action on the nervous system and by direct action on the heart. Circ J 2007;71(4):565–73.

44. Brenner R, Weilenmann D, Maeder MT, et al. Clinical characteristics, sex hormones, and long-term follow-up in swiss postmenopausal women presenting with takotsubo cardiomyopathy. Clin Cardiol 2012;35(6):340–7.

45. Manson JE, Hsia J, Johnson KC, et al. Estrogen plus progestin and the risk of coronary heart disease. N Engl J Med 2003;349(6):523–34.

46. Maekawa Y, Kawamura A, UYuasa S, et al. Direct comparison of takotsubo cardiomyopathy between Japan and USA: 3 year follow-up study. Intern Med 2012;51:6.

47. Abe Y, Tamura A, Kadota J. Prolonged cardiogenic shock caused by a high-dose intravenous administration of dopamine in a patient with takotsubo cardiomyopathy. Int J Cardiol 2010;141(1):e1–3.

48. Fujiwara S, Takeishi Y, Isoyama S, et al. Responsiveness to dobutamine stimulation in patients with left ventricular apical ballooning syndrome. Am J Cardiol 2007;100(10):1600–3.

49. De Santis V, Vitale D, Tritapepe L, et al. Use of levosimendan for cardiogenic shock in a patient with the apical ballooning syndrome. Ann Intern Med 2008; 149(5):365–7.

50. Bonacchi M, Valente S, Harmelin G, et al. Extracorporeal life support as ultimate strategy for refractory severe cardiogenic shock induced by Tako-tsubo cardiomyopathy: a new effective therapeutic option. Artif Organs 2009;33(10):866–70.

51. Hassid B, Azmoon S, Aronow WS, et al. Hemodynamic support with Tandem Heart in tako-tsubo cardiomyopathy—a case report. Arch Med Sci 2010;6(6):971–5.

52. Kurisu S, Inoue I, Kawagoe T, et al. Time course of electrocardiographic changes in patients with tako-tsubo syndrome: comparison with acute myocardial infarction with minimal enzymatic release. Circ J 2004;68(1):77–81.

53. Inoue M, Kanaya H, Matsubara T, et al. Complete atrioventricular block associated with takotsubo cardiomyopathy. Circ J 2009;73:4.

54. Mahida S, Dalageorgou C, Behr ER. Long-QT syndrome and torsades de pointes in a patient with Takotsubo cardiomyopathy: an unusual case. Europace 2009;11(3):376–8.

55. Cho SC, Kim W, Park CS, et al. Stress-induced cardiomyopathy presenting as ventricular tachycardia. Korean J Intern Med 2012;27(1):107–10.

56. Jaguszewski M, Fijalkowski M, Nowak R, et al. Ventricular rupture in Takotsubo cardiomyopathy. Eur Heart J 2012;33(8):1027.

57. Kumar S, Kaushik S, Nautiyal A, et al. Cardiac rupture in takotsubo cardiomyopathy: a systematic review. Clin Cardiol 2011;34(11):672–6.

58. Parodi G, Bellandi B, Del Pace S, et al. Natural history of tako-tsubo cardiomyopathy. Chest 2011; 139(4):887–92.

59. Sharkey SW, Windenburg DC, Lesser JR, et al. Natural history and expansive clinical profile of stress (tako-tsubo) cardiomyopathy. J Am Coll Cardiol 2010;55(4):333–41.

60. Akashi YJ, Goldstein DS, Barbaro G, et al. Takotsubo cardiomyopathy: a new form of acute, reversible heart failure. Circulation 2008;118(25):2754–62.

Takotsubo Cardiomyopathy
The Pathophysiology

Matthew H. Tranter, MRes[a], Peter T. Wright, MRes[a],
Markus B. Sikkel, MD[a], Alexander R. Lyon, MD, PhD[a,b],*

KEYWORDS

- Tako tsubo • Apical balloning • Stress • Epinephrine • Stimulus trafficking
- Beta-2 adrenergic receptor

KEY POINTS

- Available data support the hypothesis that Takotsubo cardiomyopathy (TTC) and atypical TTC-like disorders are primarily induced by catecholaminergic overstimulation, with epinephrine playing a crucial role.
- Epinephrine is a negative inotrope as high doses, such as during extreme stress, via the B2AR-Gi signalling pathway. The mammalian heart has a higher density of B2AR at the apex, which may explain the apical hypokinesia observed in typical cases.
- Future research is required to clarify different pathophysiologic elements, the mechanisms of the acute complications, and the reverse remodeling that underpins the good prognosis and recovery in TTC.
- Clinical management pathways are currently empiric, with no current evidence base to guide clinicians caring for these patients.
- Knowledge from the available preclinical models may be considered to guide development of potential clinical trials in the most severe cases, where rates of acute morbidity and mortality are highest, and also to prevent recurrence in susceptible individuals.

INTRODUCTION

Takotsubo cardiomyopathy (TTC), first described by Satoh and colleagues,[1] is an acute heart failure syndrome classically characterized by hypocontractile apical and midventricular regions of the left ventricle, with a compensatory hypercontractile base. Several conflicting hypotheses have been proposed regarding the pathophysiology of TTC. These conflicting hypotheses are understandable because apical myocardial dysfunction is a feature mimicked by several other vascular and myocardial pathologic abnormalities. Several diagnostic criteria have been proposed. The most widely quoted is the criteria proposed by the Mayo Clinic in 2004[2] and modified in 2008.[3] The criteria include the following: (1) transient hypokinesis, akinesis, or dyskinesis in the left ventricle (LV) mid segments with or without apical involvement and regional wall motion abnormality extending beyond a single epicardial vascular distribution; (2) absence of an obstructive

Mr. Tranter is supported by the National Heart and Lung Institute Foundation.
Mr. Wright is supported by the Centre for Integrative Mammalian Physiology and Pharmacology.
Dr. Sikkel is supported by the Wellcome Trust (092852).
Dr. Lyon is a British Heart Foundation Intermediate Clinical Research Fellow and is supported by the National Institute for Health Research Cardiovascular Biomedical Research Unit at the Royal Brompton Hospital.

[a] Myocardial Function Section, National Heart and Lung Institute, Imperial College London, Du Cane Road, London W12 0NN, UK; [b] Cardiovascular Biomedical Research Unit, Royal Brompton Hospital, London SW3 6LY, UK
* Corresponding author. Cardiovascular Biomedical Research Unit, Royal Brompton Hospital, Dovehouse Street, London SW3 6LY, UK.
E-mail address: a.lyon@ic.ac.uk

Heart Failure Clin 9 (2013) 187–196
http://dx.doi.org/10.1016/j.hfc.2012.12.010
1551-7136/13/$ – see front matter © 2013 Elsevier Inc. All rights reserved.

coronary lesion or evidence of acute plaque rupture; (3) new electrographic abnormalities and/or elevation in serum cardiac enzymes; and (4) absence of pheochromocytoma or myocarditis. However, the Mayo criteria have been questioned; a Swedish group has recently proposed the Gothenburg criteria.[4] Although it is widely accepted that the regional wall motion abnormalities should extend beyond a single coronary territory, and without culprit coronary disease to explain the distribution of dysfunctional myocardium, it is becoming increasingly recognized that bystander coronary disease may be present, given the predilection for an older population. Therefore, coronary disease per se should not be an exclusion criterion. Likewise, pheochromocytoma, by its very nature as a catecholamine-secreting tumor, may mimic extreme stress and trigger Takotsubo cardiomyopathy and should not be an exclusion criterion. Dysfunction may not be limited to the left ventricle but may involve the right ventricular myocardium as a primary or secondary phenomenon.

A common theme among TTC patients is a stressful event as the precipitant. This event may be either an emotional or a physical stressor (bereavement, robbery, lottery win, etc), a serious medical or surgical illness, or iatrogenic drug administration. In this review the possible pathophysiology of this disease, focusing on the initial onset of the heart failure and on the primary effect of high levels of catecholamine on the myocardium, is discussed.

Hypotheses to explain the transient and reversible apical dysfunction have included the following: (1) aborted myocardial infarction (MI) with spontaneous recanalization, particularly in the setting of a wrap-around left anterior descending coronary artery; (2) acute microvascular dysfunction; (3) multivessel coronary vasospasm; (4) acute left ventricular outflow tract obstruction (LVOTO); and (5) direct catecholamine-mediated myocardial dysfunction.

Several general pieces of evidence from both the clinical series published refute the vascular explanation as the primary cause. Endothelial function is likely to be abnormal after high catecholamine surges because of increases in shear stress, and therefore, proving causation, rather than an epiphenomenon, remains a flaw in the vascular hypotheses. First, the epidemiologic observation that TTC predominantly occurs in postmenopausal women: if atherosclerosis was the underlying cause, one would expect an elderly male predominance, matching the epidemiology of MI. Second, there is a reported summer predominance, and no winter peak nor early morning

peak in diurnal analyses, in contrast to MI. Third, myocardial perfusion studies, when performed during the acute phase, have predominantly been normal. Fourth, the coronary arteries of a series of TTC cases were studied with intravascular coronary ultrasound during the acute episode. These authors reported that plaque rupture, positive remodeling, and presumed intracoronary thrombus were absent in all cases.[5] Finally, clinical cases triggered by dobutamine, a vasodilator with no vasospastic effects, and epinephrine, which has a dominant coronary vasodilatory effect, would not support vasospasm. Indeed, in the authors' animal model (see later discussion), norepinephrine, a potent coronary vasospastic agent, did not induce apical hypokinesia.

Although it is unlikely this disease can be explained solely through a vascular pathologic abnormality, the different hypotheses are reviewed in turn, and the focus on the mechanism is explored in relation to the direct effects of high catecholamines on the myocardium.

ABORTED MI

Aborted myocardial infarction caused by plaque rupture that has subsequently recanalized has been proposed as a possible cause of TTC.[6] A brief period of ischemia can cause temporary myocardial dysfunction. However, this would have a regional distribution based on the infarct-related artery; the typical pattern of apical dysfunction in TTC does not fit with a single coronary territory. Furthermore, electrocardiographic changes differ significantly from those caused by transient coronary occlusion, which has been revascularized mechanically.[7] There are also significant differences in histopathologic features with endomyocardial biopsies taken from patients with TTC showing a pattern of myocardial abnormalities not associated with infarcted, stunned, or hibernating myocardium.[8,9]

LEFT VENTRICULAR OUTFLOW TRACT OBSTRUCTION

It has been suggested that LVOTO could be the causative factor in TTC.[10] This suggestion came from an observation of an LVOT pressure gradient in 4 cases, with a recapitulation of the gradient subsequently during dobutamine stress echocardiography. This pathophysiologic hypothesis is that patients who are prone to develop LVOTO may develop a dynamic midcavity LV obstruction under catecholamine excess. Potentially older women with smaller hearts, and prominent septal bulges, could be predisposed to acute LVOTO.

This factor would functionally separate the LV into 2 chambers: a basal chamber under normal wall stress and an apical chamber under high stress, which would reduce subendocardial flow in the apex. This reduction in apical blood flow would also be relatively self-limiting, resulting in ischemia rather than infarction because the wall stress in the apex would be subsequently reduced by the ensuing apical dysfunction. However, in a larger cohort reported, LVOTO was observed in only 25% of cases in the acute phase of TTC,[11] which suggests that although contributory in a subset of patients, LVOTO is unlikely to underlie the cause of TTC, but may be a modifier contributing to a more severe phenotype.

MULTIVESSEL VASOSPASM

Multivessel vasospasm may lead to reversible apical myocardial dysfunction if all major coronaries are affected. This phenomenon has been observed on several occasions in cases of TTC. In a case report, 3 of 30 patients were observed to have spontaneous multivessel coronary vasospasm and 43% of patients tested had vasospasm as a result of pharmacologic provocation with ergonovine or acetylcholine.[12] Another large case series revealed multivessel coronary spasm following acetylcholine provocation in 10% of patients.[13] It has been noted that location of induced vasospasm often does not correspond to the hypokinetic area in TTC, leading some authorities to state that vasospasm plays no role in the cause of the condition.[14] In addition, clinical cases[15] triggered by dobutamine, a vasodilator with no vasospastic effects, and epinephrine, which also has a dominant coronary vasodilatory effect, would not support vasospasm as the primary mediator. However after any stress and high surge in catecholamines, subsequent endothelial function may be impaired, and arteries may be prone to vasospasm on provocation. However, unless this contradictory evidence can be explained, this does not seem to be the underlying cause in most cases.

MICROVASCULAR DYSFUNCTION

Disturbance of the microcirculation has been observed in some cases of TTC and has been proposed by some authors to be central in the etiology. Such dysfunction has been investigated using several invasive and noninvasive imaging techniques. For instance, a study by Galiuto and colleagues[16] revealed areas of poorly perfused myocardium using myocardial contrast echocardiography. This poorly perfused myocardium was similar to the level of perfusion defect seen in sufferers of ST-segment elevation myocardial infarction (STEMI). In TTC but not STEMI sufferers, this was significantly reduced by the vasodilatory action of an adenosine infusion, which was fully recovered at follow-up in TTC patients but not STEMI patients. Perfusion defects in these patients seemed to form a small part of the wider akinetic region, suggesting that reduced perfusion is not essential for akinesis.[17,18] Other studies using Doppler flow wire assessment and thrombolysis in myocardial infarction frame count have also shown abnormalities in microvascular flow.[9] Other reports[19] have not found any perfusion defect at all in TTC patients.[20]

The authors think that, when present, microvascular dysfunction may be the result of apical dysfunction and its precipitants rather than its cause. Endothelial dysfunction is likely to be present after catecholamine surges with associated increases in shear stress without this necessarily being the primary cause of myocardial dysfunction. In addition, changes in muscle function may affect blood flow, particularly in the microvasculature, which would be expected in TTC and has been well documented in other causes of LV dysfunction such as dilated cardiomyopathy.[9]

DIRECT CATECHOLAMINE TOXICITY

Circulating levels of catecholamine, when measured in TTC patients, are surprisingly high even when compared with MI sufferers.[21,22] As the primary cellular receptors responsible for transducing sympatho-adrenal signals into physiologic responses, the myocardial β-adrenoceptors (βAR) are implicated in TTC. Biopsies from patients with TTC display contraction band necrosis.[23] Markers of mechanical strain, such as the natriuretic peptides, are also significantly elevated.[21] Raised levels of catecholamine may cause direct damage to the myocardium. Supraphysiologic activation of β1AR and β2AR via stimulatory G-protein (G_s) could result in cardiotoxic oxidative stress through cyclic adenosine monophosphate (cAMP)-dependent protein kinase A (PKA)-mediated calcium overload of the cellular cytoplasm and mitochondria, resulting in cell death.[24]

Stimulus Trafficking

Unlike β1AR, which couples exclusively to G_s, the β2AR is pleiotropic, coupling to both G_s and inhibitory G-protein (G_i),[25] depending on the concentration and nature of the specific agonist (biased agonism). G_i coupling causes negative inotropy by reduction in cAMP output, by direct inhibition of adenylyl cyclase. It also causes differential phosphorylation of downstream targets. In mouse cardiomyocytes, overexpressing the human β2AR, epinephrine, but not norepinephrine, can activate the G_i pathway, resulting in negative inotropy.[26] Robust βAR activation must occur as a prelude to stimulus trafficking, as an initial PKA-dependent phosphorylation of the β2AR is required (**Fig. 1**).[27,28]

Stimulus trafficking is also dependent on the G-protein receptor kinases (GRKs), which must also phosphorylate the β2AR to initiate stimulus trafficking. Epinephrine is able to cause rapid receptor phosphorylation by GRKs and consequent internalization and retrafficking to the membrane. This retrafficking to the membrane occurs much more slowly in response to stimulation with norepinephrine whereby the receptor remains internalized.[29] It is relevant to note that the only genetic polymorphism identified to date with a higher frequency in TTC patients is a GRK5 L41Q polymorphism, resulting in a constitutively active GRK5.[30] The threshold for G_i coupling would be lower in these individuals, a factor colloquially termed genetic β-blockade, with stimulus trafficking potentially occurring more rapidly at lower circulating epinephrine concentrations.

β2AR-G_i signaling following stimulus trafficking is cardioprotective: by using in vitro cell survival studies after β1AR blockade, the protection of the β2AR is lost if the PKA phosphorylation site is mutated to prevent G_s-G_i switch. The β2AR-G_i pathway has been shown to be vital in ischemic preconditioning in the isolated heart, showing that its protective effect is not limited to the prevention of catecholamine toxicity.[31] In essence, epinephrine-mediated stimulus trafficking is protecting the heart from the toxicity of excessive βAR activation following an extreme stress with the highest levels of circulating epinephrine.

Animal Models of TTC

TTC may result from high levels of serum catecholamines after an emotional or physical stressor[21] as well as catecholamines administered for medical purposes.[32] Given these possible pathways, demonstrating that catecholamines are integral to this disorder, the 2 following broad approaches have emerged to create a preclinical TTC model: (1) catecholamine infusion; or (2) psychologic stress.

In the authors' model of TTC, acute effects of intravenous catecholamine boluses are observed in rats, starting within seconds of injection, and resolving within 60 minutes. A bolus of epinephrine, but not norepinephrine, produced a reduction of apical and mid-left ventricular fractional shortening by up to 30% 20 minutes after bolus (**Fig. 2**).[28] Apical depression occurs in a G_i-dependent manner: pertussis toxin (a G_i inhibitor) pretreatment of the experimental animals prevented the depressive effects of epinephrine.

Conscious female rats restrained in dorsal recumbency are reported by Ueyama and colleagues[33] to show symptoms similar to those of TTC patients. Left ventriculography showed signs of apical ballooning or general hypokinesis, as well as a reduction in fractional shortening from 50% to 35%. This dysfunction was ameliorated by the infusion of amusalulol (an α-1 and βAR antagonist[34,35]), confirming the role of the adrenoceptors in producing acute apical dysfunction. In a later study, estrogen had a similar sympatholytic effect, reducing TTC-like symptoms.[36] These findings concur with the current opinion on the pathologic basis of TTC and its association with postmenopausal women.

Izumi and colleagues[37] acutely infused epinephrine into cynomolgus monkeys and observed acute echocardiographic, molecular, and histologic alterations. Importantly, this study assessed

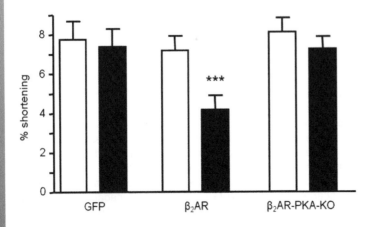

Fig. 1. Overexpression of mutant β2AR resistant to phosphorylation at PKA sites (β2AR-PKA-KO) prevents β2AR-dependent negative inotropism. ***, $P<.001$. (*From* Paur H, Wright PT, Sikkel MB, et al. High levels of circulating epinephrine trigger apical cardiodepression in a β2-adrenoceptor/Gi-dependent manner: a new model of takotsubo cardiomyopathy. Circulation 2012;126:697–706; with permission.)

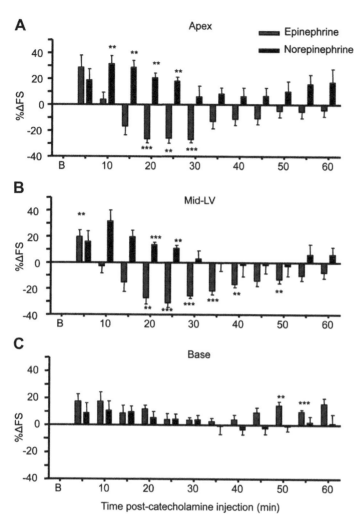

Fig. 2. Takotsubo cardiomyopathy is epinephrine specific. Apical and mid-LV specific depression was seen only after epinephrine bolus, and not norepinephrine. The basal myocardium was spared from this depression, as seen in patients with classical Takotsubo cardiomyopathy. ΔFS, change in fractional shortening; **, $P<.01$; ***, $P<.001$. (From Paur H, Wright PT, Sikkel MB, et al. High levels of circulating epinephrine trigger apical cardiodepression in a β2-adrenoceptor/Gi-dependent manner: a new model of Takotsubo cardiomyopathy. Circulation 2012;126:697–706; with permission.)

both the acute and the long-term outcomes of these animals. Acutely, systolic and diastolic blood pressures were increased and ejection fraction was reduced from 60% to 35%; heart rate was only moderately increased. This study demonstrated that the moderately β₁AR-selective β-blocker metoprolol provided some prevention. Histology showed myocytolysis, which was profound in the apical myocardium; mRNA levels of positively inotropic proteins, such as SERCA2a and RYR, were downregulated in apical tissue.

Increased Susceptibility of the Apical Myocardium to Catecholamines

To explain the regional heterogeneity seen in this disease, there must be some intrinsic heterogeneity in myocardial or vascular physiology present. Many apical-basal gradients of biologic parameters exist, and the authors hypothesized that an apicobasal gradient of βARs exists in the

mammalian heart, with a specific gradient in a relative ratio of β₂AR:β₁AR (**Fig. 3**), which may explain the predominance of apical depression in TTC.[24] The β₂AR can depress cardiac function at supraphysiologic levels of epinephrine but not norepinephrine. High-dose epinephrine, but not norepinephrine, could recapitulate the TTC phenotype with apical dysfunction in the authors' preclinical TTC model.

Izumi and colleagues[37] report that mRNA levels of ADRB2 (β₂AR) are twice as high in the apex. We used radioligand binding studies on ventricular cardiomyocytes to confirm directly an increased β₂AR:β₁AR ratio in apical rat myocytes compared with basal myocytes isolated from the same normal heart. Supporting these measurements of expression and receptor levels, functional responses are different, with basal cardiomyocytes demonstrating reduced contractile response to specific β₂AR stimulation (**Fig. 4**).[28] Although these findings have not been confirmed in

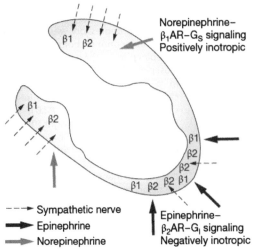

Norepinephrine–
β₁AR–Gₛ signaling
Positively inotropic

Epinephrine–
β₂AR–Gᵢ signaling
Negatively inotropic

- - -► Sympathetic nerve
──► Epinephrine
══► Norepinephrine

Fig. 3. Schematic representation of regional differences in the ventricular response to high levels of catecholamine, explaining Takotsubo cardiomyopathy. At the ventricular apex a greater β2:β1 adrenoceptor ratio causes a greater tendency for stimulus-trafficking toward Gᵢ signaling, resulting in negative inotropy. Conversely, the basal myocardium has a higher sympathetic innervation density and lower β2:β1 ratio and is less sensitive to the negative inotropic effects of circulating epinephrine. (*From* Lyon AR, Rees PS, Prasad S, et al. Stress (Takotsubo) cardiomyopathy–a novel pathophysiological hypothesis to explain catecholamine-induced acute myocardial stunning. Nat Clin Pract Cardiovasc Med 2008;5(1):22–9; with permission.)

human myocardium, the opposite basal-to-apical density gradient in sympathetic nerve terminals, reproduced across many mammalian species, has also been detected within the human myocardium.[38]

The evolutionary reasons for these apicobasal gradients are not clear; it may relate to the requirement for increased apical sensitivity to circulating catecholamines ensuring optimal ventricular ejection during moderate stress and avoiding acute LVOTO. The apex is therefore more sensitive to toxic levels of circulating catecholamines during extreme stress, and stimulus trafficking of β₂AR to the Gᵢ. TTC may represent a cardioprotective response to limit the cardiotoxicity of very high circulating levels of epinephrine during extreme stress, which may explain the reversibility of apical dysfunction and the good prognosis of patients with TTC.

Susceptibility of Postmenopausal Women

Typically TTC afflicts postmenopausal women.[39] TTC's prevalence in postmenopausal women was a feature of the early case reports and was recently confirmed in the large retrospective analysis of approximately 6800 cases from the United States.[40] Estrogens are known to have sympatholytic effects and therefore dampen the influence of stress and high levels of catecholamine on the heart.[36] Estrogen may be beneficial in the setting of childbirth, with the loss of this estrogen-mediated protection partly explaining the increased prevalence in postmenopausal women.

Atypical TTC

Atypical cases exist, with respect to the anatomic pattern of dysfunction and patient demographics. In the largest published series, approximately 10% of TTC cases occur in men or younger women, and therefore, the underlying explanation cannot solely lie with the loss of estrogen after menopause. In addition, different anatomic variants exist. The basal segment of the myocardium may be affected and hypokinetic relative to a hypercontractile apex, known

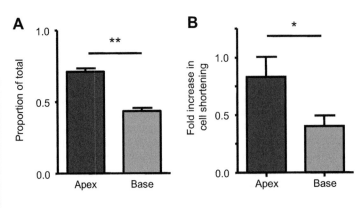

Fig. 4. Apically derived cardiomyocytes demonstrate increased levels of β2AR and responses. (*A*) Proportion of β2ARs with respect to total β2AR radioligand binding in ventricular myocytes from the apex and base of normal rat heart. (*B*) Apical cardiomyocytes show a larger increase in percentage cell shortening through the β2AR compared with basal cardiomyocytes. (*From* Paur H, Wright PT, Sikkel MB, et al. High levels of circulating epinephrine trigger apical cardiodepression in a β2-adrenoceptor/Gi-dependent manner: a new model of takotsubo cardiomyopathy. Circulation 2012; 126:697–706; with permission.)

as inverted Takotsubo cardiomyopathy. Midventricular and biventricular variants have also been reported. Atypical cases are more likely to be associated with neurologic triggers (eg, subarachnoid hemorrhage), or pheochromocytomas. A neurally mediated phenomenon may explain the inverted TTC variant, given the region of dysfunction colocalizes with the region of highest sympathetic nerve-ending density. Atypical cases may represent up to a quarter of TTC-like disorders.[41] It could be hypothesized that TTC is in fact a spectrum of disorders ranging from the most typical (postmenopausal woman, emotional stressor, and apical ballooning) to the most atypical (young man, drug induced, and basal hypokinesia).[42]

TREATMENT—INSIGHTS FROM PATHOPHYSIOLOGY

Management of individuals seeking medical attention for chest pain with electrocardiographic changes should follow local guidelines for the management of STEMI or non-ST-segment elevation myocardial infarction as appropriate. Early access to diagnostic coronary angiography is vital to confirm the diagnosis and absence of culprit coronary disease. Although long-term prognosis in survivors is excellent, TTC is not benign during the acute phase. Approximately 50% of cases have a documented cardiac complication (most commonly atrial arrhythmias). The most extreme cases may present with cardiogenic shock, hypotension, and pulmonary edema[43,44]: this presents a management conundrum. Usually patients with acute cardiogenic shock are supported pharmacologically with catecholamines or phosphodiesterase inhibitors as positive inotropes. However, given the central role of catecholamines, and cAMP-dependent pathways in the pathogenesis, using further catecholamines in treatment seems counterintuitive. In the authors' view, catecholamines and phosphodiesterase inhibitors are best avoided,[12]

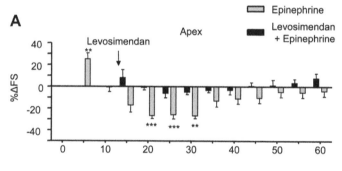

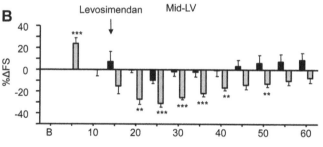

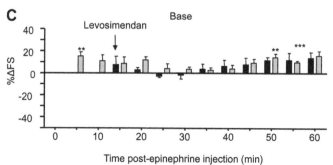

Time post-epinephrine injection (min)

Fig. 5. Levosimendan rescues the Takotsubo cardiomyopathy model. Using the same bolus as in Fig. 2, levosimendan could reverse, or markedly improve, the contractile dysfunction. ΔFS, change of fractional shortening; LV, left ventricle. (*From* Paur H, Wright PT, Sikkel MB, et al. High levels of circulating epinephrine trigger apical cardiodepression in a β2-adrenoceptor/Gi-dependent manner: a new model of takotsubo cardiomyopathy. Circulation 2012;126:697–706; with permission.)

leaving mechanical support strategies (left ventricular assist devices, extracorporeal membrane oxygenation) for life-threatening cases with deteriorating multiorgan failure.

In the authors' model, levosimendan was assessed. Levosimendan is a positive inotrope whose mechanistic action, via myofilament calcium sensitization, is independent of βARs and cAMP. Levosimendan rescued the acute epinephrine-mediated ventricular dysfunction, and this positive inotropic effect was associated with 100% survival (vs 50% in controls) (**Fig. 5**). By bypassing the β2AR-G$_i$ axis to treat this disease, contraction can be restored by sensitizing the myofilaments to calcium (levosimendan), while leaving the beneficial antiapoptotic G$_i$ signaling cascades intact. Further preclinical and clinical studies are warranted to clarify whether there is a role for levosimendan in the management of TTC.

β-Blockers have also been used in the treatment of TTC, and particularly in cases with acute LVOTO.[45,46] Propranolol has the ability to cause β$_2$AR to traffic to G$_i$ signaling independently of the presence of a catecholamine (biased agonism), which may explain why it is a strong negative inotrope. This action may overlap with epinephrine-mediated apical dysfunction, causing a worsening of the acute heart failure in the rat. Carvedilol limited basal contractility in the authors' animal model[28] and so may improve patients with LVOTO. Given the current controversy over the exact pathophysiologic mechanisms underlying TTC, the current procedures are possibly acceptable.

SUMMARY

Most data available support the hypothesis that TTC and atypical TTC-like disorders are primarily induced by catecholaminergic overstimulation, with epinephrine playing a crucial role. High levels of circulating epinephrine caused by extreme stress can trigger regional hypocontractility, primarily because of direct negative inotropic effects of epinephrine on the myocardium via stimulus trafficking of the β2AR to the cardioprotective G$_i$ pathway. Cellular damage, defects in perfusion, and altered cellular metabolism may also be present but probably act as modifiers, rather than the underlying cause, at least in the very acute phases. These conclusions are based on findings documented across human and animal studies. Future research is required to clarify different pathophysiologic elements, the mechanisms of the acute complications, and the reverse remodeling that underpins the good prognosis and recovery in TTC. Clinical management pathways are currently empiric, with no current evidence base to guide clinicians caring for these patients. Herein lies the need to utilize knowledge from the available preclinical models to guide development of potential clinical trials in the most severe cases, where rates of acute morbidity and mortality are highest and also to prevent recurrence in susceptible individuals.

REFERENCES

1. Sato H, Taiteishi H, Uchida T. Takotsubo-type cardiomyopathy due to multivessel spasm. In: Kodama K, et al, editors. Clinical aspect of myocardial injury: from ischemia to heart failure. Tokyo: Kagakuhyouronsha Co; 1990. p. 56–64.
2. Bybee KA, Kara T, Prasad A, et al. Systematic review: transient left ventricular apical ballooning: a syndrome that mimics ST-segment elevation myocardial infarction. Ann Intern Med 2004;141(11): 858–65.
3. Prasad A, Lerman A, Rihal CS. Apical ballooning syndrome (Tako-Tsubo or stress cardiomyopathy): a mimic of acute myocardial infarction. Am Heart J 2008;155(3):408–17.
4. Omerovic E. How to think about stress-induced cardiomyopathy?–Think 'out of the box'! Scand Cardiovasc J 2011;45(2):67–71.
5. Haghi D, Roehm S, Hamm K, et al. Takotsubo cardiomyopathy is not due to plaque rupture: an intravascular ultrasound study. Clin Cardiol 2010; 33(5):307–10.
6. Ibanez B, Choi BG, Navarro F, et al. Tako-tsubo syndrome: a form of spontaneous aborted myocardial infarction? Eur Heart J 2006;27(12):1509–10.
7. Ibanez B, Pinero A, Zafar MU, et al. Tako-tsubo syndrome: a new entity or new form of presentation of an old one? An electrocardiographic analysis. Int J Cardiol 2008;126(2):281–3.
8. Hoyt J, Lerman A, Lennon RJ, et al. Left anterior descending artery length and coronary atherosclerosis in apical ballooning syndrome (Takotsubo/stress induced cardiomyopathy). Int J Cardiol 2010; 145(1):112–5.
9. Nef HM, Möllmann H, Akashi YJ, et al. Mechanisms of stress (Takotsubo) cardiomyopathy. Nat Rev Cardiol 2010;7(4):187–93.
10. Merli E, Sutcliffe S, Gori M, et al. Tako-Tsubo cardiomyopathy: new insights into the possible underlying pathophysiology. Eur J Echocardiogr 2006;7(1):53–61.
11. El Mahmoud R, Mansencal N, Pilliére R, et al. Prevalence and characteristics of left ventricular outflow tract obstruction in Tako-Tsubo syndrome. Am Heart J 2008;156(3):543–8.

12. Kurisu S, Sato H, Kawagoe T, et al. Tako-tsubo-like left ventricular dysfunction with ST-segment elevation: a novel cardiac syndrome mimicking acute myocardial infarction. Am Heart J 2002;143(3):448–55.

13. Tsuchihashi K, Ueshima K, Uchida T, et al. Transient left ventricular apical ballooning without coronary artery stenosis: a novel heart syndrome mimicking acute myocardial infarction. J Am Coll Cardiol 2001;38(1):11–8.

14. Abe Y, Kondo M, Matsuoka R, et al. Assessment of clinical features in transient left ventricular apical ballooning. J Am Coll Cardiol 2003;41(5):737–42.

15. Abraham J, Mudd JO, Kapur N, et al. Stress cardiomyopathy after intravenous administration of catecholamines and beta-receptor agonists. J Am Coll Cardiol 2009;53(15):1320–5.

16. Galiuto L, De Caterina AR, Porfidia A, et al. Reversible coronary microvascular dysfunction: a common pathogenetic mechanism in Apical Ballooning or Tako-Tsubo Syndrome. Eur Heart J 2010;31(11):1319–27.

17. Burgdorf C, von Hof K, Schunkert H, et al. Regional alterations in myocardial sympathetic innervation in patients with transient left-ventricular apical ballooning (Tako-Tsubo cardiomyopathy). J Nucl Cardiol 2008;15(1):65–72.

18. Morel O, Sauer F, Imperiale A, et al. Importance of inflammation and neurohumoral activation in Takotsubo cardiomyopathy. J Card Fail 2009;15(3):206–13.

19. Salerno D, Lisi M, Gori T. The Tako-Tsubo syndrome: no evidence of peripheral endothelial or microvascular dysfunction. Int J Cardiol 2009;134(1):e23–5.

20. Akashi YJ, Nakazawa K, Sakakibara M, et al. 123I-MIBG myocardial scintigraphy in patients with 'takotsubo' cardiomyopathy. J Nucl Med 2004;45(7):1121–7.

21. Wittstein IS, Thiemann DR, Lima JA, et al. Neurohumoral features of myocardial stunning due to sudden emotional stress. N Engl J Med 2005;352(6):539–48.

22. Akashi YJ, Nakazawa K, Sakakibara M, et al. The clinical features of takotsubo cardiomyopathy. QJM 2003;96(8):563–73.

23. Nef HM, Möllmann H, Kostin S, et al. Tako-Tsubo cardiomyopathy: intraindividual structural analysis in the acute phase and after functional recovery. Eur Heart J 2007;28(20):2456–64.

24. Lyon AR, Rees PS, Prasad S, et al. Stress (Takotsubo) cardiomyopathy–a novel pathophysiological hypothesis to explain catecholamine-induced acute myocardial stunning. Nat Clin Pract Cardiovasc Med 2008;5(1):22–9.

25. Xiao RP, Ji X, Lakatta EG. Functional coupling of the beta 2-adrenoceptor to a pertussis toxin-sensitive G protein in cardiac myocytes. Mol Pharmacol 1995;47(2):322–9.

26. Heubach JF, Ravens U, Kaumann AJ. Epinephrine activates both Gs and Gi pathways, but norepinephrine activates only the Gs pathway through human β2-adrenoceptors overexpressed in mouse heart. Mol Pharmacol 2004;65(5):1313–22.

27. Wang Y, De Arcangelis V, Gao X, et al. Norepinephrine- and epinephrine-induced distinct beta2-adrenoceptor signaling is dictated by GRK2 phosphorylation in cardiomyocytes. J Biol Chem 2008;283(4):1799–807.

28. Paur H, Wright PT, Sikkel MB, et al. High levels of circulating epinephrine trigger apical cardiodepression in a β2-adrenoceptor/Gi-dependent manner: a new model of takotsubo cardiomyopathy. Circulation 2012;126:697–706.

29. Liu R, Ramani B, Soto D, et al. Agonist dose-dependent phosphorylation by protein kinase A and G protein-coupled receptor kinase regulates beta2 adrenoceptor coupling to G(i) proteins in cardiomyocytes. J Biol Chem 2009;284(47):32279–87.

30. Spinelli L, Trimarco V, Di Marino S, et al. L41Q polymorphism of the G protein coupled receptor kinase 5 is associated with left ventricular apical ballooning syndrome. Eur J Heart Fail 2010;12(1):13–6.

31. Tong H, Bernstein D, Murphy E, et al. The role of β-adrenergic receptor signaling in cardioprotection. FASEB J 2005;19:983–5.

32. Amariles P. A comprehensive literature search: drugs as possible triggers of Takotsubo cardiomyopathy. Curr Clin Pharmacol 2011;6(1):1–11.

33. Ueyama T, Kasamatsu K, Hano T, et al. Emotional stress induces transient left ventricular hypocontraction in the rat via activation of cardiac adrenoceptors: a possible animal model of 'tako-tsubo' cardiomyopathy. Circ J 2002;66(7):712–3.

34. Doggrell SA. Relaxant and beta 2-adrenoceptor blocking activities of labetalol, dilevalol, amosulalol and KF-4317 on the rat isolated aorta. J Pharm Pharmacol 1988;40(11):812–5.

35. Honda K, Takenaka T, Shiono K, et al. Autonomic and antihypertensive activity of oral amosulalol (YM-09538), a combined α- and β-adrenoceptor blocking agent in conscious rats. Jpn J Pharmacol 1985;38(1):31–41.

36. Ueyama T, Hano T, Kasamatsu K, et al. Estrogen attenuates the emotional stress-induced cardiac responses in the animal model of Tako-tsubo (Ampulla) cardiomyopathy. J Cardiovasc Pharmacol 2003;42(Suppl 1):S117–9.

37. Izumi Y, Okatani H, Shiota M, et al. Effects of metoprolol on epinephrine-induced takotsubo-like left ventricular dysfunction in non-human primates. Hypertens Res 2009;32(5):339–46.

38. Kawano H, Okada R, Yano K. Histological study on the distribution of autonomic nerves in the human heart. Heart Vessels 2003;18(1):32–9.

39. Deshmukh A, Kumar G, Pant S, et al. Prevalence of Takotsubo cardiomyopathy in the United States. Am Heart J 2012;164(1):66–71.e1.

40. Gianni M, Dentali F, Grandi AM, et al. Apical ballooning syndrome or takotsubo cardiomyopathy: a systematic review. Eur Heart J 2006;27(13): 1523–9.

41. Hsu CT, Chen CY, Chang RY, et al. Prevalence and clinical features of takotsubo cardiomyopathy in taiwanese patients presenting with acute coronary syndrome. Acta Cardiol Sin 2010;26:12–8.

42. Kaoukis A, Panagopoulou V, Mojibian HR, et al. Reverse takotsubo cardiomyopathy associated with the consumption of an energy drink. Circulation 2012;125(12):1584–5.

43. Sharkey SW, Windenburg DC, Lesser JR, et al. Natural history and expansive clinical profile of stress (tako-tsubo) cardiomyopathy. J Am Coll Cardiol 2010;55(4):333–41.

44. Previtali M, Repetto A, Panigada S, et al. Left ventricular apical ballooning syndrome: prevalence, clinical characteristics and pathogenetic mechanisms in a European population. Int J Cardiol 2009;134(1):91–6.

45. Yoshioka T, Hashimoto A, Tsuchihashi K, et al. Clinical implications of midventricular obstruction and intravenous propranolol use in transient left ventricular apical ballooning (Tako-tsubo cardiomyopathy). Am Heart J 2008;155(3):526.e1–7.

46. Migliore F, Bilato C, Isabella G, et al. Haemodynamic effects of acute intravenous metoprolol in apical ballooning syndrome with dynamic left ventricular outflow tract obstruction. Eur J Heart Fail 2010; 12(3):305–8.

Mechanisms of Stress (Takotsubo) Cardiomyopathy

Sebastian Szardien, MD[a],*, Helge Möllmann, MD[a,b],
Matthias Willmer, MD[a], Yoshihiro J. Akashi, MD[c],
Christian W. Hamm, MD[a,b], Holger M. Nef, MD[a,b]

KEYWORDS

- Stress cardiomyopathy • Takotsubo cardiomyopathy • Catecholamines • Contractile dysfunction

KEY POINTS

- Stress cardiomyopathy (SCM) is a form of reversible systolic dysfunction of the mid and apical left ventricle with pathologic changes of the electrocardiogram in absence of an obstructive coronary artery disease.
- The prevalence of SCM among patients with symptoms suggestive of myocardial infarction is 0.7% to 2.5%, and it is found predominantly in postmenopausal women (90%).
- No large studies have confirmed the etiology of SCM so far.

INTRODUCTION

Since awareness has developed of cardiac SCM, also known as takotsubo cardiomyopathy, transient apical ballooning, or broken heart syndrome, stress has become known as a major risk factor for cardiovascular morbidity and mortality.[1–4] It was first described by Dote and colleagues,[2] who named it, *takotsubo*, because the shape of the left ventricle resembles a Japanese octopus trap, with a round bottom and narrow neck. SCM is characterized by a reversible systolic dysfunction of the mid and apical segments of the left ventricle. Most commonly, postmenopausal women are affected.[5] Symptoms occur after emotional or physical stress and are similar to those seen in acute myocardial infarction, including sudden onset of chest pain associated with convex ST segment elevation and a moderate increase in creatine kinase and troponin levels.[5–7] A diagnosis of obstructive coronary artery disease can be excluded, however, in the presence of severely depressed left ventricular function. Variant forms of left ventricular dysfunction have been reported, including wall-motion abnormalities, such as mid-ventricular ballooning with sparing of the basal and apical segments or inverted Takotsubo.[8–10] Involvement of the right ventricle is common in SCM and associated with more severe left ventricular dysfunction.[11,12] Any form of contractile dysfunction is transient and reversible with resolution generally achieved within days or weeks.[1,7] The prognosis of SCM is favorable,[6] although fatal complications, such as cardiogenic shock, malignant arrhythmias, and free wall rupture of the left ventricle, have been reported.[13–16] The in-hospital disease-related mortality rate is 2% to 4%.[17,18] Although patients with SCM have a higher 4-year cardiovascular survival compared with people from the general population matched for age and gender, an association with malignancies has been demonstrated in approximately 50 patients.[17,19] No large studies have yet confirmed the cause of stress cardiomyopathy.

[a] Department of Cardiology, Kerckhoff Heart and Thorax Center, Benekestrasse 2-8, Bad Nauheim 61231, Germany; [b] Medical Department I, Cardiology, University of Giessen, Klinikstr. 33, 35392 Gießen, Germany; [c] Division of Cardiology, Department of Internal Medicine, St Marianna University School of Medicine, 2-16-1 Sugao Miyamae-ku, Kawasaki-city, Kanagawa-prefecture 216-8511, Japan
* Corresponding author. Department of Cardiology, Kerckhoff Heart and Thorax Center, Benekestrasse 2-8, Bad Nauheim 61231, Germany.
E-mail address: s.szardien@kerckhoff-fgi.de

Heart Failure Clin 9 (2013) 197–205
http://dx.doi.org/10.1016/j.hfc.2012.12.012
1551-7136/13/$ – see front matter © 2013 Elsevier Inc. All rights reserved.

HISTORICAL PATHOPHYSIOLOGIC CONCEPTS OF SCM

Several pathophysiologic concepts of SCM have been discussed in the past years. Recent research data, however, cast most of these hypotheses in doubt.

In the early stage of research activity, several investigators assumed a regional limited myocarditis as cause of SCM. Myocarditis-specific alterations, however, were excluded in numerous myocardial biopsies. Furthermore, inflammatory markers are classically not elevated in SCM and most patients do not have a history of previous infectious diseases.[1,20]

For a long time, multiple coronary vasospasms and the occurrence of SCM have been closely linked.[2] Larger cohort data, however, revealed coronary vasospasms in only 1.4% of patients with SCM.[7] In further studies, it has been tested whether vasospasms could be provoked pharmacologically in patients with SCM. Even in these studies, spontaneous vasospasms were observed in only 2% of patients and the percentage of pharmacologic provoked vasospasms varied from 0% to 43% of patients[1,6,21]; a recent meta-analysis revealed that coronary vasospasms were provocative in 27.6% of cases.[22] In summary, multiple vasospasms are unlikely to be the major trigger of SCM.

In some patients, an obstruction of the left ventricular outflow tract has been observed in the acute phase of SCM.[23,24] Therefore, it has been postulated that this obstruction may be caused by a catecholamine-induced hyperkinesia of the basal segments thereby leading to apical ballooning, which in turn leads to an impaired coronary perfusion by increased wall tension.[25] This may explain the observed regional wall abnormalities, ECG changes, and increased biomarkers.[25] Larger studies could not confirm this hypothesis, however, because in many patients no significant pressure gradient was observed.[26]

SCM is still a diagnosis by exclusion.

MORPHOLOGIC ALTERATIONS IN SCM

In recent studies, morphologic and ultrastructural alterations in SCM have been characterized systemically.[11,27] In the acute phase, a significant loss of the contractile proteins, actin and myosin, can be observed. The contractile material is partially restricted to the peripheral zone of the cell with a disarrangement of myocytes. The cytoskeletal proteins, α-actinin and titin, are significantly reduced in the acute phase of SCM, leading to changes in sarcomeric length, dissociation of myofibrils, and disturbances of the interaction between myofibrils (**Fig. 1**). The resulting functional consequence of these alterations is a reduction of contraction efficiency and relaxation capacity. A complete restoration of this myocyte arrangement can be observed after functional recovery.

Apart from the contractile apparatus, the extracellular space shows remarkable alterations. The acute phase of SCM is accompanied by an accumulation of cardiac fibroblasts and myofibroblasts.[11] Accordingly, a significant enlargement of the extracellular matrix with increased protein expression of collagen I, collagen III, and fibronectin can be observed (**Fig. 2**). The functional consequence of this enlargement of the extracellular matrix, besides a reduced systolic contraction, is an intracellular and extracellular uncoupling with consecutive affection and loss of the syncytium. After functional recovery, the amount of the extracellular proteins reveals a clear trend toward regression.[11]

TRANSCRIPTIONAL PROFILING IN SCM

After processing human biopsies, a complete transcriptional profile of patients with SCM was described for the first time in 2008.[28] Most notably, a group of genes that are controlled by the transcription factor, nuclear factor E2–related factor (Nrf-2), are significantly up-regulated during the acute phase of SCM. The Nrf-2–induced transcription plays an important role in the early cellular response to oxidative stress. Several of these Nrf-2–induced genes are involved in the so-called redox signaling.

Several genes directly controlling cellular translation are significantly up-regulated in the acute phase. In particular, ribosomal proteins 6 and 9 show a significantly increased expression. The so-called female genes are strongly expressed in the acute phase, which, given that mostly postmenopausal women are affected, is interesting.

After functional recovery, particularly mitochondrial genes as well as genes involved in respiratory chain, citrate cyle, and β-oxidation showed a significant up-regulation. Hence, signaling pathways and mechanisms responsible for energy generation in the cell in particular seem to be crucially important during the recovery phase.

DISTURBANCES OF MICROCIRCULATION

In patients with SCM, disturbances of myocardial microcirculation in the apical and midventricular myocardium were detected by using positron emission tomography, which were reversible after

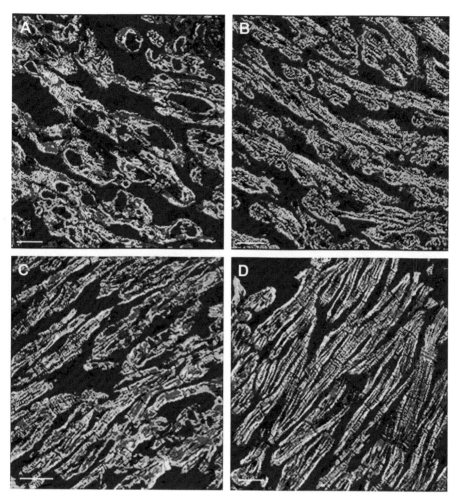

Fig. 1. Immunohistochemical staining of the cytoskeletal proteins, α-actinin (*green*) and titin (*green*). Phalloidine (*red*), nuclei (*blue*). In the acute phase, α-actinin (*A*) and titin (*C*) protein amounts were significantly reduced. After functional recovery (*B, D*), both proteins revealed a trend toward normalization.

functional recovery.[29,30] Other groups confirmed these results with the so-called Thrombolysis in Myocardial Infarction frame count method.[31] Hereby, patients revealed a decreased coronary flow velocity after exclusion of coronary stenoses, which also was reversible within a few days. Similarly, MRI studies revealed wall-motion abnormalities, which were closely similar to those seen after acute myocardial infarction.[32] The observed intracellular accumulation of ubiquitin further indicates an ischemia-triggered perturbation of protein synthesis.[11] Finally, elevation of the cardiac biomarkers, troponin and creatine kinase, presumably caused by loss of cardiomyocytes, further supports the hypothesis of an ischemia-triggered contractile dysfunction.

In summary, SCM is accompanied by disturbances in microcirculation, although they cannot be observed in all patients. It remains unclear, however, whether these microcirculation disorders are a cause or merely a consequence of SCM.

THE ROLE OF CALCIUM HOMEOSTASIS IN SCM

Disturbances of the calcium regulatory system can play a major role in the development of contractile dysfunction. The calcium regulatory protein, sarcolipin (SLN), is expressed in the left ventricle of patients in the acute phase of SCM. Physiologically, the expression of this protein is restricted to the atria. SLN regulates sarcoplasmic calcium ATPase 2a (SERCA2a) activity by reduction of its calcium affinity.[33] As previously reported, SLN can solely inhibit SERCA2a-activity as well as in combination with phospholamban (PLN).[33,34] In SCM, gene expression and protein amount were both significantly up-regulated in the acute phase,

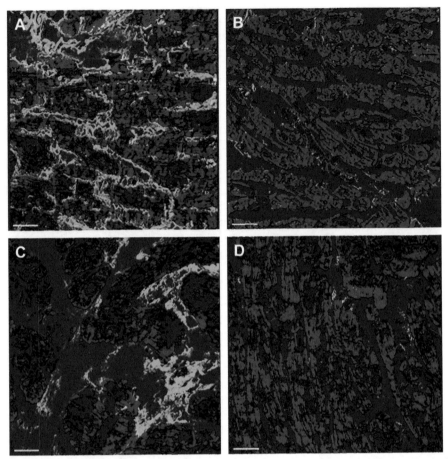

Fig. 2. Specifical immunohistochemical staining for collagen I (*green*) (*A, C*) and collagen III (*green*) (*B, D*). A significant increase of collagen I (*A*) and of collagen III was observed in the acute phase of SCM. After functional recovery (*B, D*), both proteins showed a significant decrease.

with a clear trend toward regression after functional recovery.[35] This may be one explanation for the contractile dysfunction in SCM.

Furthermore, a shift in the ratio of PLN and the SERCA2a, with increased PLN expression and reduced SERCA2a expression, was observed in the acute phase of SCM.[35] The increased PLN/SERCA2a ratio leads to a disturbed calcium reuptake and consecutively to an impaired systolic and diastolic function (**Fig. 3**). Moreover, the phosphorylation of PLN was significantly reduced. In the unphosphorylated state, PLN inhibits SERCA2a activity via reduced calcium affinity. The inhibitory function of PLN is abolished after phosphorylation. PLN can be phosphorylated at 2 positions by different protein kinases: PLN-Ser16 by the cyclic adenosine monophosphate–dependent protein kinase A and PLN-Thr17 by the calcium/calmodulin-dependent protein kinase II.[36] In the acute phase of SCM, both PLN-Ser16 and PLN-Thr17 were significantly less phosphorylated.[35] It

was also demonstrated by immunohistochemistry that the fluorescence intensity of PLN-Ser16 was apparently lower in biopsies taken from the acute phase compared with healthy myocardium.[35]

In summary, it has to assumed that the expression of SLN in the left ventricle, which in turn leads to inhibition of SERCA2a-activity, and the increased PLN protein amount with reduced PLN phosphorylation are major contributors to the contractile dysfunction in the acute phase of SCM.

THE ROLE OF CATECHOLAMINES IN SCM

Since the first description of SCM, physical and emotional stress has been a commonly accepted trigger for SCM. In this context, Wittstein and colleagues[37] showed that plasma catecholamine levels are elevated and are even higher than in patients with acute myocardial infarction in Killip class III. These results are confirmed by other groups.[11,38] Further indications of the crucial

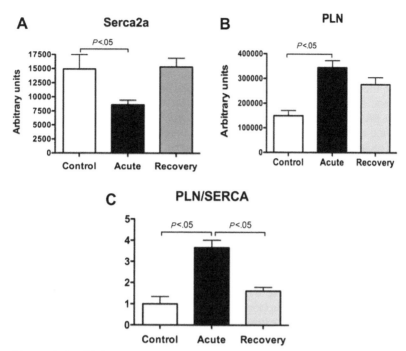

Fig. 3. Western blot analysis of (A) SERCA2a and (B) PLN. Significant increase of the PLN/SERCA2a ratio in the acute phase of SCM (C).

impact of catecholamines are the observed histologic und ultrastructural alterations in the acute phase of SCM, which are closely similar to those seen in catecholamine-induced cardiomyopathy. In both pathologies, contraction bands, unspecific vacuoles, infiltration of neutrophils, interstitial fibrosis, and a significant loss of actin and myosin can be observed (**Fig. 4**).[11] Furthermore, a displacement of the contractile apparatus into the border area of the cell was described, which might be explained by the conspicuous vacuolization in the acute phase.[11]

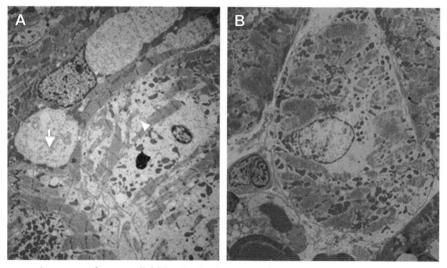

Fig. 4. Electron microscopy of myocardial biopsies in the acute phase (A) and after functional recovery (B). The acute phase of SCM is accompanied by reduction of contractile proteins, vacuolization, and a loss of cytoplasmatic structure. An enlargement of the extracellular space and increase of fibrillar structures can be observed. In the recovery phase, these alterations are nearly completely reversible. Myocytolysis (*arrowhead*); vacuolization (*arrow*).

The increased release of catecholamines results in an enhanced catecholamine degradation, which in turn causes the generation of hydrogen and tissue toxic metabolites.[39] High levels of free oxygen radicals (reactive oxygen species) develop several adverse effects in the myocardium, such as cytotoxity, arrhythmias, and reduced contractility.[40] Gene expression profiling revealed a significant increase of Nrf-2–induced genes in the acute phase of SMC.[28] Among other genes, these genes are triggered by reactive oxygen species.[41] Reactive oxygen species have the potential to injure vascular cells and cardiac myocyte directly.[42,43] In the acute phase of SCM, a significant increase of superoxide was observed, which returned to baseline values after functional recovery. Also, a significant increase of oxidative LDL has been shown in the serum of SMC patients. This indicates that oxidative stress during SCM is not a local appearance in the myocardium but a systematic reaction triggered by physical or emotional stressors, which is supported by results of animal models of SMC, where the oxidative stress-related factor, heme oxygenase-1, was up-regulated in aortic macrophages.[44]

Catecholamine overload does not lead to morphologic alterations but may lead to disturbances in intracellular calcium homeostasis. A potential calcium overload of cardiomyocytes has to be assumed due to the increased PLN/SERCA2a ratio, decreased PLN phosphorylation, and the occurrence of the SERCA-inhibiting enzyme SLN in the left ventricle. Thus, the disturbed calcium homeostasis may essentially contribute to contractile dysfunction in SCM.

Given that circulating epinephrine develops a more potent effect on the myocardium than norepinephrine,[45] it has to be assumed that the observed alterations in SCM are mainly mediated by epinephrine. This hypothesis was recently confirmed in animal experiments, which demonstrated that epinephrine but not norepinephrine leads to the development of contractile dysfunction and the typical contraction pattern of SCM.[46] Lyon and colleagues[45] reported a switch of the intracellular signaling cascade of cardiomyocytes after epinephrine stimulation. Epinephrine induces positive inotropic effects via activation of the Gs protein–coupled protein kinase A. In supraphysiologic doses, epinephrine paradoxically exerts negative inotropic effects. This depends on the switch of the stimulating Gs protein to the inhibiting Gi protein, which is called stimulus trafficking.[45] This hypothesis was confirmed in animal experiments, which demonstrated that stimulation of the β_2-adrenoceptor–G_i signaling pathway is associated with negative inotropic effects on cardiomyocytes.[47]

The typical contraction pattern of SCM can be explained by catecholaminergic effects. In the apical region, the density of β-adrenergic receptors is much higher than, for example, in the basal compartments.[48,49]

In summary, high local catecholamine levels play a major role in the pathogenesis of SCM (**Fig. 5**). The

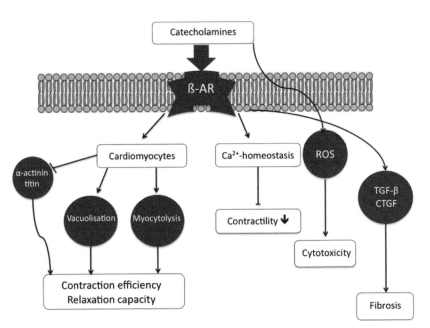

Fig. 5. Catecholamine-mediated effects in the pathogenesis of SCM. β-AR, β-adrenoceptors; ROS, reactive oxygen species; TGF-β, transforming growth factor β; CTGF, connective tissue growth factor.

contractile dysfunction can be explained by increased numbers of β-adrenergic receptors in the apical region, which lead to a higher vulnerability to catecholamine overload. Individual anatomic differences in the sympathoadrenergic system and the distribution from β-adrenergic receptors are presumably responsible for interindividual occurrence of wall-motion abnormalities in SCM.

THE ROLE OF FEMALE SEX HORMONES IN SCM

Several investigators have described the crucial role of estrogen in SCM.[50–52] Altogether, more than 90% of patients are female at the age of 50 years or older.[7] Animal experiments showed that stress-induced ventricular dysfunction and arrhythmias were significantly reduced after supplementation of estradiol.[53] The cardioprotective action of estrogen is well established and it has been shown that estrogen protects against myocardial damage during ischemia/reperfusion,[54] inhibits cardiac myofibroblast differentiation,[55] and has an important regulatory effect on the release of epinephrine in the presynaptic cardiac sympathetic nerve fibers.[56] Furthermore, the estrogen receptor is expressed on cardiomyocytes and estrogen supplementation improves calcium uptake into the cell.[57] A decreased activity of SERCA2a has been described in ovariectomized rats.[58] The complex pathogenesis of SCM, however, cannot only be explained by absence of estrogen, because men rarely develop SCM despite physiologic estrogen deficiency.

SUMMARY

SCM is characterized by an acute and in most cases completely reversible contractile dysfunction of the left ventricle with a typical contraction pattern and accounts for 1% to 2% of all acute coronary syndromes. SCM is commonly associated with preceding emotional or physical stressful events. The vast majority of patients are postmenopausal women. Despite a complete restoration of cardiac functional parameters, the prognosis of patients with SCM is comparable to those with acute myocardial infarction.

Since the first description of SCM, several pathophysiologic mechanisms have been proposed, including coronary artery vasospasm, coronary microcirculation dysfunction, obstruction of the left ventricular outflow tract, and catecholamine overload On the basis of currently available data, an excessive catecholamine release plays a key role in the pathogenesis of SCM. A systematic structural analysis revealed severe but reversible structural and morphologic alterations of heart tissue on a cellular and subcellular level.[11] Accordingly, significant morphologic disruption of sarcomeric proteins as well as an intracellular increase of vacuoles during the acute phase was documented. Increased deposition of extracellular matrix proteins also was present. Typical histologic signs of catecholamine toxicity, which are described as focal mononuclear inflammatory, areas of fibrotic response, and characteristic contraction bands, were documented. The observed alterations showed a complete reversibility after functional recovery.

After investigation of the gene expression profile in SCM by means of microarrays, increased oxidative stress, STAT3 down-regulation, and cathepsin D up-regulation could be documented, potentially triggering cardiodepressive effects.[28] In the acute phase of SCM, antioxidative genes and those genes, in particular, that regulate cell cycle and cell proliferation, were significantly up-regulated. In contrast, genes involved in the cellular energy balance were significantly down-regulated.

Furthermore, changes of the calcium-regulating system contributing to contractile dysfunction were observed. In detail, an increased PLN/SERCA2a ratio and decreased phosphorylation of PLN were observed. Furthermore, the SERCA2a-inhibiting protein, SLN, which does not exist physiologically in ventricular myocardium, was detected in left ventricular biopsies of patients with SCM.

In summary, SCM is probably caused by an excessive release of catecholamines. The ventricular dysfunction can be explained by increased numbers of β-adrenergic receptors in the apex, which leads to a higher vulnerability to catecholamine overload. Individual anatomic differences in the sympathoadrenergic system and the distribution from β-adrenergic receptors are presumably responsible for interindividual occurrence of wall-motion abnormalities in SCM.

REFERENCES

1. Akashi YJ, Nakazawa K, Sakakibara M, et al. The clinical features of takotsubo cardiomyopathy. QJM 2003;96(8):563–73.
2. Dote K, Sato H, Tateishi H, et al. Myocardial stunning due to simultaneous multivessel coronary spasms: a review of 5 cases. J Cardiol 1991;21(2):203–14 [in Japanese].
3. Nef HM, Mollmann H, Hamm CW, et al. Tako-Tsubo cardiomyopathy–a novel cardiac entity? Herz 2006; 31(5):473–9 [in German].
4. Akashi YJ, Nef HM, Mollmann H, et al. Stress cardiomyopathy. Annu Rev Med 2010;61:271–86.

5. Nef HM, Mollmann H, Elsasser A. Tako-tsubo cardio-myopathy (apical ballooning). Heart 2007;93(10): 1309–15.

6. Bybee KA, Kara T, Prasad A, et al. Systematic review: transient left ventricular apical ballooning: a syndrome that mimics ST-segment elevation myocardial infarction. Ann Intern Med 2004; 141(11):858–65.

7. Gianni M, Dentali F, Grandi AM, et al. Apical ballooning syndrome or takotsubo cardiomyopathy: a systematic review. Eur Heart J 2006;27(13): 1523–9.

8. Cacciotti L, Camastra GS, Beni S, et al. A new variant of Tako-tsubo cardiomyopathy: transient mid-ventricular ballooning. J Cardiovasc Med (Hagerstown) 2007;8(12):1052–4.

9. Botto F, Trivi M, Padilla LT. Transient left midventricular ballooning without apical involvement. Int J Cardiol 2008;127(3):e158–9.

10. Kurowski V, Kaiser A, von Hof K, et al. Apical and midventricular transient left ventricular dysfunction syndrome (tako-tsubo cardiomyopathy): frequency, mechanisms, and prognosis. Chest 2007;132(3): 809–16.

11. Nef HM, Mollmann H, Kostin S, et al. Tako-Tsubo cardiomyopathy: intraindividual structural analysis in the acute phase and after functional recovery. Eur Heart J 2007;28(20):2456–64.

12. Elesber AA, Prasad A, Bybee KA, et al. Transient cardiac apical ballooning syndrome: prevalence and clinical implications of right ventricular involvement. J Am Coll Cardiol 2006;47(5): 1082–3.

13. Donohue D, Movahed MR. Clinical characteristics, demographics and prognosis of transient left ventricular apical ballooning syndrome. Heart Fail Rev 2005;10(4):311–6.

14. Nef HM, Mollmann H, Hilpert P, et al. Severe mitral regurgitation in Tako-Tsubo cardiomyopathy. Int J Cardiol 2009;132(2):e77–9.

15. Akashi YJ, Tejima T, Sakurada H, et al. Left ventricular rupture associated with Takotsubo cardiomyopathy. Mayo Clin Proc 2004;79(6):821–4.

16. Nef HM, Mollmann H, Sperzel J, et al. Temporary third-degree atrioventricular block in a case of apical ballooning syndrome. Int J Cardiol 2006; 113(2):e33–5.

17. Elesber AA, Prasad A, Lennon RJ, et al. Four-year recurrence rate and prognosis of the apical ballooning syndrome. J Am Coll Cardiol 2007; 50(5):448–52.

18. Brinjikji W, El-Sayed AM, Salka S. In-hospital mortality among patients with takotsubo cardiomyopathy: A study of the National Inpatient Sample 2008 to 2009. Am Heart J 2012;164(2):215–21.

19. Burgdorf C, Kurowski V, Bonnemeier H, et al. Long-term prognosis of the transient left ventricular dysfunction syndrome (Tako-Tsubo cardiomyopathy): focus on malignancies. Eur J Heart Fail 2008;10(10):1015–9.

20. Abe Y, Kondo M, Matsuoka R, et al. Assessment of clinical features in transient left ventricular apical ballooning. J Am Coll Cardiol 2003;41(5):737–42.

21. Kurisu S, Sato H, Kawagoe T, et al. Tako-tsubo-like left ventricular dysfunction with ST-segment elevation: a novel cardiac syndrome mimicking acute myocardial infarction. Am Heart J 2002;143(3): 448–55.

22. Pilgrim TM, Wyss TR. Takotsubo cardiomyopathy or transient left ventricular apical ballooning syndrome: a systematic review. Int J Cardiol 2008; 124(3):283–92.

23. Merli E, Sutcliffe S, Gori M, et al. Tako-Tsubo cardiomyopathy: new insights into the possible underlying pathophysiology. Eur J Echocardiogr 2006;7(1):53–61.

24. Brunetti ND, Ieva R, Rossi G, et al. Ventricular outflow tract obstruction, systolic anterior motion and acute mitral regurgitation in Tako-Tsubo syndrome. Int J Cardiol 2008;127(3):e152–7.

25. Barriales Villa R, Bilbao Quesada R, Iglesias Rio E, et al. Transient left ventricular apical ballooning without coronary stenoses syndrome: importance of the intraventricular pressure gradient. Rev Esp Cardiol 2004;57(1):85–8 [in Spanish].

26. Desmet W. Dynamic LV obstruction in apical ballooning syndrome: the chicken or the egg. Eur J Echocardiogr 2006;7(1):1–4.

27. Fineschi V, Michalodimitrakis M, D'Errico S, et al. Insight into stress-induced cardiomyopathy and sudden cardiac death due to stress. A forensic cardio-pathologist point of view. Forensic Sci Int 2010;194(1–3):1–8.

28. Nef HM, Mollmann H, Troidl C, et al. Expression profiling of cardiac genes in Tako-Tsubo cardiomyopathy: insight into a new cardiac entity. J Mol Cell Cardiol 2008;44(2):395–404.

29. Yoshida T, Hibino T, Kako N, et al. A pathophysiologic study of tako-tsubo cardiomyopathy with F-18 fluorodeoxyglucose positron emission tomography. Eur Heart J 2007;28(21):2598–604.

30. Elesber A, Lerman A, Bybee KA, et al. Myocardial perfusion in apical ballooning syndrome correlate of myocardial injury. Am Heart J 2006;152(3): 469.e9–13.

31. Kume T, Akasaka T, Kawamoto T, et al. Relationship between coronary flow reserve and recovery of regional left ventricular function in patients with tako-tsubo-like transient left ventricular dysfunction. J Cardiol 2004;43(3):123–9 [in Japanese].

32. Sharkey SW. Electrocardiogram mimics of acute ST-segment elevation myocardial infarction: insights from cardiac magnetic resonance imaging in patients with tako-tsubo (stress) cardiomyopathy. J Electrocardiol 2008;41(6):621–5.

33. MacLennan DH, Asahi M, Tupling AR. The regulation of SERCA-type pumps by phospholamban and sarcolipin. Ann N Y Acad Sci 2003;986:472–80.

34. Asahi M, Sugita Y, Kurzydlowski K, et al. Sarcolipin regulates sarco(endo)plasmic reticulum Ca2+-ATPase (SERCA) by binding to transmembrane helices alone or in association with phospholamban. Proc Natl Acad Sci U S A 2003;100(9):5040–5.

35. Nef HM, Mollmann H, Troidl C, et al. Abnormalities in intracellular Ca2+ regulation contribute to the pathomechanism of Tako-Tsubo cardiomyopathy. Eur Heart J 2009;30(17):2155–64.

36. James P, Inui M, Tada M, et al. Nature and site of phospholamban regulation of the Ca2+ pump of sarcoplasmic reticulum. Nature 1989;342(6245):90–2.

37. Wittstein IS, Thiemann DR, Lima JA, et al. Neurohumoral features of myocardial stunning due to sudden emotional stress. N Engl J Med 2005;352(6):539–48.

38. Kume T, Kawamoto T, Okura H, et al. Local release of catecholamines from the hearts of patients with tako-tsubo-like left ventricular dysfunction. Circ J 2008;72(1):106–8.

39. Lefer DJ, Granger DN. Oxidative stress and cardiac disease. Am J Med 2000;109(4):315–23.

40. Bolli R. Mechanism of myocardial "stunning". Circulation 1990;82(3):723–38.

41. Kobayashi A, Kang MI, Watai Y, et al. Oxidative and electrophilic stresses activate Nrf2 through inhibition of ubiquitination activity of Keap1. Mol Cell Biol 2006;26(1):221–9.

42. Xu Q, Dalic A, Fang L, et al. Myocardial oxidative stress contributes to transgenic beta(2)-adrenoceptor activation-induced cardiomyopathy and heart failure. Br J Pharmacol 2011;162(5):1012–28.

43. Zhang GX, Kimura S, Nishiyama A, et al. Cardiac oxidative stress in acute and chronic isoproterenol-infused rats. Cardiovasc Res 2005;65(1):230–8.

44. Ueyama T, Kawabe T, Hano T, et al. Upregulation of heme oxygenase-1 in an animal model of Takotsubo cardiomyopathy. Circ J 2009;73(6):1141–6.

45. Lyon AR, Rees PS, Prasad S, et al. Stress (Takotsubo) cardiomyopathy—a novel pathophysiological hypothesis to explain catecholamine-induced acute myocardial stunning. Nat Clin Pract Cardiovasc Med 2008;5(1):22–9.

46. Paur H, Wright PT, Sikkel MB, et al. High levels of circulating epinephrine trigger apical cardiodepression in a beta2-Adrenoceptor/Gi-dependent manner: a new model of takotsubo cardiomyopathy. Circulation 2012;126(6):697–706.

47. Gong H, Sun H, Koch WJ, et al. Specific beta(2)AR blocker ICI 118,551 actively decreases contraction through a G(i)-coupled form of the beta(2)AR in myocytes from failing human heart. Circulation 2002;105(21):2497–503.

48. Mori H, Ishikawa S, Kojima S, et al. Increased responsiveness of left ventricular apical myocardium to adrenergic stimuli. Cardiovasc Res 1993;27(2):192–8.

49. Paur H, Wright PT, Sikkel MB, et al. High Levels of Circulating Epinephrine Trigger Apical Cardiodepression in a beta2-Adrenergic Receptor/Gi-Dependent Manner: a New Model of Takotsubo Cardiomyopathy. Circulation 2012;126(6):697–706.

50. Ueyama T, Kasamatsu K, Hano T, et al. Catecholamines and estrogen are involved in the pathogenesis of emotional stress-induced acute heart attack. Ann N Y Acad Sci 2008;1148:479–85.

51. Sclarovsky S, Nikus KC. The role of oestrogen in the pathophysiologic process of the Tako-Tsubo cardiomyopathy. Eur Heart J 2010;31(3):377 [author reply: 377–8].

52. Sclarovsky S, Nikus K. The electrocardiographic paradox of tako-tsubo cardiomyopathy-comparison with acute ischemic syndromes and consideration of molecular biology and electrophysiology to understand the electrical-mechanical mismatching. J Electrocardiol 2010;43(2):173–6.

53. Ueyama T, Hano T, Kasamatsu K, et al. Estrogen attenuates the emotional stress-induced cardiac responses in the animal model of Tako-tsubo (Ampulla) cardiomyopathy. J Cardiovasc Pharmacol 2003;42(Suppl 1):S117–9.

54. Kam KW, Qi JS, Chen M, et al. Estrogen reduces cardiac injury and expression of beta1-adrenoceptor upon ischemic insult in the rat heart. J Pharmacol Exp Ther 2004;309(1):8–15.

55. Wu M, Han M, Li J, et al. 17beta-estradiol inhibits angiotensin II-induced cardiac myofibroblast differentiation. Eur J Pharmacol 2009;616(1–3):155–9.

56. Eskin BA, Snyder DL, Roberts J, et al. Cardiac norepinephrine release: modulation by ovariectomy and estrogen. Exp Biol Med (Maywood) 2003;228(2):194–9.

57. Grohe C, Kahlert S, Lobbert K, et al. Cardiac myocytes and fibroblasts contain functional estrogen receptors. FEBS Lett 1997;416(1):107–12.

58. Bupha-Intr T, Wattanapermpool J. Regulatory role of ovarian sex hormones in calcium uptake activity of cardiac sarcoplasmic reticulum. Am J Physiol Heart Circ Physiol 2006;291(3):H1101–8.

Takotsubo Cardiomyopathy
Do the Genetics Matter?

Giuseppe Limongelli, MD, PhD, FESC[a,*],
Raffaella D'Alessandro, DSc[b], Daniele Masarone, MD[a],
Valeria Maddaloni, DSc[b], Olga Vriz, MD[c],
Rosalba Minisini, PhD[d], Rodolfo Citro, MD, FESC[e],
Paolo Calabrò, MD, PhD, FESC[a], Maria Giovanna Russo, MD[a],
Raffaele Calabrò, MD[a], Giuseppe Pacileo, MD[a],
Eduardo Bossone, MD, PhD, FESC[f,g],
Perry Mark Elliott, FRCP, MD, FESC, FACC[h]

KEYWORDS

- Takotsubo cardiomyopathy • Genetics • Adrenoceptor polymorphisms

KEY POINTS

- Takotsubo cardiomyopathy (TTC) is an enigmatic disease with a multifactorial and still unresolved pathogenesis.
- Many mechanisms have been proposed to explain transient myocardial damage, including myocardial dysfunction mediated through catecholamine-induced damage, coronary artery spasm or dysfunction, and neurally mediated myocardial stunning.
- Recently, experimental and clinical observation has suggested a role for genetics in the pathogenesis of TTC.
- Technological advances in exome capture and DNA sequencing have offered clinicians a new opportunity to discover genetics-related disease, and large prospective genetic studies using such techniques probably will shed new light on understanding the pathogenesis of this enigmatic syndrome.

INTRODUCTION

Takotsubo cardiomyopathy (TTC), also known as takotsubo syndrome, broken heart syndrome, and stress-induced cardiomyopathy, was first described in Japan in 1990[1] as transient left ventricular dysfunction with apical motion abnormalities (apical ballooning syndrome [ABS]) in the presence of angiographically normal coronary arteries. Clinical presentation includes ischemia-like chest pain, transient changes on the electrocardiogram (ECG) (ST-segment elevation in anterior leads or deep T-wave inversion), and minor cardiac biomarker elevation (troponin I, creatine kinase). Angiographic evaluation in the acute phase shows unobstructed coronary arteries and akinesis or dyskinesis of the apical one-half to two-thirds of the left ventricle consisting of "apical ballooning."

The etiology of TTC remains uncertain, and it is likely that multiple factors are involved. TTC

[a] Cardiologia SUN, Monaldi Hospital, AO Colli, Second University of Naples, Via L Bianchi, Naples 80100, Italy; [b] Genomic and Cellular Lab, Monaldi Hospital, AO Colli, Second University of Naples, Via L Bianchi, Naples 80100, Italy; [c] Department of Cardiology and Emergency Ospedale San Antonio, via Trento-Trieste, 33038, San Daniele del Friuli, Udine, Italy; [d] University of Eastern Piedmont "Amedeo Avogadro", Department of Translational Medicine, via Solaroli 17, 28100, Novara, Italy; [e] Heart Department, University Hospital "San Giovanni di Dio e Ruggi d'Aragona," Salerno, Italy; [f] Cardiology Division, "Cava de' Tirreni and Amalfi Coast" Hospital, Heart Department, University of Salerno via De Marinis, 84013 Cava de" Tirreni (SA), Italy; [g] Cardiac Surgery Department, IRCCS Policlinico San Donato, Piazza Edmondo Malan 1, 20097 San Donato Milanese, Italy; [h] The Inherited Cardiac Diseases Unit, The Heart Hospital/University College London, 16-18 Westmoreland Street, London W1H 8PH, UK
* Corresponding author. Monaldi Hospital, AO Colli, Second University of Naples, Via L Bianchi, Naples 80100, Italy.
E-mail address: limongelligiuseppe@libero.it

Heart Failure Clin 9 (2013) 207–216
http://dx.doi.org/10.1016/j.hfc.2012.12.008
1551-7136/13/$ – see front matter © 2013 Elsevier Inc. All rights reserved.

primarily occurs in postmenopausal women after physical or emotional stress.[2,3] However, variant forms such as midventricular ballooning and basal ballooning (that spares the mid left ventricular [LV] region and has paradoxic apical hyperkinesis) have recently been described even in young premenopausal women.[4] Furthermore, apical ballooning can be observed not only in the left ventricle but also in the right ventricle.[5] The etiology of TTC remains the subject of investigation, but observational data in patients, reports of its occurrence in patients with pheochromocytoma,[6] and its reproduction by infusion of epinephrine in primates[7] strongly support the hypothesis that it is caused by excessive adrenergic/catecholamine stimulation.[8] Alternative hypotheses include myocardial ischemia from multivessel coronary spasm and transient atherosclerotic plaque rupture. Ethnic as well as seasonal variation in the prevalence of TTC is well described, but it is only recently that familial cases of TTC have been reported.[9] This article explores the role of genetic mechanisms that might explain or modulate the pathogenesis of this disease.

DEFINITION

Although there is no international consensus on the diagnostic criteria for TTC, Mayo Clinic researchers proposed criteria in 2004, recently modified,[10] whereby patients must fulfill all of the following: transient hypokinesis, akinesis, or dyskinesis in the LV mid segments with apical involvement; regional wall-motion abnormalities extending beyond a single vascular distribution; a stressful trigger; the absence of obstructive coronary disease or angiographic evidence of plaque rupture; new ECG abnormalities or modest elevation in cardiac troponin; and absence of pheochromocytoma and myocarditis.

PATHOGENESIS OF TAKOTSUBO CARDIOMYOPATHY
Adrenergic Stress Hypothesis

The fact that TTC is preceded by emotional or physiologic stress in 65% of individuals, and that plasma catecholamines are elevated 2 to 3 times higher than in acute myocardial infarction, has led to the hypothesis that the syndrome is the result of a transient direct toxic effect of catecholamines on the myocardium.[11] In support of this view are myocardial biopsies that demonstrate many vacuoles of different size contributing to cellular hypertrophy, accumulation of glycogen in cytoplasma of myocytes, disorganization of contractile and cytoskeletal proteins, and an increased extracellular

matrix,[12] which nearly complete reversibility at 2 weeks.[13] This peculiar distribution of the condition may be explained by the greater adrenergic receptor β subtype density at the apex of the heart in comparison with the basal myocardium.[14] The neurohormonal response to emotional or physical stressful events is shown in **Fig. 1**.

Estrogen Deficiency

The female predominance of TTC has raised the possibility that estrogen may have a role in the pathogenesis of TTC. In a rat model of TTC, Ueyama[15] demonstrated that chronic estrogen supplementation blunted the stress-induced sympathoadrenal outflow from the brain to the heart and upregulated cardioprotective substances such as atrial natriuretic peptide and heat-shock protein 70, with prevention of stress and catecholamine-induced LV dysfunction. Kuo and colleagues[16] proposed that lack of estrogen replacement in the postmenopausal state may predispose women to TTC.

Coronary Artery and Microvascular Spasm

Coronary artery spasm, including epicardial coronary spasm, microvascular spasm, or direct injury, has been suggested as one of the triggering mechanisms of TTC. Ibañez and colleagues[17] suggested a common etiology in TTC syndrome and acute myocardial infarction secondary to left anterior descending artery occlusion, because cardiac ventriculography findings are identical. The same investigators also documented the presence of plaque rupture on intravascular ultrasonography of the left anterior descending coronary artery of patients with angiographically nonobstructive coronary artery disease and a diagnosis of TCC.[18] However, this mechanism does not entirely explain the extent of regional wall-motion abnormality seen in those without a wrap-around left anterior descending coronary artery, the presence of right ventricular dysfunction, and the preservation of apical function that occurs in some patients. It is therefore unlikely that vasospasm and atherothrombosis of a single artery underlie TTC in most patients.

The possibility of myocardial injury attributable to microvascular spasm has also been suggested. Using an intracoronary Doppler wire technique, Ako and colleagues[19] demonstrated microcirculatory impairment during transient LV hypocontraction. Daniels and Fearon[20] also reported a case of TTC with highly abnormal coronary flow reserve and microcirculatory resistance compatible with microvascular spasm. Transient and reversible coronary microcirculation dysfunction has been

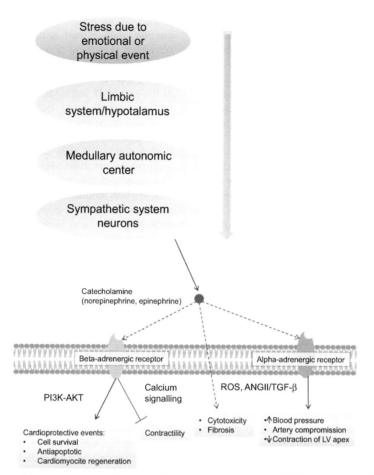

Fig. 1. Neurohormonal response to emotional or physical stressful events. ANGII, angiotensin II; LV, left ventricular; PI3K, phosphoinositide-3 kinase; ROS, reactive oxygen species; TGF, transforming growth factor.

also demonstrated using noninvasive transthoracic Doppler echocardiography.[21,22] A possible unifying hypothesis has been suggested,[23] linking estrogen deficiency in postmenopausal women with endothelial dysfunction, microvascular dysfunction, and the development of TTC during adrenergic stress.

Obstruction of the Left Ventricular Outflow Tract

Obstruction of the left ventricular outflow tract (LVOT) has been reported in about 25% of patients with TTC (particularly elderly women), associated with increased midseptal thickness, systolic anterior motion of the mitral valve, and mitral regurgitation.[24] In the presence of increased catecholaminergic tone, this feature could lead to the development of severe, transient LV midcavity obstruction, mimicking hypertrophic obstructive cardiomyopathy. However, it is likely that LVOT obstruction is a consequence rather than a cause of stress cardiomyopathy, as anteroapical ballooning is extremely rare in other situations where LVOT obstruction is common.

Coagulation Factors

A whole proteome analysis performed on serum samples was performed on 9 TTC patients, in a comparison with 12 patients with acute coronary syndrome (ACS) and 13 control patients. Proteomic evaluation revealed differences in fibrinogen γ-chain isoforms and fibrin β chains, whose level was increased in TTC patients compared with ACS patients and controls. Fibrinogen has a key role in fibrin formation and its action is influenced by thrombin, leading to plasma coagulation and platelet aggregation through glycoprotein IIb/IIIa receptors. The biological activity of fibrinogen isoforms in TTC patients might reflect an activation of the intrinsic clotting cascade.[25]

Oxidative Stress

One potential mechanism by which excess catecholamines could trigger cellular damage is through increased oxidative stress. A study conducted on animal models has shown that an increase of circulating catecholamines induced by emotional stress[26] is associated with an elevation in the levels of heme oxygenase 1 (HO-1), an enzyme involved in the first and rate-limiting step in heme degradation that seems to protect against myocardial ischemia and reperfusion injury and inhibits postmyocardial infarct remodeling. In a human study, Nef and colleagues (2008) performed microarray expression analysis on endomyocardial biopsies obtained from 3 female TTC patients and 3 (2 females and a male) donated hearts. Transcriptomic profiles demonstrated increased expression of Nrf2-induced genes, Nrf2 being a transcription factor regulating the expression of antioxidants and antioxidant enzymes. These studies link catecholamine overproduction to oxidative stress, suggesting a contribution of oxidative stress to the development of TTC.

The study performed by Nef and colleagues (2008) also showed an increase in the expression level of PI3K and DOK5 (docking protein 5, an adapter protein involved in signal transduction and phosphorylated receptor tyrosine kinases). PI3K and Akt (a serine-threonine protein kinase in the pathway of phosphoinositide-3 kinase) represent principal signaling enzymes important in cell survival, cellular proliferation, hypertrophy, and metabolic control. Akt interacts with members of the Bcl2 family (involved in apoptosis). In TTC patients, increased expression of Akt could enhance cell survival and, with nuclear factor κB, induce the expression of genes promoting cell survival. Thus, transcriptomic studies indicate a possible activation of pathways that lead to cell survival, which can result as a cardioprotective process in TTC.[27]

GENETIC DETERMINANTS OF DISEASE EXPRESSION IN TTC
Family Studies

Clinical evidence for a genetic predisposition to TTC is provided by a small number of family studies. Pison and colleagues[28] reported the case of 2 sisters affected by TTC. The first was a 44-year-old woman with chronic obstructive pulmonary disease and depression, who experienced thoracic pain and dyspnea after emotional stress. Cardiac evaluation revealed tall T waves in the anterior leads and apical akinesia, but normal coronary arteries. Laboratory examinations showed a modest increase of troponin I, creatine kinase, and creatine kinase MB levels. Her sister, at the age of 52 years, complained of dyspnea during physical exercise; she also had tall T waves

in the anterior leads, severe reduction of ejection fraction with diffuse anteroapical akinesia, and increased troponin-I concentration.

Cherian and colleagues[29] reported a familial aggregation of TTC in a mother and her daughter. At the age of 42 years, after her father's death, the mother had showed classic TTC pattern. She experienced a second clinically significant episode at the age of 55, after repeated stressful episodes. During follow-up, the clinical picture appeared completely resolved. Her daughter had severe chest pain at the age of 30 years, and cardiac examination showed negative T wave in inferior and anterior leads, a discrete midinferior-wall akinetic segment, and normal LV function (ejection fraction 55%). Troponin concentration was increased. As in her mother, there was complete normalization of the clinical picture after 6 weeks.

Finally, Kumar and colleagues[30] described the case of a female patient suffering chest pain following emotional stress. ECG analysis revealed sinus rhythm, poor R-wave progression to leads V1 through V3, mild ST-segment elevation, troponin-T elevation, normal coronary angiography, and a reduced ejection fraction, with hypokinesis of the midventricle and of the apex and hyperdynamic basal function at ventriculography. At the age of 49 years her mother, after an intense emotional stress, experienced an acute chest pain, with no angiographic evidence of obstructive coronary artery disease and wall-motion abnormalities suggestive of stress-induced cardiomyopathy.

Role of Genetic Polymorphisms in TTC

Over the last decade, several studies analyzing polymorphisms potentially involved in the pathogenesis of TTC have been published (**Table 1**), the most important of which concern those affecting adrenergic receptors located on cell membranes, which exist as several subtypes (α, β1, β2, and β3).[37] The intracellular signaling following catecholamine binding to the receptor is mediated by adrenergic receptors β1 and β2, which couple to the Ga subunit of the Gs protein complex. At the same time, catecholamines induce phosphorylation of G-protein–coupled receptor kinase, to negatively regulate the signal.[32] Common genetic polymorphisms in β-receptor subtypes include Arg389 and Ser49 in the adrenergic receptor subtype B1 (ADRB1). The first has been proposed to lead to functional alteration of the Gs-protein–coupling domain, and the presence of the arginine instead of glycine in the second is predicted to cause a gain of function of the encoded protein. Polymorphisms in the gene encoding the adrenergic receptor α2C (ADRA2C) (a receptor that regulates norepinephrine release from sympathetic cardiac nerves gene) may cause adrenergic deregulation. In particular, a deletion of 4 amino acids (protein positions starting from 322 to 325) causes an impairment of receptor coupling, leading to an alteration of the signaling to inhibition of adenylyl cyclase, stimulation of inositol phosphate accumulation, and activation of mitogen-activated protein kinase.

This polymorphism has been found to be more frequent in African Americans than in Caucasians, and its functional consequence can cause an increased response to antagonists compared with wild-type carriers, with a possible modification in drug response and disease development of deletion carriers.[38]

Animal model studies suggest the involvement of adrenergic receptor β2 in stress-induced cardiomyopathy, as an increased concentration of such receptors has been found in the apical region of dog hearts. In mice models, the overexpression of receptors belonging to the subtype β2 in the apical region of the heart has been found to be associated with increased levels of epinephrine. Taken together, these data suggest that when stress events occur, the increase in circulating epinephrine can have a major effect on the apical region of the heart because of a difference in sensitivity of β2 receptors.[26] In man, α- and β-adrenoceptor polymorphisms have been associated with the risk of cardiac injury and dysfunction after subarachnoid hemorrhage, an interesting finding given that the reversible regional LV dysfunction seen in patients with subarachnoid hemorrhage is very similar to that seen in TTC. β1AR (389 CC) and β2AR (27 CC) have been found to predict the release of cardiac troponin I, whereas α2AR deletion (del322–325) seems to be predictive of reduced LV ejection fraction.[34] However, findings in patients with TTC are contradictory. In a cohort of 61 Caucasian patients (58 women, 95%; mean age 69 ± 11 years) with TTC, Sharkey and colleagues[33] found no difference in the frequency of adrenoceptor *ADRA2C* and adrenoceptor *ADRB1* polymorphisms compared with controls, whereas Vriz and colleagues[31] found a different distribution of variation of β1 (Arg389Gly; homozygous Arg/Arg more frequent in TTC) and β2 (Gln27Glu; homozygous Gln/Gln more frequent in healthy controls) adrenergic receptors among patients and controls, but no significant difference for β2-adrenergic receptor (Arg16Gly) variation.

Spinelli and colleagues[32] investigated the presence of genetic polymorphisms in *ADRB1*, *ADRB2*, Gs-protein α subunit (*GNAS*), G-protein–coupled receptor kinase 5 (*GRK5*) genes in 22 patients, 21 of whom had a stressful event as an ascertained cause of TTC. The genetic analysis showed a similar distribution between cases and controls for most of the polymorphisms, but a significant difference for the polymorphism rs17098707 in the *GRK5* gene, with a higher prevalence among TTC subjects. The association between the polymorphism and the cardiac phenotype could be explained by the negative inotropic effect of the GRK5 L41 variant under conditions of acute catecholamine stimulation.

Finally, mouse models of stress-induced cardiomyopathy have been used to confirm unbalanced expression of significant genes in the pathologic condition. Upregulation of transcriptional factors/immediate-early genes, such as *Fos*, *Jun*, *junB*, *Egr1* (*NGFI-A*), *Nr4a1* (*NGFI-B*),[39] and other genes involved in the adaptive and protective responses to vascular and cardiac insults in the heart, has been found in such models. Some of the dysregulated transcription factors are known to be upregulated in endothelial cells when inflammation and shear stress occur, inducing the synthesis of endothelial nitric oxide synthase and thrombomodulin.

Although the studies described here are promising for the identification of genetic polymorphisms related to the development of the cardiomyopathy, a limitation in the definitive interpretation of the results is the small size of studied populations. As in all association studies, the number of subjects included in a study is a fundamental characteristic in obtaining results of a good statistical level. As described by Long and Langley,[40] analysis of polymorphisms gain sufficient power to detect the presence of causative polymorphisms of small effect when the sample studied is of at least 500 individuals, and further power is achieved if their number is increased. Moreover, Yang and colleagues[41] found that samples of 500, 1000, and 2000 subjects can provide adequate power to detect modest genetic associations in case-control studies. Given the extremely low power for studies of this size in detecting an effect of a common polymorphism, further studies will be necessary to estimate the potential clinical role of the polymorphisms studied in TTC.

GENETIC HETEROGENEITY AND ASSOCIATION WITH GENETIC SYNDROMES

TTC is likely to be a multifactorial disease caused by both genetic and environmental factors. A small number of case reports suggest an association between rare genetic syndromes and TTC.

Fragile X Syndrome

In 2009 a mutation in the *FMR1* gene, the causative gene for fragile X syndrome (a genetic disease more frequent in male patients and characterized

Table 1
Summary of polymorphisms found in patients affected by takotsubo cardiomyopathy

Protein Name	Gene Symbol	SNP ID	Protein Variation	Genetic Polymorphism	Effect	Results: Patient
β1 Adrenergic receptor	ADRB1	rs1801253 rs1801252 rs1801253	Gly389Arg Ser-49Gly Arg31Gln		Enhanced cardiac catecholamine sensitivity	Gly389Arg Homozygous for 389-Arg: 44-y-old woman with familial ABS[30] 49% homozygous for Arg-389, 49% heterozygous, 2% homozygous for Gly-389[30] Homozygous for 389-Arg 42%, homozygous for 389-Gly 12%, heterozygous 47%[31] Arg31Gln Nonsignificant difference between patients and controls[32] Ser49Gly Homozygous for 49-Ser: 44-y-old woman with familial ABS[30] 88% homozygous for Ser-49, 12% heterozygous[33]
β2 Adrenergic receptor	ADRB2	rs1042713 rs1042714 rs1800888	Arg16Gly Gln27Glu Thr164Ile		Possible increased vulnerability of the heart to adrenergic stress	Arg16Gly Wild type: 44-y-old woman with familial ABS[31,34] Homozygous for Arg-16 13%, homozygous for Gly-16 28%, heterozygous 59% Gln27Glu Homozygous for Gln-27 10%, homozygous for Glu-27 38%, heterozygous 52%[35] Thr164Ile Nonsignificant difference between patients and controls[31]

	Gene					
α2C Adrenergic receptor	ADRA2C	rs2234888	del322–325		Impaired regulation of norepinephrine release	Wild type (no deletion): 44-y-old woman with familial ABS[32] 93% wild type; 7% heterozygous[34] Nonsignificant difference between patients and controls[30]
Fragile X mental retardation	FMR1	—	Reduction of gene expression	Insertion of CGG trinucleotide	Fragile X syndrome	Female patient carrying the mutation[33]
GNAS (Gs-protein α subunit)	GNAS	rs11554276	—	g.56503898G>A	—	Nonsignificant difference between patients and controls[32]
GRK5 (G-protein–coupled receptor kinase 5)	GRK5	rs17098707 rs34679178	Gln41Leu Thr129Met	—	—	Gln41Leu Different distribution of Gln41Leu between takotsubo patients and controls; leucine[34] associated with lower heart rate in the female portion of the population[32] Thr129Met Nonsignificant difference between patients and controls[32]
CD36	CD36	rs75326924	P90S	c.268C>T Ins1159A	CD36 deficiency	One patient with TTC described with both heterozygous variations[32]

by mental retardation), was reported in a female patient with TTC. The mutation is due to the expansion of a repeated codon, normally present in a low number of copies, but which can expand to 230. The woman experienced chest pain with suspicion of acute myocardial infarction. Biochemical analysis showed an increased level of troponin T, and electrocardiographic investigation revealed anterior and lateral ischemia with negative T waves in anterolateral leads. Echocardiography and cardiac magnetic resonance imaging showed a TTC-shaped left ventricle with apical ballooning. Genetic analysis revealed that the patient was a carrier of the so-called premutation, a condition intermediate between the normal copy number of triplets and pathologic expansion of the genetic region (she had 80 copies of the codon).

Fragile X syndrome has been associated with many cardiovascular abnormalities, including low vagal tone,[42] coronary arterial-to-LV fistula,[43] cerebral perfusion abnormalities,[44] low heart-rate variability,[45] mitral valve prolapse, aortic root dilation,[46] manifestation in late childhood,[47,48] tubular hypoplasia of the aorta, and a mild coarctation.[49] Model studies have implied a role for fragile X mental retardation (FMR) in the development of cardiac phenotypes, such as abnormalities of striated muscle development, significant reduction in cardiac function, and abnormal development of cardiac embryogenesis.[50] This single case provides a possible indication of an influence of FMR on fragile X gene and TTC, which could explain the more frequent female expression of the cardiomyopathy. As such the expression of expanded FMR1 allele on the X-chromosome in a conductor of fragile X syndrome may explain the preferential occurrence of TTC in women. These patients could suffer transient cardiac events such as emotional stress–induced cardiomyopathy.[36]

CD36 Deficiency

In 2005, Kushiro and colleagues[51] reported on a 71-year-old woman suffering from chest pain and dyspnea following an argument. On admission, signs of congestive heart failure were present. Chest radiography showed cardiomegaly (cardiothoracic ratio: 56%), ECG showed negative T waves on the precordial leads, cardiac enzymes were normal, and an echo scan showed typical features of TTC (confirmed by ventriculography). Coronary angiography was normal. ^{201}Tl-labeled myocardial single-photon emission computed tomography (SPECT) showed normal accumulation at 2 weeks after admission, but ^{123}I-metaiodobenzylguanidine SPECT revealed areas of decreased accumulation at the apex at 3 weeks,

which recovered at 8 weeks. Abnormal metabolism of cardiac free fatty acids was suggested by the lack of accumulation shown by ^{123}I-β-methyl-p-iodophenyl pentadecanoic acid SPECT at 7 weeks after admission. Flow-cytometry analysis demonstrated a lack of CD36 expression in platelets, monocytes, and macrophages, and genetic analysis revealed 2 different mutations, occurring in heterozygosis: P90S and an insertion of A at nucleotide 1159. Both mutations have been previously described in patients with type I CD36 deficiency. CD36 deficiency can lead to an imbalance in the metabolism of fatty acids and oxidized low-density lipoprotein, a potential mechanism explaining the development of coronary artery disease and atherosclerosis. A possible link between CD36 deficiency and TTC is also suggested by the increased occurrence of both diseases in Japanese people in comparison with other populations.

Heart-Hand Syndrome

Danese and colleagues[52] reported an association between ABS following a quarrel and brachydactyly. The hypothesis of a link between diseases arises from the well-known recognized association between skeletal malformation and other systems involvement, and often the heart can be compromised (the so-called heart-hand syndrome).

Long-QT Syndrome

TTC has been associated with long-QT syndrome and torsades de pointes in single and recurrent episodes.[53,54] A young woman presented with TTC after a syncopal attack caused by torsades de pointes. The patient had a sporadic long-QT syndrome, and TTC was thought to arise from the syncopal attack caused by torsades de pointes.[54] Ghosh and colleagues[55] described a case of TTC cardiomyopathy causing QT prolongation and torsades de pointes in an emotionally distressed woman, with cardiac recovery in a week, and suggested TTC as the cause of long-QT syndrome and torsades de pointes. Prolongation of QT interval in TTC can be also due to an abnormality of repolarization caused by genetic variations, leading to an increase of the risk of sudden death.[56] Indeed, the association between the disease has been found in a patient carrying a mutation in the Per-Arnt-Sim domain of hERG1.[57]

SUMMARY

TTC is an enigmatic disease with a multifactorial and a still unresolved pathogenesis. To explain transient myocardial damage many mechanisms have been proposed, including myocardial dysfunction mediated through catecholamine-induced damage, coronary artery spasm or dysfunction, and neurally mediated myocardial stunning. Recent experimental and clinical observation has suggested a role for genetics in the pathogenesis of TTC. In recent years technological advances in exome capture and DNA sequencing have given clinicians a new opportunity to discover genetics-related disease.[58] Large prospective genetic studies using such techniques probably will shed new light on understanding the pathogenesis of this peculiar syndrome.

REFERENCES

1. Satoh H, Tateishi H, Uchida T. Takotsubo-type cardiomyopathy due to multivessel spasm. In: Kodama K, Haze K, Hon M, editors. Clinical aspect of myocardial injury: from ischemia to heart failure (in Japanese). Tokyo: Kagakuhyouronsya Co; 1990. p. 56–64.

2. Dorfman TA, Aqel R, Mahew M, et al. Tako-tsubo cardiomyopathy: a review of the literature. Curr Cardiol Rev 2007;3:137–42.

3. Citro R, Rigo F, Previtali M, et al. Differences in clinical features and in-hospital outcomes of older adults with tako-tsubo cardiomyopathy. J Am Geriatr Soc 2012;60:93–8.

4. Hurst RT, Prasad A, Askew JW 3rd, et al. Takotsubo cardiomyopathy: a unique cardiomyopathy with variable ventricular morphology. JACC Cardiovasc Imaging 2010;3:641–9.

5. Citro R, Caso I, Provenza G, et al. Right ventricular involvement and pulmonary hypertension in an elderly woman with tako-tsubo cardiomyopathy. Chest 2010;137:973–5.

6. Von Bergen NH, Lyon JK, Edens RE. Takotsubo-like cardiomyopathy in a 17-year-old male with a pheochromocytoma. Pediatr Cardiol 2009;30:184–7.

7. Izumi Y, Okatani H, Shiota M, et al. Effects of metoprolol on epinephrine-induced takotsubo-like left ventricular dysfunction in non-human primates. Hypertens Res 2009;32:339–46.

8. Nanda S, Pamula J, Bhatt SP, et al. Takotsubo cardiomyopathy: a new variant and widening disease spectrum. Int J Cardiol 2007;120:34–6.

9. Citro R, Previtali M, Bovelli D, et al. Chronobiological patterns of onset of Tako-Tsubo cardiomyopathy: a multicenter Italian study. J Am Coll Cardiol 2009;54:180–1.

10. Prasad A, Lerman A, Rihal CS. Apical ballooning syndrome (Tako-Tsubo or stress cardiomyopathy): a mimic of acute myocardial infarction. Am Heart J 2008;155:408–17.

11. Wittstein IS, Thiemann DR, Lima JA, et al. Neurohumoral features of myocardial stunning due to sudden emotional stress. N Engl J Med 2005;352:539–48.

12. Fineschi V, Silver MD, Karch SB. Myocardial disarray: an architectural disorganization linked with adrenergic stress? Int J Cardiol 2005;99:277–82.

13. Nef HM, Mollmann H, Kostin S, et al. Tako-tsubo cardiomyopathy: intraindividual structural analysis in the acute phase and after functional recovery. Eur Heart J 2007;28:2456–64.

14. Kawano H, Okada R, Yano K, et al. Histological study on the distribution of autonomic nerves in the human heart. Heart Vessels 2003;18:32–9.

15. Ueyama T. Emotional stress-induced Tako-tsubo cardiomyopathy: animal model and molecular mechanism. Ann N Y Acad Sci 2004;1018:437–44.

16. Kuo BT, Choubey R, Novaro GM. Reduced estrogen in menopause may predispose women to takotsubo cardiomyopathy. Gend Med 2010;7:71–7.

17. Ibañez B, Navarro F, Farré J, et al. Tako-Tsubo transient left ventricular apical ballooning is associated with a left anterior descending coronary artery with a long course along the apical diaphragmatic surface of the left ventricle. Rev Esp Cardiol 2004;57:209–16.

18. Ibañez B, Navarro F, Cordoba M, et al. Tako-tsubo transient left ventricular apical ballooning: is intravascular ultrasound the key to resolve the enigma? Heart 2005;91:102–4.

19. Ako J, Takenaka K, Uno K, et al. Reversible left ventricular systolic dysfunction—reversibility of coronary microvascular abnormality. Jpn Heart J 2001;42:355–63.

20. Daniels DV, Fearon W. The index of microcirculatory resistance (IMR) in takotsubo cardiomyopathy. Catheter Cardiovasc Interv 2011;77:128–31.

21. Citro R, Galderisi M, Maione AG, et al. Sequential transthoracic ultrasound assessment of coronary flow reserve in a patient with tako-tsubo syndrome. J Am Soc Echocardiogr 2006;19:1402–8.

22. Rigo F, Sicari R, Citro R, et al. Diffuse, marked, reversible impairment in coronary microcirculation in stress cardiomyopathy: a Doppler transthoracic echo study. Ann Med 2009;41:462–70.

23. Bugiardini R, Bairey Merz CN. Angina with "normal" coronary arteries: a changing philosophy. JAMA 2005;293:477–84.

24. El Mahmoud RN, Mansencal N, Pilliére R, et al. Prevalence and characteristics of left ventricular outflow tract obstruction in Tako-Tsubo syndrome. Am Heart J 2008;156:543–8.

25. Bang DW, Chung JW, Hyon MS, et al. Proteomic analysis of serum in patients with apical ballooning syndrome. Int J Cardiol 2011 Jan 7;146(1):118–9.

26. Lyon AR, Rees PS, Prasad S, et al. Stress (Takotsubo) cardiomyopathy—a novel pathophysiological hypothesis to explain catecholamine-induced acute myocardial stunning. Nat Clin Pract Cardiovasc Med 2008;5:22–9.

27. Nef HM, Möllmann H, Troidl C, et al. Expression profiling of cardiac genes in Tako-Tsubo

cardiomyopathy: insight into a new cardiac entity. J Mol Cell Cardiol 2008 Feb;44(2):395–404.

28. Pison L, De Vusser P, Mullens W, et al. Apical ballooning in relatives. Heart 2004;90:67–9.

29. Cherian J, Angelis D, Filiberti A, et al. Can takotsubo cardiomyopathy be familial? Int J Cardiol 2007;121:74–5.

30. Kumar G, Holmes DR Jr, Prasad A. "Familial" apical ballooning syndrome (Takotsubo cardiomyopathy). Int J Cardiol 2010;144:444–5.

31. Vriz O, Minisini R, Citro R, et al. Analysis of beta1 and beta2-adrenergic receptors polymorphism in patients with apical ballooning cardiomyopathy. Acta Cardiol 2011;66:787–90.

32. Spinelli L, Trimarco V, Di Marino S, et al. L41Q polymorphism of the G protein coupled receptor kinase 5 is associated with left ventricular apical ballooning syndrome. Eur J Heart Fail 2010;12:13–6.

33. Sharkey SW, Maron BJ, Nelson P, et al. Adrenergic receptor polymorphisms in patients with stress (tako-tsubo) cardiomyopathy. J Cardiol 2009;53:53–7.

34. Zaroff JG, Pawlikowska L, Miss JC, et al. Adrenoceptor polymorphisms and the risk of cardiac injury and dysfunction after subarachnoid hemorrhage. Stroke 2006;37:1680–5.

35. Handy AD, Prasad A, Olson TM. Investigating genetic variation of adrenergic receptors in familial stress cardiomyopathy (apical ballooning syndrome). J Cardiol 2009;54:516–7.

36. Kleinfeldt T, Schneider H, Akin I, et al. Detection of FMR1-gene in Takotsubo cardiomyopathy: a new piece in the puzzle. Int J Cardiol 2009;137:81–3.

37. Workman AJ. Cardiac adrenergic control and atrial fibrillation. Naunyn Schmiedebergs Arch Pharmacol 2010;381:235–49.

38. Small KM, Forbes SL, Rahman FF, et al. A four amino acid deletion polymorphism in the third intracellular loop of the human alpha 2C-adrenergic receptor confers impaired coupling to multiple effectors. J Biol Chem 2000;275:23059–64.

39. Ueyama T, Yoshida K, Senba E. Emotional stress induces expression of immediate early genes in rat heart via activation of α- and β-adrenoceptors. Am J Physiol Heart Circ Physiol 1999;277:1553–61.

40. Long AD, Langley CH. The power of association studies to detect the contribution of candidate genetic loci to variation in complex traits. Genome Res 2009;9:720–31.

41. Yang Y, Li SS, Chien JW, et al. A systematic search for SNPs/haplotypes associated with disease phenotypes using a haplotype-based stepwise procedure. BMC Genet 2008;22:99–100.

42. Roberts JE, Tonnsen B, Robinson A, et al. Heart activity and autistic behavior in infants and toddlers with fragile X syndrome. Am J Intellect Dev Disabil 2012;117:90–102.

43. Koganti S, Gunarathne A, Desai P, et al. A rare type of 'coronary arterial-left ventricular fistula' via thebesian veins in a Fragile X syndrome carrier. Cardiol J 2011;18:318–9.

44. Kabakus N, Aydin M, Akin H, et al. Fragile X syndrome and cerebral perfusion abnormalities: single-photon emission computed tomographic study. J Child Neurol 2006;21:1040–6.

45. Roberts JE, Boccia ML, Bailey DB Jr, et al. Cardiovascular indices of physiological arousal in boys with fragile X syndrome. Dev Psychobiol 2001;39:107–23.

46. Loehr JP, Synhorst DP, Wolfe RR, et al. Aortic root dilatation and mitral valve prolapse in the fragile X syndrome. Am J Med Genet 1986;23:189–294.

47. Crabbe LS, Bensky AS, Hornstein L, et al. Cardiovascular abnormalities in children with fragile X syndrome. Pediatrics 1993;91:714–5.

48. Sreeram N, Wren C, Bhate M, et al. Cardiac abnormalities in the fragile X syndrome. Br Heart J 1989;61:289–91.

49. Waldstein G, Hagerman R. Aortic hypoplasia and cardiac valvular abnormalities in a boy with fragile X syndrome. Am J Med Genet 1988;30:83–98.

50. Van't Padje S, Chaudhry B, Severijnen LA, et al. Reduction in fragile X related 1 protein causes cardiomyopathy and muscular dystrophy in zebrafish. J Exp Biol 2009;212:2564–70.

51. Kushiro T, Saito F, Kusama J, et al. Takotsubo-shaped cardiomyopathy with type I CD36 deficiency. Heart Vessels 2005;20:123–35.

52. Danese C, Bocchini S, Rubini G, et al. Takotsubo syndrome and brachydactyly: a new heart-hand syndrome? Clin Ter 2011;162:41–4.

53. Elkhateeb OE, Beydoun HK. Recurrent long QT syndrome and syncope in transient apical ballooning syndrome (takotsubo cardiomyopathy). Can J Cardiol 2008;24:917–9.

54. Sasaki O, Nishioka T, Akima T, et al. Association of takotsubo cardiomyopathy and long QT syndrome. Circ J 2006;70:1220–2.

55. Ghosh S, Apte P, Maroz N, et al. Takotsubo cardiomyopathy as a potential cause of long QT syndrome and torsades de pointes. Int J Cardiol 2009;136:225–7.

56. Mahida S, Dalageorgou C, Behr ER. Long-QT syndrome and torsades de pointes in a patient with Takotsubo cardiomyopathy: an unusual case. Europace 2009;11:376–88.

57. Grilo LS, Pruvot E, Grobéty M, et al. Takotsubo cardiomyopathy and congenital long QT syndrome in a patient with a novel duplication in the Per-Arnt-Sim (PAS) domain of hERG1. Heart Rhythm 2010;7:260–5.

58. Bamshad MJ, Ng SB, Bigham AW, et al. Exome sequencing as a tool for Mendelian disease gene discovery. Nat Rev Genet 2011;12:745–55.

Brain-Heart Interaction in Takotsubo Cardiomyopathy

Judith Z. Goldfinger, MD[a], Ajith Nair, MD[a],
Brett A. Sealove, MD, RPVI[b],*

KEYWORDS

- Takotsubo cardiomyopathy • Stress cardiomyopathy • Apical ballooning syndrome
- Sympathetic activation

KEY POINTS

- Takotsubo cardiomyopathy (TTC) is a novel, yet well-described, predominately reversible cardio-myopathy triggered by profound psychological or physical stress.
- Despite medical literature that spans over 25 years, much is still unknown regarding the pathogenesis of TTC.
- It seems that through a complex interaction between the brain and catecholamine-mediated stimulation, myocardial stunning and subsequent stress-related myocardial dysfunction occurs in those postmenopausal patients most susceptible to this disease.
- Insights into the mechanisms that underlie takotsubo cardiomyopathy may shed light on other cardiomyopathies and on the brain's influence on cardiac disease.

INTRODUCTION

Takotsubo cardiomyopathy was first described in 1991 in Japan as reversible myocardial stunning.[1] This cardiomyopathy, now known to be stress induced, has also been called broken heart syndrome or left ventricular apical ballooning syndrome. The original Japanese article presented 5 patients with symptoms, electrocardiographic changes, and cardiac enzymes elevations consistent with acute myocardial infarction but at cardiac catheterization were found to have segmental left ventricular akinesis on ventriculogram with angiographically normal coronaries.[2] A hallmark of takotsubo cardiomyopathy is that left ventricular wall motion abnormalities do not correspond to the distribution of a specific epicardial coronary artery, indicating that coronary perfusion is likely not a cause of the ventricular dysfunction.[3,4] An alternative explanation for the unique clinical characteristics of takotsubo cardiomyopathy has been proposed by Ibanez and colleagues.[5] They suggested that a ruptured atherosclerotic plaque and occlusion of a variant left anterior descending artery (one extending apically and diaphragmatically) followed by early reperfusion was the cause in a selected group of patients. However, this theory has been questioned by more contemporary studies.

Although takotsubo cardiomyopathy may present like a myocardial infarction, it has 2 distinctive features. First, takotsubo cardiomyopathy is more likely to affect postmenopausal women than other demographic groups.[2,4,6] Second, most patients can identify a physical or emotional stressor that preceded their symptoms.[7] Both of these features were identified in early reports and have been recognized in subsequent studies. Although the exact mechanism for left ventricular dysfunction in takotsubo cardiomyopathy has yet to be fully elucidated, the specific population that is affected and the presence of a preceding trigger have focused attention

[a] Cardiovascular Institute, Mount Sinai Medical Center, 1 Gustave L. Levy Place, Box 1030, New York, NY 10029, USA; [b] Monmouth Cardiology Associates, LLC, 301 Bingham Avenue, Suite C, Ocean, NJ 07712, USA
* Corresponding author.
E-mail address: bsealove@monmouthcardiology.com

Heart Failure Clin 9 (2013) 217–223
http://dx.doi.org/10.1016/j.hfc.2012.12.013
1551-7136/13/$ – see front matter Crown Copyright © 2013 Published by Elsevier Inc. All rights reserved.

on the connection between stress and the heart (**Fig. 1**).

In this article, the authors focus on 4 elements of the brain-heart interaction in takotsubo cardiomyopathy: the stressors that trigger takotsubo, mechanisms leading to myocardial dysfunction, factors that increase susceptibility, and psychological factors that affect the course or prognosis of the condition.

PHYSICAL OR EMOTIONAL STRESS AND TAKOTSUBO

More than 7 out of 10 patients with takotsubo cardiomyopathy describe a physical or emotional stressor that preceded the onset of their symptoms.[8–10] Acute, severe, emotional stressors, such as accidents, deaths, quarrels, and life-changing events, have classically been implicated as triggers of takotsubo cardiomyopathy, although less intense events have also been reported, such as news of an unexpected death, fear or anxiety, work-related problems, or a diagnosis of malignancy. In addition, physical stressors, such as surgery, respiratory failure, malignancy, or chemotherapy, and a variety of less common triggers, including falls, seizures, and strokes, have all been reported with varying degrees in the literature.[11,12] For example, after a series of earthquakes in Niigata, Japan in 2004, the incidence of both acute myocardial infarction and takotsubo cardiomyopathy increased dramatically.[13,14] In the 4 weeks before the earthquake, there was one case of takotsubo cardiomyopathy in the district where the earthquake occurred compared with 25 cases in the 4 weeks afterward. Similar to other cases of takotsubo cardiomyopathy, postmenopausal women were disproportionately affected.[15]

The link between stress and the development of ballooning of the left ventricle is not well understood, although the relationship is likely mediated by excess catecholamines. Pheochromocytoma can cause a takotsubolike cardiomyopathy.[16–18] Exogenous epinephrine and dobutamine can create the clinical picture of takotsubo cardiomyopathy, including electrocardiographic changes, cardiac enzyme elevation, and left ventricular dysfunction.[19,20]

In a series of experiments with rats, Ueyama and colleagues[21] showed that immobilization, a source of emotional stress for a rat led to ST segment elevations on electrocardiogram. The combination of an alpha- and beta-blocker restored the ST segments to normal. They next showed that the rat's emotional stress caused generalized left ventricular hypokinesis on ventriculography, including apical ballooning, and these changes were also reversed with the combination of an alpha- and beta-blocker.[8,21] Similarly, in patients with subarachnoid hemorrhages, those who developed ST changes

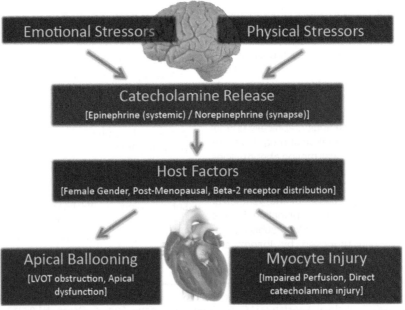

Fig. 1. Brain-heart interaction in takotsubo cardiomyopathy. Emotional and physical stressors can lead to a release of catecholamines. Susceptible patients include postmenopausal female patients. Other host factors can lead to apical cardiodepression with apical ballooning, basal hyperdynamic motion, and left ventricular outflow tract (LVOT) obstruction. Excessive catecholamines can lead to impaired perfusion and direct injury leading to myocyte necrosis.

on electrocardiograms can develop apical hypokinesis or akinesis in the absence of coronary artery disease.[22]

A phenomenon of "electrolyte–steroid–cardiomyopathy with necroses" was first described in the 1950s and includes cardiac lesions caused by specific steroids or hormones.[23] This pathologic process, also called coagulative myocytolysis or contraction band necrosis, describes a unique form of myocyte injury seen in high catecholamine states, such as pheochromocytoma and subarachnoid hemorrhage. Myocytes are hypercontracted with early myofibrillar damage and dense eosinophilic transverse banding.[12,24]

MECHANISMS LEADING TO MYOCARDIAL DYSFUNCTION

Takotsubo cardiomyopathy is one subtype of stress-related cardiomyopathies. These stress cardiomyopathies also include acute ventricular dysfunction associated with subarachnoid hemorrhages and strokes, ventricular dysfunction related to pheochromocytomas, and ventricular dysfunction in the critically ill.[25] In 1942, Dr W.B. Cannon described *voodoo death* whereby severe emotional distress could lead to sudden cardiac death.[26] Cannon and others postulated that a lasting, overwhelming stimulation of the sympathetic and adrenal system led to myocardial damage and, in some cases, sudden cardiac death. In most cases, neurocardiogenic stunning was most commonly seen with severe neurologic injury, female gender, plasma troponin release, and elevated brain natriuretic peptide levels. The insular cortex, through interactions with other centers including the amygdala and hippocampus, is thought to mediate activation of the medullary autonomic center. Through presynaptic and postsynaptic neuron excitation, there is norepinephrine release and increased adrenomedullary output leading to epinephrine release.[27,28] The role of insular activation and injury in causing adverse cardiac consequences, including ventricular arrhythmias, has been shown in patients with subarachnoid hemorrhages and lesions involving the right insular cortex.[29] In animal models of strokes, occlusion of the right middle cerebral artery resulted in neurochemical abnormalities in the ipsilateral insular cortex and amygdala and subsequent increased sympathetic output and norepinephrine release. Strokes involving the hypothalamus and experimental stimulation of the hypothalamus can also lead to sympathetic hyperstimulation.[30] In fact, roughly 20% to 30% of patients with subarachnoid hemorrhage (SAH) can develop a secondary cardiomyopathy or regional wall motion abnormalities, which is usually reversible in the absence of underlying coronary artery disease.[31] However, patients with SAH differ from those with typical takotsubo cardiomyopathy in that the most common wall motion abnormalities are hypokinesis of the basal and midventricular segments with sparing of the apical segments.[32]

Increased levels of norepinephrine and epinephrine can activate adrenergic receptors and cause enhanced myocardial adenosine 3′,5′-cyclic monophosphate production. This production can cause direct myocardial injury through calcium overload, which prolongs actin-myosin interaction and depletes ATP.[33] Further injury is mediated through oxygen free radicals. Indeed, the levels of catecholamines are two- to threefold higher in patients with takotsubo cardiomyopathy than in matched patients with myocardial infarctions.[34] Furthermore, the endomyocardial biopsy results of patients with takotsubo cardiomyopathy have demonstrated mononuclear infiltrates and contraction-band necrosis, consistent with catecholamine-associated injury.

Most of the injury involves the apex. The predominance of apical involvement is not clear, although it may be related to increased apical myocardial sensitivity to sympathetic stimulation and increased density of catecholamine receptors despite sparse sympathetic innervation.[35] A study by Paur and colleagues[36] suggested that the acute apical cardiodepression of takotsubo cardiomyopathy was predicated on the differential response of beta-2 adrenergic receptors to concentrations of epinephrine and an apical-basal gradient of beta-2 receptors. In a rat model, a rapid infusion of epinephrine reproduced the takotsubo phenotype, whereas an equivalent norepinephrine bolus did not. Furthermore, beta-2 receptor density and sensitivity was greater at the apex than at the base, and there was biased agonism of epinephrine for beta-2 receptors. Low epinephrine concentrations acted as a cardiostimulant through stimulatory G-protein–activation, whereas high epinephrine concentrations led to a cardiodepressant effect through inhibitory G-protein–activation. It was postulated that this inhibitory response likely evolved as a mechanism to attenuate catecholamine-induced myocardial injury during acute stress.

SUSCEPTIBILITY TO TAKOTSUBO CARDIOMYOPATHY

Postmenopausal women are disproportionately affected by takotsubo cardiomyopathy.[11,34,37] In a registry of patients with takotsubo, 95% were postmenopausal women.[38] In a systematic review, which included 28 case series and a total of

563 patients, 90.7% of the patients with takotsubo were women ranging from 62 to 76 years of age.[39]

Brenner and colleagues[40] studied 17 women with takotsubo cardiomyopathy, 16 age-matched controls with acute myocardial infarction, and 15 women with normal coronary arteries and measured estradiol, progesterone, luteinizing hormone, and follicle-stimulating hormone. They found that estradiol and progesterone levels were significantly higher in the patients with takotsubo during the acute event. The investigators concluded that higher levels of estrogen and progesterone provided an atheroprotective benefit but may have diverted the stress response to stress cardiomyopathy. However, conflicting results were found in an animal study. In 36 rats that had undergone ovariectomy, half were given supplemental estradiol and then all were subjected to the stress of immobilization.[41] Estrogen supplementation attenuated the tachycardia experienced by the rats. It was also associated with increases in cardioprotective mRNAs and decreases in levels of c-fos in the brain, the right and left ventricle, and adrenal glands, consistent with a decrease in sympathetic-adrenal outflow.

There has been speculation that women may have more epinephrine stores available for sudden release, which may explain the female predilection for in takotsubo cardiomyopathy.[42] Likewise, reduced estrogen levels in postmenopausal women may alter endothelial function, causing greater susceptibility to sympathetic-mediated myocardial stunning and stress-related myocardial dysfunction.[41]

Takotsubo may be more likely to occur in people with preexisting mood disorders. In a cohort of 110 patients with takotsubo cardiomyopathy, Mudd and Kass described a 40% prevalence of depression or anxiety.[43] In a retrospective case control study in Olmsted County, Minnesota, the investigators identified 25 female patients with takotsubo and compared them to 25 patients with acute myocardial infarction and 50 patients matched for age and sex. The takotsubo group had higher rates of anxiety, depression, substance abuse, and history of either physical or emotional abuse. They were also more likely to live alone.[44] In a registry of patients with takotsubo who were drawn from 2 major hospitals in Rhode Island, 37% had preexisting depression or anxiety.[38] Vidi and colleagues[45] looked at cases of takotsubo presenting to one hospital in Massachusetts and found that 21% of 34 patients with takotsubo had depression or anxiety. In many of these studies, depression and anxiety were studied as one variable. Notably, patients with takotsubo did not have a more frequent high-anxiety trait than patients presenting with ST elevation myocardial infarction.[46]

Depression may increase susceptibility to takotsubo through effects on endogenous catecholamines. Some patients with depression have high levels of systemic and cardiac catecholamines and reduced cardiac norepinephrine uptake, which leads to the accumulation of norepinephrine in the synapse.[47] Patients with depression can have an exaggerated norepinephrine response to emotional stress, with more severe depression correlating to higher plasma levels of norepinephrine.[48] Interestingly, it is not clear whether the use of antidepressants, specifically selective norepinephrine reuptake inhibitors, may contribute to takotsubo by increasing local catecholamine levels.[24] Patients with depression, thus, have a double hit of unusually high catecholamine responses and greater cardiac sympathetic sensitivity, which increases their risk for takotsubo after stress but may also increase the risk for cardiac events in general.[49]

FACTORS THAT AFFECT PROGNOSIS

Although initial imaging studies demonstrated ejection fractions from 20% to 40%, most patients normalize to 60% to 75%. Cardiac biomarkers are often only mildly elevated and are usually maximal at initial presentation. In-hospital mortality rates can be up to 8%, but patients can recover with supportive care aimed at dealing with cardiogenic shock, outflow tract obstruction, and the heightened catecholamine state associated with takotsubo cardiomyopathy.[4] Specifically, intra-aortic counterpulsation therapy or temporary mechanical support may be required in some patients with cardiogenic shock. Likewise, outflow tract obstruction may require careful fluid resuscitation in addition to beta-blocker therapy. In a rat model of takotsubo cardiomyopathy, levosimendan improved cardiac function without increasing mortality.[36] Levosimendan was effective because its mechanism of action was independent of cyclic-AMP at low doses, thus, leading to an improvement in apical function.

Although most patients recover from takotsubo, a small subset develops severe persistent heart failure. In a series of 88 patients, the overall in-hospital mortality rate was 1%. Despite this relatively benign prognosis, cardiogenic shock and ventricular fibrillation have been reported in as many as 4.2% and 1.5% of patients, respectively.[50] The benefit of implantable cardioverter-defibrillators is unclear, but routine use does not seem warranted because most patients recover myocardial function.[51]

In a retrospective study of 118 patients, the development of acute heart failure was associated with older age and having a stressor that was physical and not emotional.[3] The study's investigators suggested that physical stressors may lead to a more sustained catecholamine surge than emotional stressors. In a smaller study, among 27 patients identified with takotsubo cardiomyopathy over a 5-year period, 14 patients (52%) reached a combined end point of all-cause death, cardiogenic shock, sudden cardiac death, and rehospitalization for cardiac reasons. The patients fit the typical demographics of takotsubo cardiomyopathy because 96% were women with a mean age of 68 ± 14 years, and the study suggested a worse long-term outcome than what was previously reported.[52] The overall recurrence rate of apical ballooning syndrome was shown to be 11.4% in a series of 100 patients with a confirmed diagnosis of takotsubo cardiomyopathy by angiography.[53]

SUMMARY

Takotsubo cardiomyopathy is a novel, yet well-described, predominately reversible cardiomyopathy triggered by profound psychological or physical stress. Despite medical literature that spans over 25 years, much is still unknown regarding the pathogenesis of this disease. It seems, however, that through a complex interaction between the brain and catecholamine-mediated stimulation, myocardial stunning and subsequent stress-related myocardial dysfunction occurs in those postmenopausal patients most susceptible to this disease. Insights into the mechanisms that underlie takotsubo cardiomyopathy may shed light on other cardiomyopathies and on the brain's influence on cardiac disease.

REFERENCES

1. Sealove BA, Tiyyagura S, Fuster V. Takotsubo cardiomyopathy. J Gen Intern Med 2008;23(11):1904–8.
2. Dote K, Sato H, Tateishi H, et al. Myocardial stunning due to simultaneous multivessel coronary spasms: a review of 5 cases. J Cardiol 1991;21(2):203–14 [in Japanese].
3. Madhavan M, Rihal CS, Lerman A, et al. Acute heart failure in apical ballooning syndrome (TakoTsubo/stress cardiomyopathy): clinical correlates and Mayo Clinic risk score. J Am Coll Cardiol 2011;57(12):1400–1.
4. Bybee KA, Kara T, Prasad A, et al. Systematic review: transient left ventricular apical ballooning: a syndrome that mimics ST-segment elevation myocardial infarction. Ann Intern Med 2004;141(11):858–65.
5. Ibanez B, Navarro F, Cordoba M, et al. Tako-tsubo transient left ventricular apical ballooning: is intra-vascular ultrasound the key to resolve the enigma? Heart 2005;91(1):102–4.
6. Akashi YJ, Nakazawa K, Sakakibara M, et al. The clinical features of takotsubo cardiomyopathy. QJM 2003;96(8):563–73.
7. Seth PS, Aurigemma GP, Krasnow JM, et al. A syndrome of transient left ventricular apical wall motion abnormality in the absence of coronary disease: a perspective from the United States. Cardiology 2003;100(2):61–6.
8. Akashi YJ, Musha H, Kida K, et al. Reversible ventricular dysfunction takotsubo cardiomyopathy. Eur J Heart Fail 2005;7(7):1171–6.
9. Eitel I, von Knobelsdorff-Brenkenhoff F, Bernhardt P, et al. Clinical characteristics and cardiovascular magnetic resonance findings in stress (takotsubo) cardiomyopathy. JAMA 2011;306(3):277–86.
10. Tsuchihashi K, Ueshima K, Uchida T, et al. Transient left ventricular apical ballooning without coronary artery stenosis: a novel heart syndrome mimicking acute myocardial infarction. Angina Pectoris-Myocardial Infarction Investigations in Japan. J Am Coll Cardiol 2001;38(1):11–8.
11. Vieweg WV, Hasnain M, Mezuk B, et al. Depression, stress, and heart disease in earthquakes and takotsubo cardiomyopathy. Am J Med 2011;124(10):900–7.
12. Wittstein IS. Apical-ballooning syndrome. Lancet 2007;370(9587):545–7.
13. Tagawa M, Nakamura Y, Ishiguro M, et al. Transient left ventricular apical ballooning developing after the Central Niigata Prefecture earthquake: two case reports. J Cardiol 2006;48(3):153–8.
14. Watanabe H, Kodama M, Okura Y, et al. Impact of earthquakes on takotsubo cardiomyopathy. JAMA 2005;294(3):305–7.
15. Sato M, Fujita S, Saito A, et al. Increased incidence of transient left ventricular apical ballooning (so-called 'takotsubo' cardiomyopathy) after the mid-Niigata Prefecture earthquake. Circ J 2006;70(8):947–53.
16. Agarwal V, Kant G, Hans N, et al. Takotsubo-like cardiomyopathy in pheochromocytoma. Int J Cardiol 2011;153(3):241–8.
17. Chia PL, Foo D. Tako-tsubo cardiomyopathy precipitated by pheochromocytoma crisis. Cardiol J 2011;18(5):564–7.
18. Lassnig E, Weber T, Auer J, et al. Pheochromocytoma crisis presenting with shock and tako-tsubo-like cardiomyopathy. Int J Cardiol 2009;134(3):e138–40.
19. Abraham J, Mudd JO, Kapur NK, et al. Stress cardiomyopathy after intravenous administration of

catecholamines and beta-receptor agonists. J Am Coll Cardiol 2009;53(15):1320–5.

20. Lubitz SA, Duvall WL, Kim MC, et al. Dobutamine-induced myocardial infarction with normal coronary arteries during stress SPECT myocardial perfusion imaging. J Nucl Cardiol 2007;14(4):613–6.

21. Ueyama T, Yoshida K, Senba E. Stress-induced elevation of the ST segment in the rat electrocardiogram is normalized by an adrenoceptor blocker. Clin Exp Pharmacol Physiol 2000;27(5–6):384–6.

22. Novitzky D, Wicomb WN, Cooper DK, et al. Prevention of myocardial injury during brain death by total cardiac sympathectomy in the Chacma baboon. Ann Thorac Surg 1986;41(5):520–4.

23. Samuels MA. The brain-heart connection. Circulation 2007;116(1):77–84.

24. Wittstein IS. Stress cardiomyopathy: a syndrome of catecholamine-mediated myocardial stunning? Cell Mol Neurobiol 2012;32:847–57.

25. Bybee KA, Prasad A. Stress-related cardiomyopathy syndromes. Circulation 2008;118(4):397–409.

26. Cannon WB. "Voodoo" death. American Anthropologist, 1942;44(new series):169-181. Am J Public Health 2002;92(10):1593–6 [discussion: 1594–5].

27. Cheshire WP Jr, Saper CB. The insular cortex and cardiac response to stroke. Neurology 2006;66(9):1296–7.

28. Cheung RT, Hachinski V. The insula and cerebrogenic sudden death. Arch Neurol 2000;57(12):1685–8.

29. Mayer SA, Lin J, Homma S, et al. Myocardial injury and left ventricular performance after subarachnoid hemorrhage. Stroke 1999;30(4):780–6.

30. Samuels MA. Neurogenic heart disease: a unifying hypothesis. Am J Cardiol 1987;60(18):15J–9J.

31. Banki N, Kopelnik A, Tung P, et al. Prospective analysis of prevalence, distribution, and rate of recovery of left ventricular systolic dysfunction in patients with subarachnoid hemorrhage. J Neurosurg 2006;105(1):15–20.

32. Zaroff JG, Rordorf GA, Ogilvy CS, et al. Regional patterns of left ventricular systolic dysfunction after subarachnoid hemorrhage: evidence for neurally mediated cardiac injury. J Am Soc Echocardiogr 2000;13(8):774–9.

33. Richard C. Stress-related cardiomyopathies. Ann Intensive Care 2011;1(1):39.

34. Wittstein IS, Thiemann DR, Lima JA, et al. Neurohumoral features of myocardial stunning due to sudden emotional stress. N Engl J Med 2005;352(6):539–48.

35. Mori H, Ishikawa S, Kojima S, et al. Increased responsiveness of left ventricular apical myocardium to adrenergic stimuli. Cardiovasc Res 1993;27(2):192–8.

36. Paur H, Wright PT, Sikkel MB, et al. High levels of circulating epinephrine trigger apical cardiodepression in a beta2-adrenergic receptor/Gi-dependent manner: a new model of takotsubo cardiomyopathy. Circulation 2012;126(6):697–706.

37. Eitel I, Schuler G, Gutberlet M, et al. Biventricular stress-induced (takotsubo) cardiomyopathy with left midventricular and right apical ballooning. Int J Cardiol 2011;151(2):e63–4.

38. Regnante RA, Zuzek RW, Weinsier SB, et al. Clinical characteristics and four-year outcomes of patients in the Rhode Island Takotsubo Cardiomyopathy Registry. Am J Cardiol 2009;103(7):1015–9.

39. Pilgrim TM, Wyss TR. Takotsubo cardiomyopathy or transient left ventricular apical ballooning syndrome: a systematic review. Int J Cardiol 2008;124(3):283–92.

40. Brenner R, Weilenmann D, Maeder MT, et al. Clinical characteristics, sex hormones, and long-term follow-up in Swiss postmenopausal women presenting with takotsubo cardiomyopathy. Clin Cardiol 2012;35(6):340–7.

41. Ueyama T, Ishikura F, Matsuda A, et al. Chronic estrogen supplementation following ovariectomy improves the emotional stress-induced cardiovascular responses by indirect action on the nervous system and by direct action on the heart. Circ J 2007;71(4):565–73.

42. Lyon AR, Rees PS, Prasad S, et al. Stress (takotsubo) cardiomyopathy–a novel pathophysiological hypothesis to explain catecholamine-induced acute myocardial stunning. Nat Clin Pract Cardiovasc Med 2008;5(1):22–9.

43. Mudd JO, Kass DA. Reversing chronic remodeling in heart failure. Expert Rev Cardiovasc Ther 2007;5(3):585–98.

44. Summers MR, Lennon RJ, Prasad A. Pre-morbid psychiatric and cardiovascular diseases in apical ballooning syndrome (tako-tsubo/stress-induced cardiomyopathy): potential pre-disposing factors? J Am Coll Cardiol 2010;55(7):700–1.

45. Vidi V, Rajesh V, Singh PP, et al. Clinical characteristics of tako-tsubo cardiomyopathy. Am J Cardiol 2009;104(4):578–82.

46. Del Pace S, Parodi G, Bellandi B, et al. Anxiety trait in patients with stress-induced cardiomyopathy: a case-control study. Clin Res Cardiol 2011;100(6):523–9.

47. Barton DA, Dawood T, Lambert EA, et al. Sympathetic activity in major depressive disorder: identifying those at increased cardiac risk? J Hypertens 2007;25(10):2117–24.

48. Mausbach BT, Dimsdale JE, Ziegler MG, et al. Depressive symptoms predict norepinephrine response to a psychological stressor task in Alzheimer's caregivers. Psychosom Med 2005;67(4):638–42.

49. Ziegelstein RC. Depression and tako-tsubo cardiomyopathy. Am J Cardiol 2010;105(2):281–2.

50. Gianni M, Dentali F, Grandi AM, et al. Apical ballooning syndrome or takotsubo cardiomyopathy: a systematic review. Eur Heart J 2006;27(13):1523–9.

51. Goldfinger JZ, Choi AD, Adler ED. Implantable cardiac defibrillators and cardiac resynchronization therapy for heart failure in older adults. Geriatrics 2009;64(8):20–9.

52. Ionescu CN, Aguilar-Lopez CA, Sakr AE, et al. Long-term outcome of tako-tsubo cardiomyopathy. Heart Lung Circ 2010;19(10):601–5.

53. Elesber AA, Prasad A, Lennon RJ, et al. Four-year recurrence rate and prognosis of the apical ballooning syndrome. J Am Coll Cardiol 2007; 50(5):448–52.

Drug-induced Takotsubo Cardiomyopathy

Yasukatsu Izumi, MD, PhD

KEYWORDS

- Drug-induced • Iatrogenic • Inotropic agents • Stress cardiomyopathy
- Takotsubo cardiomyopathy

KEY POINTS

- Reports have been made about some drugs associated with direct or indirect overstimulation of the sympathetic nervous system that may cause Takotsubo cardiomyopathy (TTC).
- The common characteristic of almost all the drugs that may cause TTC is thought to be catecholamines or sympathetic excess.
- Given the limited information available, clinicians should be on the alert to suspect and recognize the possible development of drug-associated TTC.

INTRODUCTION

Takotsubo cardiomyopathy (TTC) or stress cardiomyopathy was first reported in 1991. Emotional or physical stress may play a key role in Takotsubo cardiomyopathy. Currently, left ventricular (LV) systolic dysfunction has been identified as transient LV apical ballooning syndrome and apical cardiomyopathy. TTC is an acquired, reversible cardiomyopathy that is characterized by a transient decrease in the ejection fraction without significant coronary artery disease, and by reversible LV dysfunction accompanied by akinesia involving the apical or midventricular segments.[1,2] TTC is not a rare disease and accounts for 1% of acute coronary syndrome with elevated biomarkers, such as atrial natriuretic peptide and brain natriuretic peptide. Although the etiologic mechanism of TTC remains unclear, a dramatic increase in catecholamines, such as epinephrine and norepinephrine, has been recognized as a possible causative factor in catecholamine-induced myocardial stunning and an exacerbation factor of this syndrome.[3,4] In fact, high levels of catecholamine are often seen in patients with TTC. High doses of epinephrine may be directly toxic to myocardial cells and may cause damage by inducing spasm of the coronary microvasculature or stunning of the cardiomyocytes.[3] Repeated intravenous infusion of epinephrine overdose in cynomolgus monkeys induced Takotsubo-like cardiomyopathy, characterized by severe hypokinesia in the LV apical region and hyperkinesia in the basal region.[5] Furthermore, TTC is most often seen in postmenopausal women, suggesting that estrogen deficiency may be a risk factor in the development of stress cardiomyopathy. Ueyama and colleagues[6] have reported that estrogen supplementation therapy would be a possible preventative of stress-induced TTC in postmenopausal women. Excessive sympathetic stimulation is a trigger to the pathogenesis of this disease. The aim of this article is to summarize the drugs that have been recognized as possible triggers of drug-induced TTC. The drugs that are used independently include epinephrine, norepinephrine, dobutamine, ergonovine, oxymetazoline, atropine, nortriptyline, duloxetine, venlafaxine, flourouracil (5-FU), combretastatin, cefotiam, pazopanib, anagrelide, levothyroxine, lumiracoxib, dipyridamole, and potassium chloride.[7] Commonly used drug combinations include dobutamine and atropine, epinephrine and ketamine,

Conflict of Interest: The author declares no conflict of interest.
Department of Pharmacology, Osaka City University Medical School, 1-4-3 Asahimachi, Abeno-ku, Osaka 545-8585, Japan
E-mail address: izumi@msic.med.osaka-cu.ac.jp

Heart Failure Clin 9 (2013) 225–231
http://dx.doi.org/10.1016/j.hfc.2012.12.004

epinephrine and isoproterenol, ephedrine and atropine, epinephrine and norepinephrine, ephedrine, atropine, and phenylephrine, and ephedrine, norepinephrine, and vasopressin.[7] Drug withdrawal drugs are metoprolol and oxycodone (**Table 1**).

DRUG-INDUCED TTC
Catecholamine-induced TTC

Many of the drugs that may induce TTC are believed to act secondarily to a catecholamine surge. In fact, most cases of iatrogenic TTC that have been reported are associated with sympathomimetic drugs with direct action on the sympathetic nervous system, such as epinephrine, dobutamine, ephedrine, ergonovine, and oxymetazoline, or indirect actions, such as atropine, duloxetine, nortriptyline, and venlafaxine.[7]

Sympathomimetic drugs with direct action
Much of the evidence comes from observational and case-control studies that have found an association between elevated levels of catecholamine and disease onset.[2,3,8] Direct evidence for the role of catecholamines in disease pathogenesis was obtained from animal studies that have shown that iatrogenic administration of catecholamines can lead to reversible LV apical ballooning.[5,9–11]

Although the detailed mechanism by which epinephrine can induce transient LV dysfunction is unclear, a possible mechanism is that high doses of epinephrine are directly toxic to myocardial cells. This direct toxicity is supported by histologic findings from animal studies and autopsy findings from Takotsubo patients who document myofibrillar degeneration, contraction band necrosis, and leukocyte infiltration.[5,10,11] Furthermore, in vitro studies in cultured cardiomyocytes

Table 1
Drug-induced Takotsubo cardiomyopathy

Drug	Dose	Route	Disease	Ref No.
Sympathomimetic drug with direct-acting				
Epinephrine	0.5–40 mg	IV/IM/SC/inhalator	Anaphylaxis/asthma/cervix uteri biopsy	5,9,10
			Colonscopy/keloid repair/nasal surgery	11,17
Dobutamine	6–40 µg/kg/min	IV	Dobutamine echocardiography	18,19
Ephedrine	10–50 mg	IV	Bradicardia and hypotension	20,21
Ergonovine	0.2 mg	IV	Prevention of postpartum hemorrhage	22,23
Oxymetazoline	0.05% solution	Rhinenchysis	Allergic rhinitis	24,25
Sympathomimetic drug with indirect-acting				
Atropine	0.5 mg	IV	Symptomatic bradycardia	26
Duloxetine	60 mg/d	Oral	Diabetic neuropathy	28
Nortriptyline	1000 mg	Oral	Unknown	27
Venlafaxine	Overdose	Oral	Major depression	29
Nonsympathomimetic drug				
Fluorouracil	375–750 mg/d	IV	Colon/rectal/colorectal cancer	30–32
Combretastatin	45 mg/m²	IV	Anaplastic thyroid carcinoma	34,35
Pazopanib	800 mg	Oral	Renal cell carcinoma	37
Anagrelide	1.5 mg/d	Oral	Essential thrombocytopenia	38
Levothyroxine	200 mg	Oral	Thyroid nodules	39,40
Potassium chroride	15% solution	Epidural anesthesia	Anesthesia for caesarean	41
Drug withdrawal				
Metoprolol	100 mg/d	Oral	Hypertension	42
Oxycodone	40 mg twice a day	Oral	Degenerative osteoarthritis	43

Abbreviations: IM, intramuscular; IV, intravenous; SC, subcutaneous.

have shown that high doses of epinephrine are directly toxic to the cells and result in a dramatic rise in cyclic AMP and levels of calcium that then trigger the formation of free oxygen radicals, initiation of expression of stress response genes, and induction of apoptosis in a subset of cells.[12] In response to the stress induced by catecholamines, the heart upregulates immediate early genes, heat shock proteins, and intracellular signal transduction pathways, such as mitogen-activated protein kinase pathways.[13–15] Furthermore, after a few hours of the administration of the stressor, cardiac atrial natriuretic peptide and brain natriuretic peptide mRNA expressions are upregulated as secondary responses to heart failure.[15,16] Thus, in the animal models, the molecular injury caused by catecholamines leads to an impairment of myocardial function that may persist for hours to days in the affected individual. Treatment with α-adrenoceptor and β-adrenoceptor blockers could attenuate the above gene expression significantly in response to stress in cells and animals.[5,15]

Epinephrine has been proposed to cause damage by inducing spasms of the coronary microvasculature or stunning of cardiac myocytes directly. A set of studies in animals documents that the local administration of vasodilators, such as bradykinin, improves LV function in a dog model, whereas local injection of the vasodilator nicorandil into the coronary arteries during the acute phase of the disease reduces the extent of ST-segment elevation in human patients.[9,17]

Dobutamine is a β1-selective synthetic catecholamine with a positive inotropic effect that produces an increase in myocardial contractility without significantly altering blood pressure. TTC was induced in patients without emotional or stress trigger. The only apparent initiation factor would seem to be dobutamine infusion at dobutamine-stress echocardiography (DSE). Increased apical responsiveness to adrenergic stimulation may offer a potential mechanism as to how DSE could culminate in transient apical ballooning. In addition to overstimulation of the apical adrenoceptors, dobutamine may have worsened the hyperdynamic basal systolic function, creating an artificial LV outflow tract gradient, and further stressing the myocardium. DSE is a widely performed test and is largely safe, although induction of myocardial infarction is well recognized. DSE has the potential to induce transient apical ballooning, through a combination of adrenergic overstimulation and LV midcavity obstruction.[18,19]

Ephedrine combined with phenylephrine, epinephrine, or atropine directly interacts with and activates adrenoceptors and enhances the ability to displace catecholamines from storage sites in noradrenergic nerves—thus causing sympathetic nervous system hyperactivity.[20,21] Phenylephrine, ephedrine, norepinephrine, and vasopressin likely all contribute to the patient developing TTC and ultimately to heart failure.

Like other ergot alkaloids, ergonovine generates arterial vasoconstriction by both stimulation of α-adrenergic and serotonin receptors and inhibition of endothelial-derived relaxation factor release. Ergonovine induces vasospasm and causes vasoconstriction of coronary arteries, and as a result, may induce vascular spasm and myocardial ischemia.[22,23]

Oxymetazoline belongs to the imidazoline class. With vasoconstrictive action, it is frequently used as a component of nasal decongestants and is an over-the-counter medication. It primarily stimulates the α2-adrenergic receptors of the central nervous system at low serum levels, whereas peripheral α-adrenoceptors are predominantly stimulated at higher doses. At typical doses, the major side effects are neurologic manifestations, and at higher doses, hypertension caused by vasoconstriction and tachyarrhythmias arises. Because of its vasoconstriction effect, the temporal relationship with acute coronary syndrome, and the absence of critical coronary lesions on both coronary angiography and ultrasound cardiography, a cause-and-effect relationship is suggested. Several reports correlate vasoconstrictors with acute coronary syndrome[24] and coronary spasm as the most probable mechanism in the literature.[25]

Sympathomimetic drug abuse primarily causes blood pressure elevation because of the vasoconstriction effect of these drugs. In general, intravenous medications, such as sodium nitroprusside, are mandatory for managing the event. α-Adrenoceptor blockers have also proven to be effective. In the management of tachyarrhythmias, β-adrenoceptor blockers may not be used alone, because α-adrenoceptor-mediated effects may be exacerbated. Myocardial ischemia is caused by coronary vasoconstriction in most of these cases. When the nasal decongestant is discontinued, patients report improvement of these symptoms, demonstrating a probable causal relationship between the use of sympathomimetic drugs and TTC.

Sympathomimetic drugs with indirect action

The most widely accepted underlying mechanism for atropine-mediated myocardial damage is stunning as a result of enhanced sympathetic activity. The withdrawal of parasympathetic drive should exacerbate sympathetic activity, leading to the genesis or worsening of disease activity.[26] After atropine was administered intravenously for symptomatic bradycardia to a patient with substernal chest discomfort, the patient subsequently complained of worsening chest pain and developed new T-wave inversions on the electrocardiogram. Cardiac catheterization revealed normal coronary arteries but akinesis of the apical segment.

Duloxetine, nortriptyline, and venlafaxine inhibit the reuptake of catecholamines into the presynaptic neuron, leaving a net gain in the concentration of epinephrine (nortriptyline[27]) or epinephrine and serotonin (duloxetine[28] and venlafaxine[29]) in the synapse, increasing the probability and frequency of neurotransmitter binding to postsynaptic neurotransmitter receptors. Similarly, there are some case reports of TTC in patients associated with an abuse of recreational drug use producing a similar effect to nortriptyline and duloxetine. In general, these substances are associated with a state of hyperactivity of the sympathetic nervous system caused by an increase of epinephrine and other neurotransmitters (norepinephrine, dopamine, and serotonin) by inhibiting their reuptake into the presynaptic cells.

Nonsympathomimetic Drug-induced TTC

Fluorouracil-induced TTC

The pyrimidine analogue 5-FU is the foundation of adjuvant chemotherapy for colorectal cancer. It is also frequently used in the treatment of gastric, esophageal, pancreatic, breast, bladder, and prostate cancer. By inhibiting thymidylate synthase in malignant cells, 5-FU disrupts DNA synthesis and promotes cell death. Cardiotoxicity is a known adverse effect of 5-FU and occurs in 1.2% to 18% of patients who receive the agent. Although the mechanism of cardiotoxicity caused by 5-FU is not well established, some reports of cardiotoxicity describe coronary ischemia that is thought to result from vasospasm. In recent years, there have been accounts of 5-FU-associated TTC. Exaggerated sympathetic stimulation is thought to play a role in the development of TTC.[29] TTC is transient and patients frequently improve to baseline with supportive care.

Although vasospasm is a theorized mechanism for TTC that occurs with 5-FU, other potential mechanisms have been proposed. In 1 report of 5-FU-related TTC, a negative methylergometrine test excluded coronary spasm as the cause for cardiomyopathy.[30] Both human autopsy and animal studies show that myocarditis can be responsible for cardiomyopathy in patients who receive 5-FU.[31,32] In addition, recent data also suggest that 5-FU induces global reversible endothelial injury.[33] Given the tendency toward global

hypokinesis in 5-FU-related TTC, myocarditis may be a more possible mechanism for cardiomyopathy than vascular causes. It is important for physicians to monitor for and recognize TTC because this disease is a reversible syndrome and because 5-FU is a frequently administered agent for colorectal and other cancers.

Combretastatin-induced TTC

Combretastatin A-4 phosphate is an antitumor vascular targeting agent. Combretastatin A-4 phosphate is a prodrug and is rapidly dephosphorylated to the active compound combretastatin A-4. Combretastatin has a broad range of cytotoxicity against several tumor cell lines and is effective in mouse xenograft models. However, the precise mechanism of action of combretastatin is unknown. Combretastatin may precipitate acute coronary syndrome.[34] Although cardiovascular toxicities following combretastatin are known, the findings of regional wall-motion abnormalities, cardiac biomarker elevations, and angiographically normal coronary arteries suggest a new toxicity for combretastatin.[34]

Combretastatin induces cytoskeletal changes in endothelial cells, increases vascular permeability, and inhibits blood flow. Some patients receiving combretastatin complain of chest pain within 6 hours, which resolves in 1 day.[35] Combretastatin causes endothelial cell apoptosis. Positron emission tomography revealed decreased cardiac output, attributable to the increased peripheral vascular resistance induced by combretastatin and not to myocardial toxicity. Combretastatin induces apoptosis of human proliferating endothelial cells and umbilical vein endothelial cells and disrupts the endothelial networks formed in type I collagen.[36] Positron emission tomography demonstrated decreased blood flow to spleen and kidney. Combretastatin enhances endothelial toxicity, which may be further enhanced by cisplatin, another known endothelial-damaging agent. Combretastatin may increase myocardial radiosensitivity.

β-Adrenoceptor blockers and verapamil, a calcium-channel blocker, may be beneficial. The benefit of calcium-channel blockers is supported by the role of diffuse coronary microvascular spasm. The deleterious effects of elevated catecholamines suggest that vasopressors and inotropes may be harmful.

Pazopanib-induced TTC

Pazopanib is a vascular endothelial growth factor receptor antagonist that acts through inhibition of endothelial nitric oxide synthase. Vascular endothelial growth factor antagonism may have an important role in the development of the TTC through its modulation of nitric oxide and catecholamine effects. Thus, a reduction of nitric oxide may cause an increase in the response to catecholamines in some tissues and organs, including the heart.[37]

Anagrelide-induced TTC
Anagrelide is a phosphodiesterase III inhibitor used in the treatment of essential thrombocythemia. Anagrelide exhibits a positive inotropic and chronotropic effect in the myocardium. Moreover, it can induce vasospasm directly on the epicardial coronary arteries. The development of TTC was determined by the accumulated drug dose, through an intensive inotropic stimulation and an overstimulation of the sympathetic nervous system in a susceptible myocardium.[38]

Levothyroxine-induced TTC
Levothyroxine, a thyroid hormone, is known to have cardiovascular effects similar to catecholamine-mediated stimulation of β-adrenoceptors, such as the effects of dobutamine.[39,40] In thyrotoxicosis there is increased expression of β-adrenoceptors and considerable improvement of cardiovascular symptoms with the use of β-blockers such as propranolol. However, a plausible pharmacologic explanation is unclear.

Because some cases are not related to sympathomimetic drugs, it is possible that the cause of TTC is multifactorial, in which drugs with a sympathomimetic effect may be one of the factors.

Potassium chloride-induced TTC
When a pregnant woman presented for her first Caesarean section, the epidural anesthetic agent was inadvertently diluted with potassium chloride instead of normal saline. This solution was injected through an epidural catheter into the epidural space. A few hours later, pulmonary edema, requiring mechanical ventilatory support occurred because of TTC. The patient was stabilized after the placement of an intra-aortic balloon pump.[41]

Drug Withdrawal-induced TTC

Metoprolol withdrawal-induced TTC
TTC is induced by the drugs mentioned thus far. On the other hand, withdrawal of the β-adrenoceptor blocker, metoprolol, also precipitates TTC.[42]

Oxycodone withdrawal-induced TTC
Oxycodon is typically prescribed for chronic pain. The opioid in oxycodone is slowly released over 12 hours, providing safe and effective pain relief. It was prescribed in the hospital to a patient for long-term opioid dependence associated with the treatment of multijoint degenerative osteoarthritis.

The patient presented to the emergency department 1 day after discharge from the hospital following total knee arthroplasty revision with acute-onset dyspnea and chest pain. Although emergency coronary angiography revealed no major coronary atherosclerosis, the LV ejection fraction was severely decreased and new regional wall motion abnormalities typical of broken heart syndrome were noted.[43]

SUMMARY

There are some reports of drugs, associated with direct or indirect overstimulation of sympathetic nervous system, that may cause TTC. The common characteristic of almost all of these drugs is thought to be catecholamines or sympathetic excess.[44] It is necessary to alert clinicians to suspect and recognize the possibility of the development of drug-associated TTC, given the limited information available.

REFERENCES

1. Bybee KA, Prasad A. Stress-related cardiomyopathy syndromes. Circulation 2008;118(4):397–409.
2. Kurowski V, Kaiser A, von Hof K, et al. Apical and midventricular transient left ventricular dysfunction syndrome (tako-tsubo cardiomyopathy): frequency, mechanisms, and prognosis. Chest 2007;132(3):809–16.
3. Litvinov IV, Kotowycz MA, Wassmann S. Iatrogenic epinephrine-induced reverse Takotsubo cardiomyopathy: direct evidence supporting the role of catecholamines in the pathophysiology of the "broken heart syndrome". Clin Res Cardiol 2009; 98(7):457–62.
4. Prasad A, Madhavan M, Chareonthaitawee P. Cardiac sympathetic activity in stress-induced (Takotsubo) cardiomyopathy. Nat Rev Cardiol 2009;6(6):430–4.
5. Izumi Y, Okatani H, Shiota M, et al. Effects of metoprolol on epinephrine-induced takotsubo-like left ventricular dysfunction in non-human primates. Hypertens Res 2009;32(5):339–46.
6. Ueyama T, Kasamatsu K, Hano T, et al. Catecholamines and estrogen are involved in the pathogenesis of emotional stress-induced acute heart attack. Ann N Y Acad Sci 2008;1148:479–85.
7. Amariles P. A comprehensive literature search: drugs as possible triggers of Takotsubo cardiomyopathy. Curr Clin Pharmacol 2011;6(1):1–11.
8. Sealove BA, Tiyyagura S, Fuster V. Takotsubo cardiomyopathy. J Gen Intern Med 2008;23(11):1904–8.
9. Kinugawa S, Post H, Kaminski PM, et al. Coronary microvascular endothelial stunning after acute pressure overload in the conscious dog is caused by oxidant processes: the role of angiotensin II type 1

receptor and NAD(P)H oxidase. Circulation 2003; 108(23):2934–40.

10. Lee JC, Downing SE. Ventricular function in norepinephrine-induced cardiomyopathic rabbits. Am J Physiol 1982;242(2):H191–6.

11. Movahed A, Reeves WC, Mehta PM, et al. Norepinephrine-induced left ventricular dysfunction in anesthetized and conscious, sedated dogs. Int J Cardiol 1994;45(1):23–33.

12. Lyon AR, Rees PS, Prasad S, et al. Stress (Takotsubo) cardiomyopathy–a novel pathophysiological hypothesis to explain catecholamine-induced acute myocardial stunning. Nat Clin Pract Cardiovasc Med 2008;5(1):22–9.

13. Senba E, Ueyama T. Stress-induced expression of immediate early genes in the brain and peripheral organs of the rat. Neurosci Res 1997;29(3):183–207.

14. Snoeckx LH, Cornelussen RN, Van Nieuwenhoven FA, et al. Heat shock proteins and cardiovascular pathophysiology. Physiol Rev 2001;81(4):1461–97.

15. Ueyama T, Senba E, Kasamatsu K, et al. Molecular mechanism of emotional stress-induced and catecholamine-induced heart attack. J Cardiovasc Pharmacol 2003;41(Suppl 1):S115–8.

16. Ueyama T. Emotional stress-induced Tako-tsubo cardiomyopathy: animal model and molecular mechanism. Ann NY Acad Sci 2004;1018:437–44.

17. Ito K, Sugihara H, Kawasaki T, et al. Assessment of ampulla (Takotsubo) cardiomyopathy with coronary angiography, two-dimensional echocardiography and 99mTc-tetrofosmin myocardial single photon emission computed tomography. Ann Nucl Med 2001;15(4):351–5.

18. Cherian J, Kothari S, Angelis D, et al. Atypical takotsubo cardiomyopathy: dobutamine-precipitated apical ballooning with left ventricular outflow tract obstruction. Tex Heart Inst J 2008;35(1):73–5.

19. Margey R, Diamond P, McCann H, et al. Dobutamine stress echo-induced apical ballooning (Takotsubo) syndrome. Eur J Echocardiogr 2009;10(3):395–9.

20. Crimi E, Baggish A, Leffert L, et al. Images in cardiovascular medicine. Acute reversible stress-induced cardiomyopathy associated with cesarean delivery under spinal anesthesia. Circulation 2008;117(23): 3052–3.

21. Littlejohn FC, Syed O, Ornstein E, et al. Takotsubo cardiomyopathy associated with anesthesia: three case reports. Cases J 2008;1(1):227.

22. Citro R, Pascotto M, Provenza G, et al. Transient left ventricular ballooning (tako-tsubo cardiomyopathy) soon after intravenous ergonovine injection following caesarean delivery. Int J Cardiol 2010;138(2):e31–4.

23. Keskin A, Winkler R, Mark B, et al. Tako-tsubo cardiomyopathy after administration of ergometrine following elective caesarean delivery: a case report. J Med Case Rep 2010;4:280.

24. Forte RY, Precoma-Neto D, Chiminacio Neto N, et al. Myocardial infarction associated with the use of a dietary supplement rich in ephedrine in a young athlete. Arq Bras Cardiol 2006;87(5):e179–81.

25. Wang R, Souza NF, Fortes JA, et al. Apical ballooning syndrome secondary to nasal decongestant abuse. Arq Bras Cardiol 2009;93(5):e75–8.

26. Sandhu G, Servetnyk Z, Croitor S, et al. Atropine aggravates signs and symptoms of Takotsubo cardiomyopathy. Am J Emerg Med 2010;28(2):258, e255-7.

27. De Roock S, Beauloye C, De Bauwer I, et al. Takotsubo syndrome following nortriptyline overdose. Clin Toxicol (Phila) 2008;46(5):475–8.

28. Bergman BR, Reynolds HR, Skolnick AH, et al. A case of apical ballooning cardiomyopathy associated with duloxetine. Ann Intern Med 2008;149(3): 218–9.

29. Christoph M, Ebner B, Stolte D, et al. Broken heart syndrome: tako Tsubo cardiomyopathy associated with an overdose of the serotonin-norepinephrine reuptake inhibitor Venlafaxine. Eur Neuropsychopharmacol 2010;20(8):594–7.

30. Basselin C, Fontanges T, Descotes J, et al. 5-Fluorouracil-induced Tako-Tsubo-like syndrome. Pharmacotherapy 2011;31(2):226.

31. Grunwald MR, Howie L, Diaz LA Jr. Takotsubo cardiomyopathy and Fluorouracil: case report and review of the literature. J Clin Oncol 2012;30(2):e11–4.

32. Tsibiribi P, Bui-Xuan C, Bui-Xuan B, et al. Cardiac lesions induced by 5-fluorouracil in the rabbit. Hum Exp Toxicol 2006;25(6):305–9.

33. Jensen SA, Sorensen JB. 5-fluorouracil-based therapy induces endovascular injury having potential significance to development of clinically overt cardiotoxicity. Cancer Chemother Pharmacol 2012;69(1): 57–64.

34. Bhakta S, Flick SM, Cooney MM, et al. Myocardial stunning following combined modality combretastatin-based chemotherapy: two case reports and review of the literature. Clin Cardiol 2009;32(12):E80–4.

35. Dark GG, Hill SA, Prise VE, et al. Combretastatin A-4, an agent that displays potent and selective toxicity toward tumor vasculature. Cancer Res 1997;57(10):1829–34.

36. Grosios K, Loadman PM, Swaine DJ, et al. Combination chemotherapy with combretastatin A-4 phosphate and 5-fluorouracil in an experimental murine colon adenocarcinoma. Anticancer Res 2000;20(1A):229–33.

37. White AJ, LaGerche A, Toner GC, et al. Apical ballooning syndrome during treatment with a vascular endothelial growth factor receptor antagonist. Int J Cardiol 2009;131(3):e92–4.

38. Proietti R, Rognoni A, Ardizzone F, et al. Atypical Takotsubo syndrome during anagrelide therapy. J Cardiovasc Med (Hagerstown) 2009;10(7):546–9.

39. Kwon SA, Yang JH, Kim MK, et al. A case of Takotsubo cardiomyopathy in a patient with iatrogenic thyrotoxicosis. Int J Cardiol 2010;145(3):e111–3.

40. van de Donk NW, America YG, Zelissen PM, et al. Takotsubo cardiomyopathy following radioiodine therapy for toxic multinodular goitre. Neth J Med 2009;67(10):350–2.

41. Parodi G, Antoniucci D. Transient left ventricular apical ballooning syndrome after inadvertent epidural administration of potassium chloride. Int J Cardiol 2008;124(1):e14–5.

42. Jefic D, Koul D, Boguszewski A, et al. Transient left ventricular apical ballooning syndrome caused by abrupt metoprolol withdrawal. Int J Cardiol 2008; 131(1):e35–7.

43. Rivera JM, Locketz AJ, Fritz KD, et al. "Broken heart syndrome" after separation (from OxyContin). Mayo Clin Proc 2006;81(6):825–8.

44. Arora S, Alfayoumi F, Srinivasan V. Transient left ventricular apical ballooning after cocaine use: is catecholamine cardiotoxicity the pathologic link? Mayo Clin Proc 2006;81(6):829–32.

Chemotherapy-Induced Takotsubo Cardiomyopathy

Sakima A. Smith, MD*, Alex J. Auseon, DO

KEYWORDS

- Chemotherapy • Takotsubo cardiomyopathy • Stress cardiomyopathy

KEY POINTS

- Stress cardiomyopathy may be more common than is reported in the literature.
- Although several different drugs have been associated with chemotherapy-induced takotsubo cardiomyopathy, fluorouracil appears to be the most common agent.
- Chemotherapy-induced takotsubo cardiomyopathy needs to be considered in all patients with chest pain, electrocardiographic changes, or abnormal cardiac biomarkers while receiving a chemotherapeutic agent.

CASE VIGNETTE

A 60-year-old woman was admitted to the hospital for chemotherapy for gray-zone lymphoma. During infusion of rituximab, ST-segment elevations in leads V1 to V6 were seen on telemetry and confirmed with an electrocardiogram (ECG). She was asymptomatic at the time of the event. A stat troponin level was 2.67 ng/mL. A bedside transthoracic echocardiogram revealed apical ballooning with hyperdynamic basal segments and an ejection fraction of 20% to 25%. An echo 3 days before chemotherapy was normal. Coronary angiography revealed no stenosis. Rituximab was subsequently discontinued. She remained asymptomatic, received a different regimen, and was discharged home with an angiotensin-converting enzyme (ACE) inhibitor and β-blocker. A multigated acquisition scan revealed her left ventricular ejection fraction (LVEF) to be 42% 1 month later. This case highlights the growing evidence that chemotherapeutic agents can be causative agents of stress cardiomyopathy (SC) and that this subject requires greater attention.

BACKGROUND

SC, also known as takotsubo cardiomyopathy, broken heart syndrome, or apical ballooning syndrome, is a rapidly reversible form of acute heart failure reported to be triggered by stressful events and associated with a distinctive left ventricular (LV) contraction pattern classically described as apical akinesis/ballooning with hyperdynamic contraction of the basal segments (**Fig. 1**) in the absence of obstructive coronary artery disease (>50% luminal stenosis). Dote and colleagues[1] first described this phenomenon in 5 patients who had chest pain and had ECG abnormalities matching the symptoms of acute myocardial infarction (**Fig. 2**), but had no coronary artery stenoses on angiography. LV angiograms revealed akinesis in the apical, diaphragmatic, and/or anterolateral segments, with hyperkinesis in the basal segments; the akinesis was transient and resolved in 7 days.[1] This syndrome was initially given the name takotsubo cardiomyopathy (TC) because the classic apical ballooning shape resembles that of a Japanese octopus trap.

Conflict of Interest: None declared.

Division of Cardiovascular Medicine, Davis Heart & Lung Research Institute, The Ohio State University Medical Center, Suite 200, 473 West 12th Avenue, Columbus, OH 43210-1252, USA

* Corresponding author.

E-mail address: sakima.smith@osumc.edu

Heart Failure Clin 9 (2013) 233–242

http://dx.doi.org/10.1016/j.hfc.2012.12.009

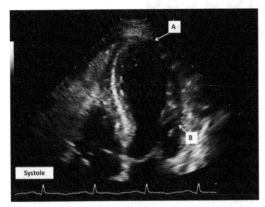

Fig. 1. Representative echocardiographic image of stress cardiomyopathy in a 4-chamber view at end-systole. The apex (A) displays classic akinesis/ballooning seen in stress cardiomyopathy (*arrow*). The base (B) reveals the typical hyperdynamic contraction (*arrow*).

Although SC has traditionally been associated with a known precipitating stressor or event, reports of chemotherapy-induced SC have been increasing in incidence. While studies of chemotherapeutic agents have generated copious data regarding their inherent cardiotoxic effects, conjecture on their role in causing SC is becoming increasingly more common, and is the focus of this review.

TRADITIONAL CLINICAL PRESENTATION
Causal Events

Classically SC presents in postmenopausal women encountering some degree of stress. A recent study revealed that in a large cohort the most common presenting cardiovascular symptoms were substantial chest pain (63%), exertional dyspnea (18%), and syncope (3%). SC was precipitated by intensely stressful emotional (47%) or physical (42%) events, including 22 cases associated with sympathomimetic drugs or medical/surgical procedures, whereas 15 other patients (11%) had no evident stress trigger. Twenty-five patients (18%) were taking β-blockers at the time of SC events. The stressors were diverse, ranging from an emotional divorce, to hip surgery, to failure to keep up with a daughter during a bicycle race.[2] On October 23, 2004, a town in Japan was shaken by a series of 3 strong earthquakes. Takotsubo cardiomyopathy increased in the 4 weeks after the earthquake to 25 cases, compared with only 1 case reported in the 4 weeks before the earthquake, none in 2003, and 1 in 2002.[3]

Appearance of the Presenting Electrocardiogram

Usually the ECG will reveal ST-segment elevations, but there are a variety of ECG abnormalities that may be present with SC. Dib and colleagues[4] demonstrated that ST-segment elevation is absent in two-thirds of patients with SC. ST-segment elevation or new left bundle branch block were seen 34.2% of the time, T-wave inversions in 30.4% of the time, and nonspecific ST-segment changes 35.2% of the time. Thus, the

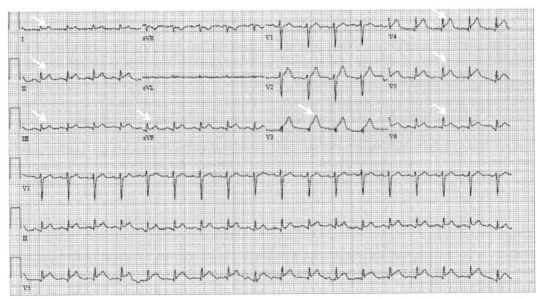

Fig. 2. An electrocardiogram during an acute case of stress cardiomyopathy, showing diffuse ST-segment elevations (*arrows*).

cardiomyopathy may mimic either ST-segment elevation or non–ST-segment elevation myocardial infarction.[4]

Complications of the Syndrome

Associated complications of SC are uncommon but include hemodynamic instability, atrial and ventricular arrhythmias, heart failure, cardiogenic shock and, rarely, death. A minor elevation in creatine kinase MB or cardiac troponins is common, but usually quite low in proportion to the amount of myocardium involved. Cardiac angiography reveals no identifiable obstructive epicardial coronary artery disease despite the pronounced wall-motion abnormalities usually present.[1–3] There is also a rat model of SC. Ueyama and colleagues[5] performed left ventriculograms on rats experiencing emotional stress (immobilization) and were able to induce reversible LV apical ballooning, which was normalized by pretreatment with β-adrenoceptor blockade.

Appearance During Diagnostic Imaging

Three distinct patterns of LV contraction abnormalities characterized by cardiovascular magnetic resonance have been described. One pattern revealed combined midventricular and distal (apical) LV akinesis. Another demonstrated midventricular to LV akinesis only, and another showed distal (apical) LV akinesis. Whereas 95% of patients ultimately showed follow-up LVEF values of greater than 50%, normalization was delayed for 2.5 to 12 months in 5% of patients. Severe apical akinesis should raise consideration for prophylactic anticoagulation in patients with apical akinesis and systolic dysfunction that persists at discharge, as this group of individuals may be more susceptible to thrombus formation and embolization.

General Principles of Management

Treatment of SC should be carried out according to current guidelines for acute coronary syndromes, and should include β-blockers and ACE inhibitors. Anywhere from 5% to 10% of patients may have recurrence of the syndrome.[2,6] A study by Lee and colleagues[7] suggested that SC has a higher in-hospital mortality rate than previously reported. In their study, 9 deaths (16%) occurred during hospitalization at a large tertiary referral center. The absence of recovery of LV function was independently associated with increased mortality. During clinical follow-up up to 6 months, 3 more patients died, 2 of whom had recurrences of SC. The actual long-term prognosis and outcomes of SC is still being defined.

MECHANISMS OF STRESS CARDIOMYOPATHY

The most commonly accepted explanation revolves around excessive catecholamine stimulation caused by a significant physiologic stressor. Mann and colleagues[8] examined the potential lethal effects that norepinephrine can have on cardiac myocytes. Norepinephrine stimulation resulted in a concentration-dependent decrease in cardiac myocyte viability. Norepinephrine-mediated cell toxicity was attenuated significantly by β-adrenoceptor blockade. The norepinephrine-induced toxic effect is thought to be the result of cyclic adenosine monophosphate (AMP)-mediated calcium overload of the cell, which appears to be an important early event in the process of catecholamine-induced cardiac injury. The fact that norepinephrine-mediated cell toxicity was somewhat ameliorated by β-adrenoceptor blockade led to the rationale that β-blockers would provide marked benefit in SC.

Another study by Wittstein and colleagues[9] evaluated 19 patients who presented with LV dysfunction after sudden emotional stress. All of the patients underwent coronary angiography and serial echocardiography, and had plasma catecholamine levels drawn, and some had endomyocardial biopsies, which showed mononuclear infiltrates and contraction-band necrosis. Plasma catecholamine levels at presentation were markedly higher among patients with SC. Histologically catecholamines have been associated with contraction-band necrosis, a unique form of myocyte injury characterized by hypercontracted sarcomeres, dense eosinophilic transverse bands, and an interstitial mononuclear inflammatory response that is distinct from the polymorphonuclear inflammation seen with infarction.

Abraham and colleagues[10] observed 9 cases of SC precipitated immediately by the intravenous administration of epinephrine or dobutamine. Patients were evaluated with coronary angiography and with serial echocardiography, electrocardiography, and cardiac enzymes. The median ejection fraction on admission was 35%. During follow-up (from 4 to 13 days) there was recovery of LV systolic function in all patients (median ejection fraction 55%). These observations strongly support the excessive sympathetic stimulation/catecholamine hypothesis.

Another study by Ueyama and colleagues[11] lends insight into the observed female preponderance of SC. Estrogen supplementation in immobilized mice partially attenuated the cardiac changes in SC. Estrogen treatment also upregulated the levels of cardioprotective substances, such as atrial natriuretic peptide, in the heart. Because the ERα and ERβ estrogen receptors are expressed in the cardiac cells, estrogen can directly act to reduce the reactivity of the heart to catecholamines. Administration of estrogen reduced isoproterenol-induced tachycardia as well as the incidence of ischemia/reperfusion-induced arrhythmia and production of cyclic AMP in rat hearts. These data suggest that reduction of estrogen levels following menopause might be involved in the primary cause of SC both by indirect action on the nervous system and by direct action on the heart.[11]

There may also be upregulation of certain cardiac genes during the acute and recovery phase of SC. Nef and colleagues[12] performed a systematic expression profiling of genes by microarray analysis in the acute phase and after functional recovery during SC. In the acute phase of SC there is an increase of Nrf2-induced genes, which are activated in the presence of reactive oxygen species (ROS). These ROS, when stimulated by catecholamines, have the potential to directly injure vascular cells and cardiac myocytes, initiating a series of local chemical reactions and genetic alterations that ultimately result in an amplification of the initial ROS-mediated cardiomyocyte dysfunction and/or cytotoxicity. The significant upregulation of genes that are involved in energy, fatty acid, and carbohydrate metabolism after functional recovery of SC might represent a compensatory mechanism that contributes to the restoration of contractile function.

Lyon and colleagues[13] recently hypothesized that SC is a variant form of myocardial stunning, with cellular mechanisms different to those traditionally seen during transient episodes of ischemia secondary to coronary stenoses. Lyon and colleagues believe that high levels of circulating epinephrine trigger a switch in intracellular signal trafficking in ventricular cardiomyocytes, from Gs protein to Gi protein signaling via the β2-adrenoceptor. This switch to β2-adrenoceptor–Gi protein signaling protects against the proapoptotic effects of intense activation of β1-adrenoceptors, but it is also negatively inotropic. This effect is most pronounced at the apical myocardium, where β-adrenoceptor density is greatest, and may in part explain apical ballooning.

There are several potential hypotheses regarding the unique apical ballooning that is present in SC. Tsuchihashi and colleagues[14] proposed that several anatomic and physiologic factors might contribute to LV apical wall-motion abnormalities: (1) the fact that the LV apex does not have a 3-layered myocardial structure; (2) the easy loss of elasticity of LV apex after excessive expansion; (3) the fact that the LV apex is the border zone of the perfusion area of major coronary arteries; and (4) the delay of functional recovery from global dysfunction. Compensatory transient basal hypercontraction may produce midventricular obstruction and plays an important role in amplifying apical ballooning, which might contribute to secondary ischemia through increased wall tension.

STRESS CARDIOMYOPATHY AND CANCER

There has been a steady increase in the literature linking SC to cancer and chemotherapeutic agents. Burgdorf and colleagues[15] examined 50 patients with SC and 50 age-matched and gender-matched control patients with acute anterior myocardial infarction. On follow-up (2.9 ± 1.6 years), 7 malignancies were newly diagnosed in the SC cohort, whereas no new case of malignancy was found in the control group. Their entire cohort to date consists of 191 patients with SC and in this population, 23.6% had cancer, which greatly exceeds the expected prevalence of cancer in age-matched populations in the United States and Europe.[16] Recent work by Song and colleagues[17] demonstrated a substantial overall long-term mortality with SC, although cardiac mortality was low. In their cohort 40% of the nonsurvivors died of cancer during follow-up. Cancer is accompanied by increased psychological stress and elevated sympathetic nervous tone, so the investigators hypothesize it might trigger SC in susceptible persons. In addition, paraneoplastic mediators may directly alter cardiac adrenoceptors, and cancer is a chronic inflammatory state associated with excess levels of cytokines, free radicals, prostaglandins, and catecholamines.[15,16] Beyond associated links between malignancy itself and SC, there are specific cancer medications that are known to provoke the syndrome. The chemotherapeutic agent cited most often in the literature is 5-fluorouracil (5-FU), but there are additional data implicating rituximab, vascular endothelial growth factor antagonists, and vascular disrupting agents in SC.

RITUXIMAB AND CARDIOTOXICITY
Pathophysiology

Rituximab, a human/mouse chimeric anti-CD20 antibody, has become part of standard therapy for patients with CD20-expressing B-cell lymphoma and is used in autoimmune diseases, such as rheumatoid arthritis. Rituximab is generally well tolerated. Most patients experience mild to moderate infusion-related reactions during the first administration of rituximab, but the incidence decreases markedly with subsequent infusions. Rituximab induces a rapid depletion of normal CD20-expressing B cells in the peripheral blood, and levels remain low or undetectable for 2 to 6 months before returning to pretreatment levels within 12 months. Serum immunoglobulin levels remain largely stable.

Reported Cases

As of 2008, more than 540,000 patients worldwide have received rituximab, with serious adverse reactions in a small minority of patients.[18] One of the first cases, reported in the literature in 2001, described the case of a 41-year-old man with end-stage, nonischemic dilated cardiomyopathy of 11 years' duration. The patient had been deemed ineligible for transplantation when he was diagnosed with non-Hodgkin lymphoma 7 years prior. Rituximab was initiated as salvage therapy, but the patient was unable to tolerate it and his clinical condition deteriorated rapidly, eventually leading to his death. The investigators surmised that his cardiorenal compromise was in part due to "cytokine release" syndrome overwhelming his advanced heart failure.[19] Poterucha and colleagues[20] reported a case of symptomatic polymorphic ventricular tachycardia that occurred during an initial infusion of rituximab. Kanamori and colleagues[21] reported 3 cases of reduced cardiac function with complications in patients with non-Hodgkin lymphoma who were treated with rituximab. During autopsy, patients' cardiac myocytes were observed to have diffuse amounts of reticulin fiber, and levels of transforming growth factor β were elevated. The investigators suggest that the continuous elevation of transforming growth factor β promotes the growth of reticulin fiber in cardiac myocytes, which may affect both myocardial contractility and conduction. Armitage and colleagues[22] reported 3 cases of acute coronary syndromes during infusion of rituximab. All 3 patients experienced fairly typical chest pain syndromes and experienced elevations of cardiac enzymes consistent with myocardial ischemia. Millward and colleagues[23] described a case of cardiogenic shock that occurred during rituximab therapy for thrombotic thrombocytopenic purpura.

Despite these case reports, there are 2 studies suggesting that these are merely isolated events and that rituximab does not have serious adverse cardiovascular effects. Kilickap and colleagues[24] reported that the addition of rituximab to standard CHOP chemotherapy (cyclophosphamide/adriamycin/vincristine/prednisone) for lymphoma did not significantly increase the risk of doxorubicin-induced cardiotoxicity as measured by the LVEF and fractional shortening. One of the largest prospective studies to assess the risk of rituximab on cardiac function was conducted by Provencio and colleagues.[25] The investigators measured the LVEF of 42 patients with non-Hodgkin lymphoma treated with rituximab-based chemotherapy in a 1-hour infusion. A drop in the posttreatment ejection fraction of more than 10% from the pretreatment base figure was found in 13 patients (31% of the total of the series, with 39% of those receiving adriamycin-based chemotherapy). None of the patients without adriamycin had a decrease in LVEF. Although the data in this study suggest that rapid-infusion rituximab does not cause relevant cardiac toxicity, there was a high percentage of reductions in LVEF of more than 10%, but mostly in patients receiving adriamycin, a well-known cardiotoxic chemotherapeutic agent. At present the data regarding the cardiotoxic effects of rituximab are still unclear, but it appears to have an association with SC, and to the best of the authors' knowledge the case vignette described earlier is the only known case of SC attributable to rituximab.

5-FLUOROURACIL AND CARDIOTOXICITY
Pathophysiology

5-FU is a pyrimidine analogue widely used in systemic cytostatic treatment of solid tumors, especially colorectal tumors. By inhibiting thymidylate synthase in malignant cells, 5-FU disrupts DNA synthesis and promotes cell death. Common toxicities include diarrhea, mucositis, neurotoxicity, palmoplantar dysesthesia, and myelosuppression.[26] Clinical manifestations include chest pain, diaphoresis, and nausea as well as electrocardiographic changes in myocardial injury. The first case of an adverse cardiovascular event related to 5-FU was described in 1975.[27] The incidence of cardiotoxicity may be around 1.6%,[26] but a more recent retrospective study suggests it may be as high as 4.3%.[28] Proposed mechanisms for 5-FU cardiotoxicity include direct myocardial ischemia, coronary spasm, and toxic myocarditis from impurities in the preparation.[29] Pathologic studies also suggest that toxic myocarditis leads to LV dysfunction.[30] There are case reports that 5-FU can cause an acute and reversible cardiomyopathy with apical thrombus development.[31] Arterial vasoconstriction is believed to be another adverse effect of 5-FU. In an elegant study using high-resolution ultrasonography of the brachial artery in patients with malignant tumors, 50% of the patients showed vessel contraction at completion of 5-FU application, whereas no single contraction was noticed in 30 patients following non–5-FU-based chemotherapy.[26] In one of the only prospective studies on this topic, 644 patients who received 5-FU–based therapy were monitored for cardiac events. Overall, 4% developed clinical signs of a cardiac event (angina) or ECG/laboratory evidence of cardiotoxicity.[32] This study suggests that patients with continuous 5-FU infusion may have a higher incidence of cardiotoxicity and that the toxic effects of 5-FU on the myocardium may be schedule dependent.

Reported Cases

5-FU has been implicated in several cases of SC (**Table 1**). In 2009, Gianni and colleagues[33] described a 79-year-old woman with metastatic rectal cancer who received 5-FU and presented with typical ischemic chest pain, elevated cardiac enzymes, and significant ST-segment abnormalities on her electrocardiogram. Echocardiography revealed a wall-motion abnormality, involving the apical and periapical segments, which appeared akinetic. Coronary angiography revealed no obstructive coronary lesions. Four weeks later after being stabilized on medical therapy she remained completely asymptomatic. A repeat echocardiogram revealed a normal ejection fraction and a resolution of the apical akinesis. In 2009, a group in Japan[34] described a case of SC in a 63-year-old woman with rectal adenocarcinoma who received 5-FU. Her initial LVEF during admission was 28%, and 10 days later after medical therapy it normalized to 67%. She had received weekly intravenous 5-FU for 6 weeks. More recent reports describe a case of SC in an 81-year-old woman with stage III colorectal cancer and no history of cardiac disease or emotional precipitant,

who presented with acute onset of chest pain after 5-FU therapy and an LVEF of 35% seen during catheterization that revealed nonobstructive coronary disease. One week later it normalized at 60% after β-blockers and ACE inhibitors were provided.[35] Another case report reported similar findings in a 60-year-old woman with stage III colon cancer. During an infusion of 5-FU she developed severe chest pain, and 40 hours later presented to the hospital. She was found to be tachycardic, with mildly elevated biomarkers and no significant lesions on catheterization. However, marked LV dysfunction with an ejection fraction estimated at 10% to 15% was noted. Treatment with aspirin, carvedilol, lisinopril, simvastatin, and furosemide was begun. A repeat echocardiogram 4 weeks later revealed normal LV systolic function with an estimated ejection fraction of 55% to 60%.[36] This collection of case reports and the previous studies demonstrating the cardiotoxicity of 5-FU clearly demonstrate that this agent may be a legitimate precipitate of SC.

VASCULAR ENDOTHELIAL GROWTH FACTOR ANTAGONISTS AND VASCULAR DISRUPTING AGENTS
Bevacizumab

Pathophysiology
Bevacizumab is a monoclonal antibody that inhibits vascular endothelial growth factor (VEGF). VEGF is a diffusible glycoprotein produced by normal and neoplastic cells, and is an important regulator of physiologic and pathologic angiogenesis. In addition to its direct antiangiogenic effects, bevacizumab may also improve the delivery of chemotherapy by altering tumor vasculature and

Table 1
Cases of 5-fluorouracil stress cardiomyopathy

Authors,[Ref.] Year	Age (y)	Sex	Cancer	LVEF (%) or Description	ECG Abnormality	Chest Pain (Yes/No)	Survived (Yes/No)	Follow-up LVEF (%)/Interval
Gianni et al,[33] 2009	79	Female	Rectal	Abnormal	ST-segment elevations	Yes	Yes	Normal/4 wk
Kobayashi et al,[34] 2009	63	Female	Rectal	28	ST-segment elevations	Yes	Yes	67/10 d
Stewart et al,[35] 2010	81	Female	Colorectal	35	T-wave inversions	Yes	Yes	60/1 wk
Grunwald et al,[36] 2012	60	Female	Colorectal	10–15	ST-segment elevations	Yes	Yes	55–60/4 wk

decreasing the elevated interstitial pressure in tumors.[37] Bevacizumab is a novel chemotherapeutic agent initially approved as part of combination chemotherapy for metastatic colorectal cancer.[38] The package insert states that arterial thrombosis, including cerebral infarction, transient ischemic attacks, myocardial infarction, and angina, are common, occurring in 4.4% of patients whose regimen includes bevacizumab (vs 1.9% on regimen without bevacizumab).[39] In animal models, VEGF antagonists as a category have been linked to heart failure after initially providing compensatory LV hypertrophy.[40] in addition, high levels of inflammatory cytokines and chemoattractant proteins have been isolated in the plasma and myocardial tissue of mice that were exposed to bevacizumab, and are speculated to cause cardiotoxicity.[41] A recent meta-analysis suggests a link between bevacizumab and arterial thrombosis. Data pooled from 5 randomized controlled trials including a total of 1745 patients showed that combination treatment with bevacizumab and chemotherapy, compared with chemotherapy alone, was associated with a 2-fold increased risk of arterial thromboembolism.[42]

Reported cases

There have been several cases of VEGF-related SC documented in the literature. White and colleagues[43] describe the case of a 61-year-old man who developed SC during treatment with a VEGF receptor antagonist. He was a participant in a phase II clinical trial and had been taking the drug for 8 weeks, at a dose of 800 mg daily. He had no prior history of coronary artery disease. The patient's 12-lead ECG showed widespread nonspecific ST-segment elevation, and he presented with hypotension. Cardiac catheterization revealed no coronary artery stenoses. There was akinesis of the mid to apical regions of all walls and compensatory hyperkinesis of the basal myocardial segments, consistent with a diagnosis of SC. A transthoracic echocardiogram was performed, which was notable for a severe outflow tract gradient caused by marked basal septal LV thickening and systolic anterior motion of the anterior leaflet of the mitral valve. The chemotherapeutic agent was discontinued and oral β-blockers were started. A repeat echocardiography 3 weeks later showed normalization of LV function and resolution of the LV outflow tract gradient. The investigators hypothesized that VEGF antagonism may have an important mechanistic role in SC through its modulation of nitric oxide and catecholamine effects.[43]

Specifically, bevacizumab has been implicated in 2 cases of SC (**Table 2**).[44] In a case report by Franco and colleagues,[44] both cases of SC with bevacizumab occurred in men that did not have chest pain. In the first case, a 76-year-old man with colon cancer presented to the emergency room with fever and hypotension 2 days after initiating chemotherapy with bevacizumab. His ECG revealed ST-segment elevations in the anterior and inferior leads. Angiography revealed no significant stenosis, and he had moderate LV dysfunction. Three weeks later during a subsequent admission, his LVEF normalized. In the second case, a 61-year-old man with metastatic non–small cell lung cancer presented to the emergency room with hemoptysis and tachycardia. He had a left heart catheterization following ST-segment elevation on his ECG, which demonstrated no significant stenoses but severe LV dysfunction. Two weeks later his LVEF returned to normal.

Combretastatin

Pathophysiology and reported cases

Combretastatin is a tubulin-depolymerizing agent structurally related to colchicines.[45] Combretastatin has been shown to increase tumor hypoxia within 1 hour of administration. In a study assessing the cardiovascular profile of this agent, combretastatin was found to prolong the QTc interval on the ECG, and there was a temporal relationship with the combretastatin infusion and with ECG

Table 2
Cases of bevacizumab stress cardiomyopathy

Authors,[Ref.] Year	Age (y)	Sex	Cancer	LVEF Description	ECG Abnormality	Chest Pain (Yes/No)	Survived (Yes/No)	Follow-up LVEF/Interval
Franco et al,[44] 2008	76	Male	Colon	Decreased	ST-segment elevations	No (fevers)	Yes	Normal/3 wk
Franco et al,[44] 2008	61	Male	Colon	Severely decreased	ST-segment elevations	No (hemoptysis)	Yes	Normal/2 wk

Table 3
Cases of combretastatin stress cardiomyopathy

Authors,[Ref.] Year	Age (y)	Sex	Cancer	LVEF (%)	ECG Abnormality	Chest Pain (Yes/No)	Survived (Yes/No)	Follow-up LVEF (%)/Interval
Bhakta et al,[47] 2009	71	Female	Thyroid	40–50	T-wave inversions	No (nausea)	Yes	55–65/4 wk
Bhakta et al,[47] 2009	78	Female	Thyroid	50–55	T-wave inversions	Yes	Yes	60–65/4 wk

changes consistent with an acute coronary syndrome in 2 patients.[46] Bhakta and colleagues[47] reported 2 cases of SC following combined-modality therapy with combretastatin (**Table 3**). In this series the syndromes were not preceded by an acute emotional stressor. Moreover, after developing ECG and echocardiographic abnormalities both patients remained asymptomatic and, despite decreased LVEF and significant wall-motion abnormalities, both patients remained stable and uncomplicated.[47]

SUMMARY

Although the exact mechanisms behind cardiotoxic effects of chemotherapeutic agents remain unclear, there is a clear association with a small cohort of medications. There appears to be a complex interconnection between the stressors of cancer, inflammation, cytokine release, and excessive catecholamines that result in the syndrome of chemotherapy-associated stress, or takotsubo, cardiomyopathy. 5-FU seems to have the most definitive association with SC, requiring clinicians to be cognizant of this adverse effect during routine use. All patients who are receiving rituximab, 5-FU, and bevacizumab should be closely monitored and placed on telemetry because of the possible risk of adverse arrhythmias and the potential for significant ECG changes, including those seen in SC. As chest pain may not be a reliable presenting symptom, one must have a heightened sense of awareness of other more subtle signs of cardiac complications.

REFERENCES

1. Dote K, Sato H, Tateishi H, et al. Myocardial stunning due to simultaneous multivessel coronary spasms: a review of 5 cases. J Cardiol 1991;21(2):203–14.
2. Sharkey SW, Windenburg DC, Lesser JR, et al. Natural history and expansive clinical profile of stress (tako-tsubo) cardiomyopathy. J Am Coll Cardiol 2010;55(4):333–41.
3. Watanabe H, Kodama M, Okura Y, et al. Impact of earthquakes on Takotsubo cardiomyopathy. JAMA 2005;294:305–7.
4. Dib C, Asirvatham S, Elesber A, et al. Clinical correlates and prognostic significance of electrocardiographic abnormalities in apical ballooning syndrome (Takotsubo/stress-induced cardiomyopathy). Am Heart J 2009;157(5):933–8.
5. Ueyama T, Kasamatsu K, Hano T, et al. Emotional stress induces transient left ventricular hypocontraction in the rat via activation of cardiac adrenoceptors: a possible animal model of 'tako-tsubo' cardiomyopathy. Circ J 2002;66(7):712–3.
6. Bybee KA, Prasad A. Stress-related cardiomyopathy syndromes. Circulation 2008;118(4):397–409.
7. Lee PH, Song JK, Sun BJ, et al. Outcomes of patients with stress-induced cardiomyopathy diagnosed by echocardiography in a tertiary referral hospital. J Am Soc Echocardiogr 2010;23(7):766–71.
8. Mann DL, Kent RL, Parsons B, et al. Adrenergic effects on the biology of the adult mammalian cardiocyte. Circulation 1992;85(2):790–804.
9. Wittstein IS, Thiemann DR, Lima JA, et al. Neurohumoral features of myocardial stunning due to sudden emotional stress. N Engl J Med 2005;352(6):539–48.
10. Abraham J, Mudd JO, Kapur NK, et al. Stress cardiomyopathy after intravenous administration of catecholamines and beta-receptor agonists. J Am Coll Cardiol 2009;53(15):1320–5.
11. Ueyama T, Kasamatsu K, Hano T, et al. Catecholamines and estrogen are involved in the pathogenesis of emotional stress-induced acute heart attack. Ann N Y Acad Sci 2008;1148:479–85.
12. Nef HM, Möllmann H, Troidl C, et al. Expression profiling of cardiac genes in Tako-Tsubo cardiomyopathy: insight into a new cardiac entity. J Mol Cell Cardiol 2008;44(2):395–404.
13. Lyon AR, Rees PS, Prasad S, et al. Stress (Takotsubo) cardiomyopathy—a novel pathophysiological hypothesis to explain catecholamine-induced acute

myocardial stunning. Nat Clin Pract Cardiovasc Med 2008;5(1):22–9.

14. Tsuchihashi K, Ueshima K, Uchida T, et al. Transient left ventricular apical ballooning without coronary artery stenosis: a novel heart syndrome mimicking acute myocardial infarction. Angina Pectoris-Myocardial Infarction Investigations in Japan. J Am Coll Cardiol 2001;38(1):11–8.

15. Burgdorf C, Kurowski V, Bonnemeier H, et al. Long-term prognosis of the transient left ventricular dysfunction syndrome (Tako-Tsubo cardiomyopathy): focus on malignancies. Eur J Heart Fail 2008;10(10):1015–9.

16. Burgdorf C, Nef HM, Haghi D, et al. Tako-tsubo (stress-induced) cardiomyopathy and cancer. Ann Intern Med 2010;152(12):830–1.

17. Song BG, Hahn JY, Cho SJ, et al. Clinical characteristics, ballooning pattern, and long-term prognosis of transient left ventricular ballooning syndrome. Heart Lung 2010;39(3):188–95.

18. Kimby E. Tolerability and safety of rituximab (MabThera). Cancer Treat Rev 2005;31(6):456–73.

19. Nikolaidis LA. When cancer and heart failure cross paths: a case report of severe cardiorenal compromise associated with the anti-CD20 monoclonal antibody rituximab in a patient with dilated cardiomyopathy. Congest Heart Fail 2001;7(4):223–7.

20. Poterucha JT, Westberg M, Nerheim P, et al. Rituximab-induced polymorphic ventricular tachycardia. Tex Heart Inst J 2010;37(2):218–20.

21. Kanamori H, Tsutsumi Y, Mori A, et al. Delayed reduction in left ventricular function following treatment of non-Hodgkin's lymphoma with chemotherapy and rituximab, unrelated to acute infusion reaction. Cardiology 2006;105(3):184–7.

22. Armitage JD, Montero C, Benner A, et al. Acute coronary syndromes complicating the first infusion of rituximab. Clin Lymphoma Myeloma 2008;8(4):253–5.

23. Millward PM, Bandarenko N, Chang PP, et al. Cardiogenic shock complicates successful treatment of refractory thrombotic thrombocytopenia purpura with rituximab. Transfusion 2005;45(9):1481–6.

24. Kilickap S, Yavuz B, Aksoy S, et al. Addition of rituximab to chop does not increase the risk of cardiotoxicity in patients with non-Hodgkin's lymphoma. Med Oncol 2008;25(4):437–42.

25. Provencio M, Sanchez A, Maximiano C, et al. A prospective study of left ventricle function after treatment with rapid-infusion rituximab in patients with non-Hodgkin lymphoma. Leuk Lymphoma 2009;50(10):1642–6.

26. Südhoff T, Enderle MD, Pahlke M, et al. 5-Fluorouracil induces arterial vasocontractions. Ann Oncol 2004;15(4):661–4.

27. Roth A, Kolari C, Popovic S. Cardiotoxicity of 5-FU. Cancer Chemother Rep 1975;59:1051–2.

28. Labianca R, Beretta G, Clerici M, et al. Cardiac toxicity of 5-fluorouracil: a study on 1,083 patients. Tumori 1982;68:505–10.

29. Jensen SA, Sørensen JB. Risk factors and prevention of cardiotoxicity induced by 5-fluorouracil or capecitabine. Cancer Chemother Pharmacol 2006; 58(4):487–93.

30. Robben NC, Pippas AW, Moore JO. The syndrome of 5-fluorouracil cardiotoxicity: an elusive cardiopathy. Cancer 1993;71:493–509.

31. Sasson Z, Morgan CD, Wang B, et al. 5-Fluorouracil related toxic myocarditis: case reports and pathological confirmation. Can J Cardiol 1994;10(8): 861–4.

32. Kosmas C, Kallistratos MS, Kopterides P, et al. Cardiotoxicity of fluoropyrimidines in different schedules of administration: a prospective study. J Cancer Res Clin Oncol 2008;134(1):75–82.

33. Gianni M, Dentali F, Lonn E. 5 fluorouracil-induced apical ballooning syndrome: a case report. Blood Coagul Fibrinolysis 2009;20(4):306–8.

34. Kobayashi N, Hata N, Yokoyama S, et al. A case of Takotsubo cardiomyopathy during 5-fluorouracil treatment for rectal adenocarcinoma. J Nippon Med Sch 2009;76(1):27–33.

35. Stewart T, Pavlakis N, Ward M. Cardiotoxicity with 5-fluorouracil and capecitabine: more than just vasospastic angina. Intern Med J 2010;40(4):303–7.

36. Grunwald MR, Howie L, Diaz LA Jr. Takotsubo cardiomyopathy and fluorouracil: case report and review of the literature. J Clin Oncol 2012;30(2): e11–4.

37. Willett CG, Boucher Y, di Tomaso E, et al. Direct evidence that the VEGF-specific antibody bevacizumab has antivascular effects in human rectal cancer. Nat Med 2004;10:145–7.

38. Hurwitz H, Fehrenbacher L, Novotny W, et al. Bevacizumab plus irinotecan, fluorouracil, and leucovorin for metastatic colorectal cancer. N Engl J Med 2004; 350(23):2335–42.

39. Genentech, Inc. 2008. Bevacizumab Prescribing Information [online]. Available at: http://www.gene. com/gene/products/information/pdf/avastin-prescribing.pdf. Accessed April 30, 2012.

40. Izumiya Y, Shiojima I, Sato K, et al. Vascular endothelial growth factor blockade promotes the transition from compensatory cardiac hypertrophy to failure in response to pressure overload. Hypertension 2006;47(5):887–93.

41. Drímal J, Zúrová-Nedelcevová J, Knezl V, et al. Cardiovascular toxicity of the first line cancer chemotherapeutic agents: doxorubicin, cyclophosphamide, streptozotocin and bevacizumab. Neuro Endocrinol Lett 2006;27(Suppl 2):176–9.

42. Scappaticci FA, Skillings JR, Holden SN, et al. Arterial thromboembolic events in patients with metastatic carcinoma treated with chemotherapy

and bevacizumab. J Natl Cancer Inst 2007;99(16): 1232–9.

43. White AJ, LaGerche A, Toner GC, et al. Apical ballooning syndrome during treatment with a vascular endothelial growth factor receptor antagonist. Int J Cardiol 2009;131(3):e92–4.

44. Franco TH, Khan A, Joshi V, et al. Takotsubo cardiomyopathy in two men receiving bevacizumab for metastatic cancer. Ther Clin Risk Manag 2008;4(6): 1367–70.

45. Dachs GU, Steele AJ, Coralli C, et al. Anti-vascular agent Combretastatin A-4-P modulates hypoxia

inducible factor-1 and gene expression. BMC Cancer 2006;6:280.

46. Cooney MM, Radivoyevitch T, Dowlati A, et al. Cardiovascular safety profile of combretastatin a4 phosphate in a single-dose phase I study in patients with advanced cancer. Clin Cancer Res 2004; 10(1 Pt 1):96–100.

47. Bhakta S, Flick SM, Cooney MM, et al. Myocardial stunning following combined modality combretastatin-based chemotherapy: two case reports and review of the literature. Clin Cardiol 2009;32(12):E80–4.

Takotsubo Cardiomyopathy
Japanese Perspective

Kenichi Aizawa, MD, PhD[a], Toru Suzuki, MD, PhD[a,b],*

KEYWORDS

- Takotsubo cardiomyopathy • Stress • Postmenopause

KEY POINTS

- Although takotsubo cardiomyopathy (TC) has a variety of names—TC, apical ballooning syndrome, ampulla cardiomyopathy, and broken heart syndrome—it is commonly agreed that the disease is likely induced by stress and that postmenopausal women account for the majority of patients.
- Several questions about TC remain unanswered, including why it is induced by stress, what differentiates the stress that induces this disease from other types of stress that do not induce it, why women are more likely to develop this disease, why the apical part of the heart is affected, and how it is different from the subtype in which the base and middle parts are affected.
- Although TC is uncommon, clinicians should be aware that this disease can commonly develop in wider areas including noncardiac complications and general operations.

HISTORICAL ASPECTS—TAKOTSUBO CARDIOMYOPATHY WAS FIRST DISCOVERED IN JAPAN

TC is a disease concept first presented by Dote and colleagues[1] in 1990. The name is derived from the image on left ventriculography at the end-systolic stage, which presents a takotsubo-like shape due to excessive contraction of the base of heart that compensates for the extensive lack of contraction occurring mainly at the left ventricular apex. *Takotsubo* refers to a vase-like contraption used to fish for octopus (**Fig. 1**). The entry or neck area is narrower than the body; therefore, once an octopus enters the contraption through the narrow entry, it is trapped inside the wider body area. Hence, the term takotsubo is used to refer to this distinct angiographic finding with a similar shape.

Dote and colleagues[1] proactively started to perform urgent cardiac catheter examination for cases with suspicion of acute myocardial infarction (AMI), judging from chest symptoms or electrocardiographic changes, beginning in 1981 at Hiroshima City Hospital. In 1983, they came across an unusual case that presented with a strange systolic abnormality that reminded them of a takotsubo. Until 2003, they performed approximately 1800 cases of diagnosis/treatment of AMI; 1.7% (30 cases) of the patients were diagnosed as having TC that met the above mentioned conditions (extensive lack of contraction at the left ventricular apex and excessive contraction of the base of heart). In the late 1990s, this symptom, which presents a takotsubo-like shape caused by the left ventriculography at the end-systolic stage, began to be reported as TC in Japanese medical conferences and medical journals. At first, this uniquely named disease was regarded as a locally ubiquitous peculiar pathologic condition or an endemic disease. At a multicenter institute in Japan, 88 cases of TC were compiled in 2001.[2] The name,

a Department of Cardiovascular Medicine, Graduate School of Medicine, The University of Tokyo, 7-3-1 Hongo, Bunkyo-ku, Tokyo 113-8655, Japan; b Department of Ubiquitous Preventive Medicine, Graduate School of Medicine, The University of Tokyo, 7-3-1 Hongo, Bunkyo-ku, Tokyo 113-8655, Japan
* Corresponding author. Department of Cardiovascular Medicine, Graduate School of Medicine, The University of Tokyo, 7-3-1 Hongo, Bunkyo-ku, Tokyo 113-8655, Japan.
E-mail address: torusuzu-tky@umin.ac.jp

Heart Failure Clin 9 (2013) 243–247
http://dx.doi.org/10.1016/j.hfc.2012.12.001
1551-7136/13/$ – see front matter © 2013 Elsevier Inc. All rights reserved.

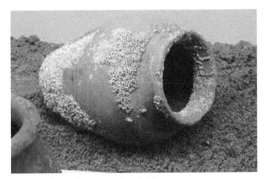

Fig. 1. Takotsubo used for fishing octopus.

takotsubo, was not accepted by the review committee. As a result, the morphologic features were considered a bulging left ventricular apex and reported as transient left ventricular ballooning. Currently, it is established as a pathologic entity. It was not until a report by Desmet and colleagues[3] in 2003 that this disease began to be known to develop in persons other than the Japanese.

A debate is under way over the involvement of pathologic conditions, such as coronary artery multivessel spasm, catecholamine toxicity, and microcirculatory disorder, but much remains unclear. Some Western researchers, who were exposed to this disease via the report by Tsuchihashi and colleagues,[2] see this disease from a standpoint other than that of stunned myocardium and continue to conduct research into the underlying mechanisms of the condition.

PATIENT CARE IN JAPAN

The discovery of TC in Japan resulted from many coincidences, such as low examination expense supported by the compliant national health insurance system, proliferation and progress of coronary intervention, and rise in inspection/operation age and because most acute coronary syndromes were examined at an early stage via coronary angiography/left ventriculography examination. The left ventricular wall motion abnormalities usually normalize in a short period of time. Therefore, if left unrecognized, they might have been misunderstood as cases of normal coronary artery with left ventricular function recovering in a short period of time or as typical clinical cases of stunned myocardium, if acute stages of contrast examination had not been conducted.

NATIONWIDE SURVEY IN JAPAN

A multicenter nation-wide research questionnaire, conducted by the Idiopathic Cardiomyopathy Research Committee in Japan, revealed that the prevalence rate was 2.3% of patients with suspicion of AMI who underwent emergency coronary angiography (0.3% - 6.25%; average 1.4% [96/6774 cases]). Because male patients usually account for the overwhelming majority of emergency coronary angiography cases, it is estimated that the onset frequency would be several times higher than 2.3% if confined to female patients. According to a report by institutes that presented actual numbers, the prevalence rate of TC exceeds 8%.[4] Globally, it is reported as 1.0%, but the basis for the estimation is not always clear.[5] It is also estimated that the prevalence rate is less than 2.3% of ST segment elevation acute coronary syndromes.[6]

ETIOLOGY OF TAKOTSUBO CARDIOMYOPATHY

Wittstein and colleagues[7] compared 13 cases with left ventricular function abnormality that occurred after an acute emotional stress with 7 cases of cardiac infarction in the Killip class III. Because high levels of plasma catecholamine, small round cell infiltration, and contraction band necrosis were observed, they concluded that emotional stress as a trigger factor could induce reversible severe functional deterioration of the left ventricular apex through sympathetic stimulation. The following were indicated as pathogenic mechanisms: (1) stunned myocardium due to multivessel spasm, (2) intramyocardial microvascular contraction, (3) myocarditis, (4) myocardium injury due to catecholamine (pheochromocytoma), (5) orthosympathetic myocardial injury (subarachnoid hemorrhage), and (6) high level of β-adrenergic receptor concentration due to the apical myocardium. Ueyama and colleagues[8] experimented using an akinesia restriction test for rats, 40% of which developed apical ballooning and another 40% showed decreased diffuse contraction, and demonstrated that the onset of the disease could be prevented by prior administration of adrenergic receptor antagonist. TC shows a higher β-receptor concentration that compensates for the poor sympathetic nerve fiber concentration at the left ventricular apex and high level of myocardium reactivity for the sympathetic stimulation. These are believed the causes of myocardial injury/functional deterioration under a variety of stresses.

GUIDELINES FOR DIAGNOSIS

In Japan, guidelines for diagnosis were issued in 2004 by a TC (takotsubo myocardial damage) research study group of the Research Committee of Idiopathic Cardiomyopathy funded by the Japanese Ministry of Health, Labour and Welfare (**Box 1**). Further investigation of the pathologic condition of this disease and development of a therapeutic method are expected.[9] A questionnaire was sent to 203 institutes that had applied with a TC-related presentation subject for the academic meetings hosted by the Japanese Circulation Society from 1989 to 2002. Among them, 33 doctors who had experience with presentation on this disease replied, 21 of whom participated in drafting the guidelines. In 2003, the draft of the diagnostic criteria was completed, and the guidelines for diagnosis TC were formally approved at the annual meeting of the Japanese Circulation Society in 2004 (Intractable Disease Conquest Study supported by subsidies for Health and Labor Scientific Research of the Health, Labour and Welfare Ministry. Research Study Group on the Idiopathic Cardiomyopathy; 2002~2004 General Research Paper [p. 97, issued in 2005]). The guidelines consist of 3 parts: (1) definition, (2) exclusion criteria, and (3) references for diagnosis. The guidelines refer to definition, diagnostic guidelines, clinical characteristics, and pathologic conditions. Further reading of these guidelines is suggested for clarification of the Japanese perspective on this condition because details are beyond the scope of this article. Furthermore, it is important to exclude coronary lesions and acute myocarditis in the diagnosis of TC. Myocardial disorder that occurs after head injury, brain hemorrhage, and pheochromocytoma is considered a takotsubo-like cardiomyopathy and distinguished from special cases.

Internationally, the Mayo criteria issued in 2004 are well known.[10] The Mayo criteria specify that the disease is a transient myocardial disorder that develops mainly in the left ventricular apex unaccompanied by any coronary lesion but accompanied by unfamiliar electrocardiogram changes (increase of ST or negative T wave).

EFFECTS OF THE GREAT EARTHQUAKES ON ONSET OF TAKOTSUBO CARDIOMYOPATHY IN JAPAN

A discernible relationship between natural disasters, such as earthquakes and onset of heart disease, has been seen in Japan. From a historical point of view, there is an inextricable relation between an earthquake and risk of myocardial infarction. Inspection of the data from the great Hanshin-Awaji earthquake in 1995 revealed that there was a rapid increase of AMI in the afflicted areas, and 13 cases were confirmed as affected by the disease, with 53% of them in women.[11,12]

Women had a higher percentage, which doubled from nondisaster times. Considering that 3 cases of coronary lesions were involved, there might be a possibility that TC was latent (overlooked) because the recognition of this disease was limited at that time in Japan. Onset of this disease rapidly increased after the Niigata Chuetsu earthquake in 2004 and as many as 11 patients were confirmed even on the first night of the earthquake.[13] Later, 16 patients in the first week and 25 patients in the first 3 weeks were confirmed, most of whom were women (24/25 cases). In addition to the stress caused by the first hit of the earthquake, life at evacuation centers as well as subsequent aftershocks that inflicted a tremendous stress on elderly women were believed the causes of the condition in Japan.[14] This was also true even after the great East Japan earthquake in 2011.

REPORT ON RECENT INSTANCES OF TAKOTSUBO CARDIOMYOPATHY IN JAPAN

Of the patients who were sent to a Tokyo coronary care unit network, a network of 67 institutes having a coronary care unit facility in Tokyo, those with TC accounted for 0.5% of the total in 2010, 4.7% of which later turned out to be recurrent cases and of which approximately 40% developed a serious cardiac event during the hospital stay.[15] According to the report, 23,063 patients were taken to a hospital in the network by ambulance in 2010. TC accounted for 107 cases, 82 cases (76.6%) of which were women, the average age of whom was 74 years, the average height of whom was 153 cm, and the average weight of whom was 49 kg. Apical ballooning-type accounted for 91.6% and anticipatory stress was confirmed in 68.2% of cases. Recurrent cases accounted for 4.7% (5 cases). In-hospital mortality TC amounted to 9 cases (8.4%), 4 cases of which were cardiac death (heart failure, cardiogenic cerebral infarction, and cardiogenic shock). Aside from 5 cases of noncardiac deaths, most of the deaths were complicated with shock or heart failure, which was considered as the result of being affected by takotsubo cardiomyopathy. It may be possible that the result of being affected by TC. In addition, most of the cardiac deaths occurred within 1 week after transfer to a hospital, whereas noncardiac deaths occurred approximately 2 months after transfer to a hospital. It was concluded that it was not unusual for patients with TC to have complications with cardiac disease during the hospital stay, from which many of them died. A long-term follow-up survey of the Japanese patients is necessary in the future.

Box 1
Japanese guidelines for diagnosis of takotsubo cardiomyopathy

Definition

TC (ampulla cardiomyopathy) is a disease exhibiting an acute left ventricular apical ballooning of unknown cause. In this disease, the left ventricle takes on the shape of a takotsubo (Japanese octopus trap). There is nearly complete resolution of the apical akinesis in the majority of the patients within a month. The contraction abnormality occurs mainly in the left ventricle, but involvement of the right ventricle is observed in some cases. A dynamic obstruction of the left ventricular outflow tract (pressure gradient difference, acceleration of blood flow, or systolic cardiac murmurs) is also observed. Note: there are patients, such as cerebrovascular patients, who have an apical systolic ballooning similar to that in TC but with a known cause; such patients are diagnosed as having cerebrovascular disease with takotsubo-like myocardial dysfunction and are differentiated from idiopathic cases.

1. Exclusion criteria

    The following lesions and abnormalities from other diseases must be excluded in the diagnosis of TC (ampulla cardiomyopathy):

    a. Significant organic stenosis or spasm of a coronary artery; in particular, AMI due to a lesion of the anterior descending branch of the left coronary artery, which perfuses an extensive territory, including the left ventricular apex (an urgent coronary angiogram is desirable for imaging during the acute stage, but coronary angiography is also necessary during the chronic stage to confirm the presence or absence of a significant stenotic lesion or a lesion involved in the abnormal pattern of ventricular contraction)

    b. Cerebrovascular disease

    c. Pheochromocytoma

    d. Viral or idiopathic myocarditis

Note: for the exclusion of coronary artery lesions, coronary angiography is required. Takotsubo-like myocardial dysfunction could occur with diseases, such as cerebrovascular disease and pheochromocytoma.

2. References for diagnosis

    a. Symptoms: chest pain and dyspnea similar to those in acute coronary syndrome. TC can occur without symptoms.

    b. Triggers: emotional or physical stress may trigger TC, but it can also occur without any apparent trigger.

    c. Age and gender differences: known tendency to increase in the elderly, particularly in women.

    d. Ventricular morphology: apical ballooning and its rapid improvement in the ventriculogram and echocardiogram.

    e. Electrocardiogram: ST segment elevations might be observed immediately after the onset. Thereafter, in a typical case, the T wave becomes progressively more negative in multiple leads, and the QT interval prolongs. These changes improve gradually, but a negative T wave may continue for several months. During the acute stage, abnormal Q waves and changes in the QRS voltage might be observed.

    f. Cardiac biomarkers: in a typical case, there are only modest elevations of serum levels of cardiac enzymes and troponin.

    g. Myocardial radionuclear study: abnormal findings in myocardial scintigraphy are observed in some cases.

    h. Prognosis: the majority of the patients rapidly recover, but some patients suffer pulmonary edema and other sequelae or death.

From Kawai S, Kitabatake A, Tomoike H. Guidelines for diagnosis of takotsubo (ampulla) cardiomyopathy. Circ J 2007;71(6):990–2; with permission.

SUMMARY

Twenty years have passed since this peculiar syndrome was discovered, and it has attracted much attention from Western clinicians and researchers. Although it has a variety of names— TC, apical ballooning syndrome, ampulla cardiomyopathy, and broken heart syndrome—it is commonly agreed that the disease is likely induced by stress and that postmenopausal women account for the majority of patients. There has not been an unequivocal answer, however, as to why it is induced by stress, what differentiates the stress that induces this disease from other types of stress that do not induce it, why women are more likely to develop this disease, why the apical part is affected, and how it is different from the subtype in which the base and middle parts are affected. Further accumulation/examination of clinical data and intervention via experimental mechanistic studies are needed. Although uncommon, this is not a disease that only cardiovascular doctors and emergency physicians encounter. Clinicians should keep in their mind that this disease can commonly develop in wider areas, such as noncardiac complications and general operations are good cases in point.

REFERENCES

1. Dote K, Sato H, Tateishi H, et al. Myocardial stunning due to simultaneous multivessel coronary spasms: a review of 5 cases. J Cardiol 1991;21(2):203–14 [in Japanese].

2. Tsuchihashi K, Ueshima K, Uchida T, et al. Transient left ventricular apical ballooning without coronary artery stenosis: a novel heart syndrome mimicking acute myocardial infarction. Angina Pectoris-Myocardial Infarction Investigations in Japan. J Am Coll Cardiol 2001;38(1):11–8.

3. Desmet WJ, Adriaenssens BF, Dens JA. Apical ballooning of the left ventricle: first series in white patients. Heart 2003;89(9):1027–31.

4. Kawai S. [Takotsubo-like left ventricular dysfunction]. Annual Review Cardiology. Chugai-igakusha Co, Tokyo 2003;2003:77–82. [in Japanese].

5. Pina-Oviedo S, De Leon-Bojorge B, Cuesta-Mejias T, et al. Glioblastoma multiforme with small cell neuronal-like component: association with human neurotropic JC virus. Acta Neuropathol 2006; 111(4):388–96.

6. Bybee KA, Prasad A, Barsness GW, et al. Clinical characteristics and thrombolysis in myocardial infarction frame counts in women with transient left ventricular apical ballooning syndrome. Am J Cardiol 2004;94(3):343–6.

7. Wittstein IS, Thiemann DR, Lima JA, et al. Neurohumoral features of myocardial stunning due to sudden emotional stress. N Engl J Med 2005; 352(6):539–48.

8. Ueyama T, Kasamatsu K, Hano T, et al. Emotional stress induces transient left ventricular hypocontraction in the rat via activation of cardiac adrenoceptors: a possible animal model of 'tako-tsubo' cardiomyopathy. Circ J 2002;66(7):712–3.

9. Kawai S, Kitabatake A, Tomoike H. Guidelines for diagnosis of takotsubo (ampulla) cardiomyopathy. Circ J 2007;71(6):990–2.

10. Bybee KA, Kara T, Prasad A, et al. Systematic review: transient left ventricular apical ballooning: a syndrome that mimics ST-segment elevation myocardial infarction. Ann Intern Med 2004; 141(11):858–65.

11. Suzuki S, Sakamoto S, Koide M, et al. Hanshin-Awaji earthquake as a trigger for acute myocardial infarction. Am Heart J 1997;134(5 Pt 1):974–7.

12. Suzuki S, Sakamoto S, Miki T, et al. Hanshin-Awaji earthquake and acute myocardial infarction. Lancet 1995;345(8955):981.

13. Satoh H, Tateishi H, Uchida T, et al. Stunned myocardium with specific (tsubo-type) left ventriculographic configuration due to multivessel spasm. In: Kodama K, Haze K, Hori M, editors. Clinical aspect of myocardial injury: from ischemia to heart failure. Kagakuhyouronsya Co, Tokyo 1990. p. 56-64. [in Japanese].

14. Watanabe H, Kodama M, Okura Y, et al. Impact of earthquakes on Takotsubo cardiomyopathy. JAMA 2005;294(3):305–7.

15. Dr. Tsutomu Murakami of Sakakibara Heart Institute (Fuchu, Tokyo), a member of Tokyo CCU Network Scientific Committee, made a presentation of characteristics of takotsubo cardiomyopathy at the 76th Annual Scientific Meeting of the Japanese Circulation Society, 2012. Fukuoka, Japan, June 16–18, 2012.

Takotsubo Cardiomyopathy
Overview

Eduardo Bossone, MD, PhD, FESC[a,b], Gianluigi Savarese, MD[c],
Francesco Ferrara, MD[b,d], Rodolfo Citro, MD, FESC[b],
Susanna Mosca, MD[c], Francesca Musella, MD[c],
Giuseppe Limongelli, MD, PhD, FESC[e],
Roberto Manfredini, MD[f], Antonio Cittadini, MD, PhD[d],
Pasquale Perrone Filardi, MD, PhD[c],*

KEYWORDS

- Takotsubo cardiomyopathy • Apical ballooning • Stress cardiomyopathy

KEY POINTS

- Takotsubo cardiomyopathy (TTC) is a unique acute syndrome characterized by transient left ventricular (LV) systolic dysfunction in the absence of significant coronary artery disease.
- TTC occurs mostly in postmenopausal women after an emotional and/or physical stress.
- Because the symptoms and signs are nonspecific, a high clinical index of suspicion is necessary to detect the disease in different clinical settings.
- Noninvasive multimodality imaging (ie, echocardiography, CT, and magnetic resonance) may be useful to promptly distinguish TTC from other acute cardiac and thoracic diseases; however, coronary angiography remains mandatory to differentiate TTC from acute coronary syndromes (ACSs).
- Despite the often dramatic clinical presentation, prognosis is generally favorable, with a rapid recovery of ventricular function within few weeks.

INTRODUCTION

Takotsubo cardiomyopathy (TTC) is an acute reversible clinical condition mimicking an acute myocardial infarction (AMI).[1] It is also known as stress cardiomyopathy, transient LV apical ballooning syndrome (ABS), or broken heart syndrome (**Box 1**). The popular and original term, *takotsubo*, first described in Japan by Sato and colleagues[2] in 1990 and reported in 5 patients by Dote and coworkers in 1991,[3] was coined on the basis of similarities between LV morphologic features observed on left ventriculography and the shape of a fishing pot takotsubo (round bottom and narrow neck) used in Japan to trap octopuses. TTC is usually characterized by transient LV systolic dysfunction, represented by a balloon-like apical akinesia with compensatory

Funding Sources: None.
Conflict of Interest: None.
[a] Department of Cardiac Surgery, IRCCS Policlinico San Donato, Piazza Edmondo Malan 1, 20097 San Donato Milanese, Italy; [b] Department of Cardiology and Cardiac Surgery, University Hospital "Scuola Medica Salernitana", Via De Marinis - 84013 Cava de' Tirreni, Salerno, Italy; [c] Department of Advanced Biomedical Sciences, Federico II University, Via Pansini, 5 - 80131 Naples, Italy; [d] Department of Medical Translational Sciences, Federico II University, Via Pansini, 5 - 80131 Naples, Italy; [e] Department of Cardiology, Monaldi Hospital, Second University of Naples, Via L. Bianchi - 80100 Naples, Italy; [f] Section of Clinica Medica, Department of Clinical and Experimental Medicine, University of Ferrara, Via Aldo Moro - 44020 Ferrara, Italy
* Corresponding author. Department of Advanced Biomedical Sciences, Federico II University; Via Pansini, 5 - 80131 Naples, Italy.
E-mail address: fpperron@unina.it

Heart Failure Clin 9 (2013) 249–266
http://dx.doi.org/10.1016/j.hfc.2012.12.015
1551-7136/13/$ – see front matter © 2013 Elsevier Inc. All rights reserved.

| Box 1 |
| Names tabulated from published reports |

Apical ballooning

ABS

Acute LV ABS

LV ABS

Transient LV ABS

Primary apical ballooning

Transient apical ballooning

Transient ABS

Transient cardiac ABS

Transient left ABS

Transient cardiac ballooning

Left ABS

Acute ABS

Cardiac ABS

Apical ballooning

Apical ballooning without apical ballooning

Apical ballooning cardiomyopathy

Reversible apical ballooning of left ventricle

LV ballooning syndrome

Midventricular variant of transient apical ballooning

Midventricular ballooning syndrome

Transient LV midportion ballooning

Transient midventricular ballooning

Transient midventricular ballooning cardiomyopathy

Transient LV nonapical ballooning

Reverse or inverted LV ABS

Inverted LV ABS

Transient basal ballooning

Stress cardiomyopathy

Acute stress cardiomyopathy

Human stress cardiomyopathy

Acute and reversible cardiomyopathy provoked by stress

Stress-induced cardiomyopathy

Stress-induced TTC

Stress-induced ABS

Stress-related left ventricular dysfunction

Stress-related cardiomyopathy

Stress-related cardiomyopathy syndrome

Stress TTC

Emotional stress-induced ampulla cardiomyopathy

Midventricular stress cardiomyopathy

Atypical transient stress-induced cardiomyopathy

Stress-induced myocardial stunning

Emotional stress-induced TTC

Stress-associated catecholamine induced cardiomyopathy

Neurogenic stress syndrome

Other

Neurogenic stunned myocardium

Adrenergic cardiomyopathy

Broken heart syndrome

Ampulla cardiomyopathy

Ampulla-shaped cardiomyopathy

Chestnut-shaped transient regional left ventricular hypokinesia

Ball-shaped spherical dilation of LV apex

The artichoke heart

Transient midventricular akinesia

Transient anteroapical dyskinesia

Takotsubo

TTC

Takotsubo-like cardiomyopathy

Takotsubo syndrome

Takotsubo disease

Takotsubo LV dysfunction

Takotsubo-like LV dysfunction

Takotsubo-like transient biventricular dysfunction

Takotsubo-like transient LV ballooning

Takotsubo-shaped cardiomyopathy

Takotsubo-shaped hypokinesia of left ventricle

Takotsubo-type cardiomyopathy

Takotsubo transient LV apical ballooning

Midventricular TTC

Midventricular form of TTC

Inverted takotsubo contractile pattern

Inverted TTC

Inverted takotsubo pattern

Atypical TTC

Reverse takotsubo syndrome

Atypical basal type TTC

Reproduced from Sharkey SW, Lesser JR, Maron MS, et al. Why not just call it tako-tsubo cardiomyopathy: a discussion of nomenclature. JACC 2011;57:1496–500; with permission.

Box 2
Proposed Mayo Clinic criteria for takotsubo cardiomyopathy

1. Transient hypokinesis, akinesis, or dyskinesis of the LV midsegments with or without apical involvement; the regional wall motion abnormalities extend beyond a single epicardial vascular distribution; a stressful trigger is often, but not always, present.[a]

2. Absence of obstructive coronary disease or angiographic evidence of acute plaque rupture.[b]

3. New ECG abnormalities (either ST-segment elevation and/or T-wave inversion) or modest elevation in cardiac troponin.

4. Absence of pheochromocytoma or myocarditis.

In both of above circumstances, the diagnosis of TTC should be made with caution, and a clear stressful precipitating trigger must be sought.

[a] There are rare exceptions to these criteria, such as those patients in whom the regional wall motion abnormality is limited to a single coronary territory.
[b] It is possible that a patient with obstructive coronary atherosclerosis may also develop TTC. This is rare, however, in the authors' experience and in the published literature, perhaps because such cases are misdiagnosed as an ACS.

hyperkinesis of the basal segments[4] in absence of significant coronary artery disease, occurring mostly in postmenopausal women after an emotional and/or physical stress (**Box 2**). Despite the frequent dramatic clinical presentation, however, the prognosis is generally favorable, with a rapid improvement of LV systolic function in a period of days or few weeks.[5] This review discusses the epidemiology, pathophysiology, clinical features, prognosis, and management of TTC.

PATHOPHYSIOLOGY

The pathophysiology of TTC is not well understood. The broad clinical spectrum suggests heterogeneous and multifactorial pathophysiologic mechanisms are involved.[6,7] A rapid elevation of circulating catecholamine levels triggered by emotional and/or physical stress may play a key pathogenic role.[8] The direct effects of catecholamines on the myocardium (cellular damage, contraction band necrosis, defects in perfusion, altered cellular metabolism, and negative inotropic effects of epinephrine via stimulation of the cardioprotective β_2-adrenergic receptors–G_i signaling pathway) may represent the major determinants

of myocardial reversible dysfunction.[6,9–11] Moreover, in the apical ventricular region, a greater $\beta_2:\beta_1$ adrenoceptor ratio may lead to a higher responsiveness and vulnerability to sympathetic stimulation. Interindividual anatomic differences in the sympathoadrenergic system and in the distribution of β-adrenergic receptors may be responsible for the different occurrence of wall motion abnormalities (**Fig. 1**).[7]

Experimental and clinical observations suggest a role of genetics in the pathogenesis of TTC.[7,12–16] Recently, familial cases of TTC have been reported.[12–14] Over the past decade, several studies analyzing polymorphisms potentially involved in the pathogenesis of TTC have been published, the most relevant concerning those affecting adrenergic receptors.[7,15–18] Although the described studies are promising for the identification of genetic polymorphisms related to the development of the cardiomyopathy, a limitation in the definitive interpretation of the results is the small size of studied populations. In the past few years, a new opportunity to discover the genetic nature and molecular mechanisms of cardiovascular diseases comes from technologic advances in exome capture and DNA sequencing.[18–20] Large prospective genetic studies using these techniques probably will shed light in understanding the pathogenesis of this peculiar syndrome.

EPIDEMIOLOGY

Although TTC is still misdiagnosed, it is more often recognized in daily routine clinical practice and thus increasingly reported in literature.[4,21] The TTC current prevalence estimate is approximately 1% to 3% of patients (up to 6%–9% if only women are considered) with suspicion of ACSs.[1,22–26] It occurs mostly in postmenopausal women (90% of overall TTCs).[27] The mean age ranges from 62 to 76 years in absence of significant differences between men and women.[28] Recently, in the Nationwide Inpatient Sample discharge database of the United States for the year 2008, TTC was diagnosed in approximately 0.02% of all hospitalizations (6.837 diagnosed with TTC among 33,506,402 patients), mostly in elderly women (90% female; mean age ranging from 66 to 80 years), with histories of smoking, alcohol abuse, anxiety states, and hyperlipidemia. A peak incidence of hospitalization during summer was registered. Whites had a higher frequency of TTC compared with African Americans and Hispanics (67.4% vs 4.4 and 4.3%, respectively).[29]

A chronobiologic pattern of the occurrence of TTC has been described, with most events occurring during the morning and summer.[30,31] A higher

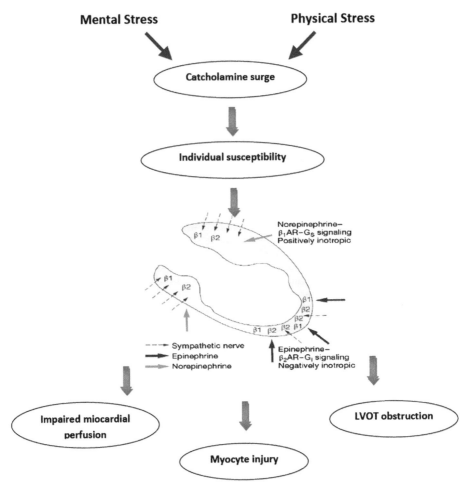

Fig. 1. Proposed pathophysiology of TTC. AR, AdrenoReceptor; LVOT, Left Ventricular Outflow Tract. (*Adapted and Modified from* Prasad A, Lerman A, Rihal CS. Apical ballooning syndrome [Tako-Tsubo or stress cardiomyopathy]: a mimic of acute myocardial infarction. Am Heart J 2008;155:408–17, with permission; and Lyon AR, Rees PS, Prasad S, et al. Stress [Takotsubo] cardiomyopathy—a novel pathophysiological hypothesis to explain catecholamine-induced acute myocardial stunning. Nat Clin Pract Cardiovasc Med 2008;5:22–9; with permission.)

frequency of TTC onset on Monday has been also reported.[32] Due to the limited number of studies and small sample size, however, definite conclusions cannot be drawn, and time of onset is not a useful tool in diagnosing TTC.[33] On one hand, the morning frequency of TTC is similar to that of AMI, and it is possible that they share concurrent underlying risk factors, with a pivotal role operated by circadian rhythms and stress. On the other hand, the summer preference is different from the well-known winter peak of AMI, but underlying causes are still unknown. Nevertheless, the identification of temporal frames characterized by highest frequency of onset, if confirmed, could allow tailored appropriate therapy, especially during vulnerable periods.[34]

CLINICAL PRESENTATION

The most common presenting clinical symptoms of TTC are chest pain and dyspnea, reported in 70% to 80% and 20% of patients, respectively.[28,35] Uncommon presenting symptoms include syncope, palpitations, hypotension and cardiogenic shock, nausea and vomiting, serious ventricular arrhythmias (ventricular fibrillation), and/or cardiac arrest.[5,28,36] In a small proportion of patients, symptoms may be atypical or absent, and TTC is identified accidentally after ischemic ECG changes and/or cardiac biomarkers elevation, during hospitalization to ICU for noncardiac physical illnesses.[5,28,36,37] Cerebrovascular accidents, drug abuse, anxiety disorders, mood disorders, malignancy, chronic liver disease, and sepsis represent the most common comorbidities. Cardiovascular risk factors (obesity, hypertension, diabetes, previous coronary artery disease, and smoking), however, are reported less common in TTC than in patients with AMI.[38] The clinical onset is usually preceded by an emotional and/or physical stress with a similar distribution in approximately two-thirds of the patients.[5,35,36] Physical stress is more frequent in men, whereas emotional stress or no identifiable trigger is more prevalent in female patients.[37,39] Several emotional stressors have been reported, including the death of a relative, loved one, or friend; domestic abuse; confrontational arguments; catastrophic medical diagnosis; devastating business; earthquakes; social events; and public speaking or a surprise party.[28] Physical stressors include acute critical illness, severe pain, subarachnoid hemorrage and posterior reversible encephalopathy syndrome, asthma attack, gastric endoscopy, stress testing, cocaine use, and thyrotoxicosis.[28] In up of 30% of patients, however, no preceding emotional or physical stressful events can be identified.[35]

DIAGNOSTIC METHODS AND IMAGING TECHNIQUES

Given the nonspecific symptoms and signs, a high clinical index of suspicion followed by laboratory tests (troponin and BNP), ECG, and imaging study (echocardiography or MRI) is essential for prompt diagnosis of TTC. Coronary angiography remains, however, mandatory to differentiate TTC from AMI (**Table 1**).

Cardiac Biomarkers and Laboratory Findings

Elevation of cardiac troponin (peak within 24 hours), creatine kinase, and creatine kinase–MB are reported approximately in 85%, 53%, and 38% of TTC patients, respectively.[28] In general, the magnitude of cardiac biomarkers elevation is less than in ST-segment elevation myocardial infarction (STEMI) but similar in non-STEMI and disproportionately lower than the extent of LV dysfunction.[40,41] These findings may reflect the underlying pathophysiologic mechanism of myocardial stunning with less myonecrosis. Conversely, the plasma levels of B-type natriuretic peptide (BNP) and/or of precursor N-terminal proBNP are more markedly elevated than those observed in patients with ACS.[41,42] The BNP peak level occurs over the first 24 hours and remains elevated for several days (≥10 days), with incomplete resolution during the 3 months thereafter, despite the reported rapid resolution of wall motion abnormalities.[43] Wittstein and colleagues[8] also reported higher plasma catecholamine levels (within 1–2 days of symptoms

onset and persisting for 5–7 days) in TTC patients compared with ACS. Other studies, however, reported conflicting and different results, for which hormones routine, such as catecholamine and/or cortisol levels, are not validated in diagnostic assessment of TTC.[41,44] Recently, Neil and colleagues[45] reported that the extent of slowly reversible myocardial edema from T2-weighted cardiac MRI correlates with regional wall motion abnormalities and both catecholamines and peak N-terminal proBNP but not with systemic inflammatory markers. In conclusion, extreme elevation of BNP out of proportion to increase in troponin (ratio BNP/troponin T) could be considered a useful additional diagnostic tool to distinguish TTC from STEMI.[41]

Electrocardiography

The ECG findings on clinical presentation of TTC are heterogeneous. The most common ECG abnormalities are ST-segment elevation (71%–81%) and T-wave inversion (61%–64%). Pathologic Q waves, reported approximately in 31% of patients, are usually transient.[28,35] Compared with AMI, ST-segment elevation in TTC often involves the precordial leads (predominantly V3–V6 vs V1–V3)[46] with a smaller ST elevation magnitude.[40,47] Furthermore, transient prolonged QT interval may occur within 24 to 48 hours from the acute onset, improving within few days, rarely triggering malignant arrhythmia.[48] Instead, T-wave abnormalities can take from days to months to normalize.[49] Other uncommon ECG findings include atrial arrhythmia, sinus or atrioventricular nodal dysfunction, and left bundle branch block.[50,51]

Echocardiography

Echocardiography has the advantage of being widely available, cost-effective, safe, and easily performed in emergency settings. It provides key diagnostic and prognostic information regarding LV morphology (typical vs variant forms) and regional and global systolic/diastolic function. LV wall motion abnormalities typically extend beyond the distribution of any single coronary artery, with circumferential pattern, which symmetrically involves opposite walls of the LV.[52] Typical TTC form is characterized by akinesis of the LV mid and apical segments (compensatory basal hyperkinesis may be observed) (**Figs. 2** and **3**). Atypical variants have been reported, including midventricular akinesis, with preserved function of the apex (apical sparing variant).[53] Rarely, basal akinesis with normal contractility of the apical and midventricular segments (inverted TTC) has also been

Table 1
Relative strengths and weaknesses of noninvasive multimodality imaging in takotsubo cardiomyopathy

	Echocardiography	CCTA	MRI	Nuclear Imaging
Availability	++++	+++	++	++
Portability	++++	—	—	—
Cost	Low	Medium	High	Medium
Speed of acquisition	++++	++++	+	+
Radiation risk	—	++++	—	++++
Suitability for sick or claustrophobic patients	++++	++++	±	±
Contrast agents	—	++++	+[a]	—
Temporal resolution	++++	++	+++	—[b]
Spatial resolution	++	++++	+++	+
Cardiac structure	+++	++	++++	—
Ventricular function quantification	+++	—	++++	+++
Regional function assessment	++++	—	++++	+
Tissue characterization	+	+	++++	+
Myocardial viability	+	+	++++	++++
First-pass perfusion	++	—	++++	++++
Coronary artery imaging	++	++++	+++	—
Assessment of pressure gradients	++++	—	+	—
Clinical Application	• Widespread use in the emergency room • Assessment of reversible wall motion abnormalities • Detection of cardiac complications	• Ruling out underlying coronary disease non-invasively in emergency room • "Triple out" strategy of major acute thoracic disease	• Differential diagnosis between TTC and other cardiac disease (myocardial infarction or myocarditis) • Higher sensitivity to detect thrombi and RV involvement	• Evaluation of myocardial sympathetic activity (^{123}I-MIBG SPECT) and metabolism (^{18}F-FDG PET)

[a] Renal insufficiency (GFR<30 mL/min) contraindicates the use of gadolinium contrast agents.
[b] Temporal resolution for nuclear techniques is variable and depends on the radiotracer and counts.

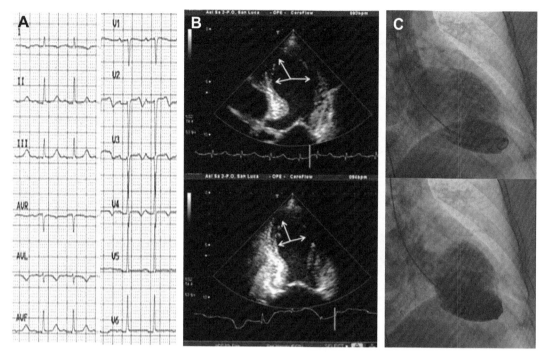

Fig. 2. TTC cardiomyopathy in a 69-year-old woman triggered by emotional stress. (*A*) ECG on admission; note the slight ST-segment elevation in the anterior precordial leads despite an extensive area of myocardial dysfunction as demonstrated in (*B*) by transthoracic echocardiography (*arrows*) along with reduced ejection fraction (38%). (*C*) Left ventriculography: diastolic frame (*top*) and systolic frame (*bottom*). Typical morphology of LV apical ballooning that in systole resembles the shape of a Japanese pot (takotsubo) with a narrow neck and wide base can be appreciated.

described.[54] Echocardiography also plays an important role in the early detection of severe potential complications, such as right ventricular (RV) involvement (biventricular ballooning),[55] LV outflow tract obstruction, thrombus formation, mitral regurgitation, and ventricular rupture.[56,57] Impaired LV ejection fraction detected by echocardiography has been related to adverse in-hospital outcome, especially in elderly patients.[58] Finally, nonconventional echocardiographic techniques (namely, tissue Doppler, strain imaging, and real-time 3-D echocardiography), coronary flow velocity reserve, and myocardial contrast echocardiography may provide new insights in the assessment of LV and RV myocardial function and coronary microcirculation physiopathology.[59–61]

acute plaque rupture, a nontrivial number of patients (up to 10%) may present critical stenosis (≥50%) in epicardial coronary arteries not supplying the dysfunctional myocardium. The presence of significant CAD should not be considered an unexpected finding: the vast majority of patients with TTC are postmenopausal old women with comorbidities and a high prevalence of the common risk factors for atherosclerotic diseases, such as advanced age, diabetes, and family history of CAD.

Contrast left ventriculography remains an useful test in patients with suspected TTC to better define the degree of systolic dysfunction along with regional wall motion abnormalities observed by a previous TTE study.

Coronary Angiography and Left Ventriculography

Cardiac catheterization remains the gold standard test in the differential diagnosis between TTC and an ACS and assessing coronary anatomy and LV wall motion abnormalities. Although the diagnosis of TTC usually implies the absence of obstructive coronary disease or angiographic evidence of

Cardiac MRI

Cardiac MRI provides important diagnostic and prognostic insights in the evaluation of cardiomyopathies.[62,63] It may be helpful to distinguish TTC from other cardiac diseases, such as AMI (characterized by intense late gadolinium enhancement [LGE], predominantly subendocardial or transmural in a vascular territory) and myocarditis (defined

A   **B**

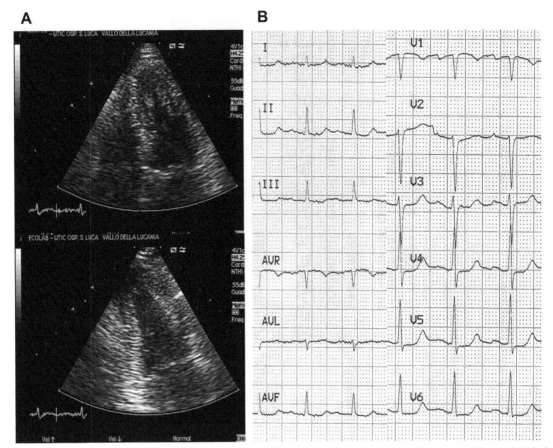

Fig. 3. (*A*) Transthoracic echocardiography at 1-month follow-up showing recovery of LV contractility and global systolic function (ejection fraction 65%). (*B*) ECG at the same time was completely normalized.

by myocardial inflammation edema, and intramyocardial and/or subepicardial LGE without a clear vascular distribution).[63–65] Diagnostic MRI criteria for TTC are (1) severe LV dysfunction in a noncoronary regional distribution pattern, (2) myocardial edema (high signal intensity with a transmural distribution reversible after few weeks) located in segments with wall motion abnormalities, (3) absence of high-signals area (>5 SD above normal) in LGE images, and (4) increased early myocardial gadolinium uptake (**Fig. 4**).[66–70] Cardiovascular MRI may be also more sensitive than echocardiography and left ventriculography for evaluation of intraventricular thrombi and RV involvement, reported approximately in 2% to 5%[66,71,72] and 26 to 34 of overall TTC patients, respectively.[66,73] Recently, in a large multicenter population of 256 patients (89% female; mean age 69 ± 12) with TTC from North America and Europe, Eitel and colleagues[66] define the clinical spectrum and evolution of TTC using a comprehensive, state-of-the-art cardiac MRI protocol. Cardiac MRI data (available for 239 patients

[93%]) revealed 4 distinct patterns of regional ventricular ballooning: apical (n = 197 [82%]), biventricular (n = 81 [34%]), midventricular (n = 40 [17%]), and basal (n = 2 [1%]). Follow-up cardiac MRI at 6 months showed complete normalization of LV ejection fraction and inflammatory markers in the absence of significant fibrosis in all patients. Further investigations, however, are required to define the prognostic role of cardiac MRI in TTC.

Nuclear Imaging

The assessment of myocardial perfusion with single-photon emission CT (SPECT), positron emission tomography (PET), and assessment of glucose metabolism with fludeoxyglucose F 18 (^{18}F-FDG) have been used to evaluate TTC patients in several studies.[74] Typically, the early/acute phase of TTC is characterized by reduced uptake of the structural analog of norepinephrine metaiodobenzyl guanidine I 123 (^{123}I-MIBG) SPECT and of ^{18}F-FDG PET (caused probably by sympathetic-induced insulin resistance), suggesting a neurogenic stunned

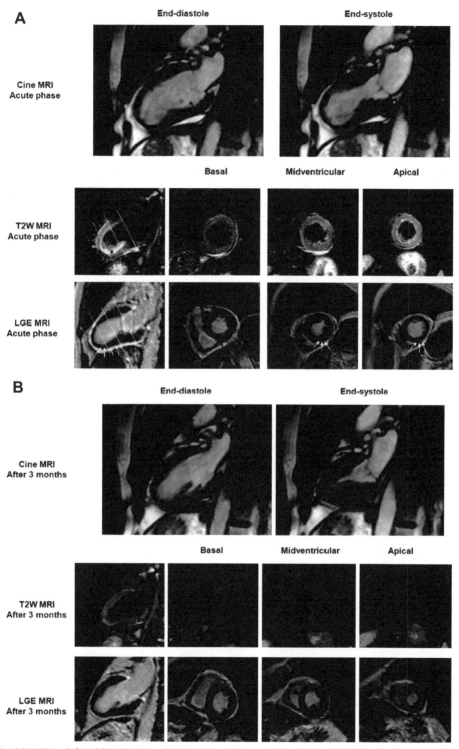

Fig. 4. Cine MRI, T2-weighted (T2W) MRI and LGE MRI in a 69-year-old patient with TTC in (*A*) the acute phase and (*B*) the chronic phase. Apical ballooning and myocardial edema are observed on T2W MRI in the acute state (*red arrows*); (*asterisk*) slow flow artifact. LGE MRI reveals slightly increased myocardial signal intensity in the inferior wall (*yellow arrows*). Myocardial edema, LGE, and wall motion abnormality disappeared after 3 months. (*Adapted from* Nakamori S, Matsuoka K, Onishi K, et al. Prevalence and signal characteristics of late gadolinium enhancement on contrast-enhanced magnetic resonance imaging in patients with takotsubo cardiomyopathy. Circ J 2012;76:914–21; with permission.)

myocardium etiology.[75–79] Usually the regional reduction of ^{123}I-MIBG uptake and impairment of glucose metabolism have the tendency to improve few months after the acute phase of the TTC (**Fig. 5**).[79] Thus, nuclear imaging may be a useful tool for the evaluation of TTC pathophysiology assessing myocardial perfusion, sympathetic nervous activity, and metabolism.

Cardiac CT Angiography

Cardiac CT angiography (CCTA) may be used in the emergency setting to diagnose and/or exclude major acute thoracic disease, such as ACS, aortic dissection, and pulmonary embolism (triple rule-out strategy).[80,81] Normal findings on CCTA have high negative predictive value for ruling out

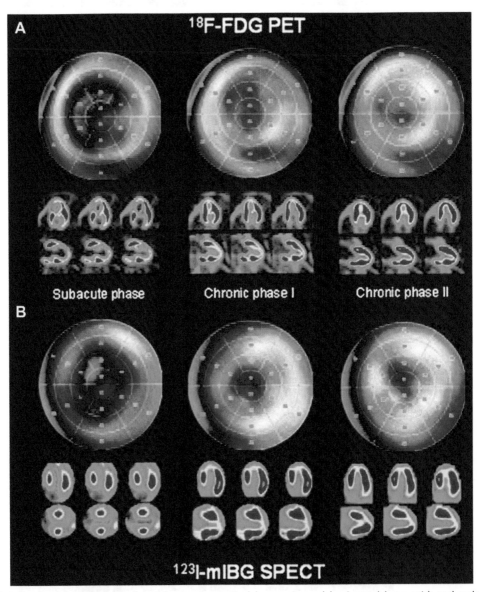

Fig. 5. Left ventricle transaxial slices (short axis, vertical long-axis, and horizontal long-axis) and polar map presentation (17-segment model) SPECT with ^{18}F-FDG PET (*A*) and ^{123}I-MIBG SPECT (*B*) were performed in the subacute and chronic phases in 2 patients with TTC. Remarkably reduced uptake in the apical region of the left ventricle was found on both the ^{18}F-FDG and ^{123}I-MIBG images in the subacute phase. Despite a significant improvement, the uptake of ^{18}F-FDG and ^{123}I-MIBG in the apex was not completely normalized 6 months after the onset of symptoms. (*From* Cimarelli S, Sauer F, Morel O, et al. Transient left ventricular dysfunction syndrome: patho-physiologic bases through nuclear medicine imaging. Int J Cardiol 2010;144:212–8; with permission.)

ACS.[82–85] Few case studies, however, have reported the use of CCTA in the acute diagnosis of TTC, demonstrating high sensitivity and specificity for the assessment of coronary artery anatomy and systolic LV dysfunction (**Fig. 6**).[86–89] Further investigations are needed to well establish the noninvasive potential role of CCTA, along with biomarkers assays (BNP/troponin), in the acute differential diagnosis between TTC and ACS.

THERAPY

The optimal management of TTC is usually supportive, leading to spontaneous recovery. Because the differential diagnosis between TTC and AMI usually cannot be established prior coronary angiography, in the emergency setting, standard treatment of ACS should be implemented (aspirin, heparin, clopidogrel, and/or fibrinolytic drugs). In general, patients with TTC are treated with

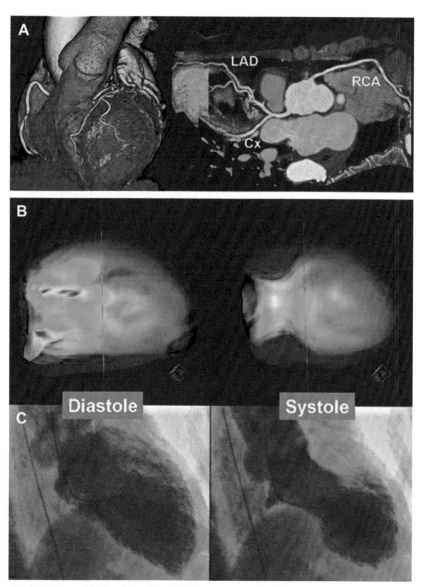

Fig. 6. Diagnosis of TTC in an elderly subject (age 70s) that presented with acute chest pain after dead of spouse. (*A*) CCTA revealed normal coronary arteries. (*B*) Functional analysis showed LV apical hypokinesis with systolic ballooning prompting a diagnosis of TTC. (*C*) Left heart catheterization confirmed TTC diagnosis showing normal coronary arteries and persistent LV apical hypokinesis with systolic ballooning. LAD, Left Anterior Descending; Cx, Circumflex; RCA, Right Coronay Artery. (*Adapted from* Nance JW, Schoepf UJ, Ramos-Duran L. Tako-tsubo cardiomyopathy: findings on cardiac CT and coronary catheterisation. Heart 2010;96:406–7; with permission.)

Table 2
Takotsubo cardiomyopathy: overview of studies (≥30 cases) from 2000 to present

Author Year	Patients/Female (%) Age (Mean ± SD)	Region	TTC/ACS TTC/ Angiography (%)	In-Hospital Mortality CV Death, n (%)	Follow-Up Months (Mean ± SD)	Recurrences (n) (%)	Long-Term Mortality CV Death, n (%)
Tsuchihashi et al,[97] 2001	88/76 (86) 67 ± 13	Japan	— —	1 (1)	13 ± 14	2/72 (2.7)	1 (1.3) 1 (1.3)
Abdulla et al,[22] 2006	35/34 (97) 68 ± 13	Australia	2.6 —	—	6–66	4 (11)	— —
Hertting et al,[98] 2006	32/29 (91) 67.5 (40–85)	Europe	— 0.18	0	6 (2–30)	—	2 (6.2) 0
Elesber et al,[5] 2007	100/95 (95) 66 ± 13	United States	—	2 (1)	26 ± 12	10 (11.4)	17 (17) 7 (7)
Kurowski et al,[23] 2007	35/33 (94) 72 ± 9	Europe	1.2 —	3 (8.6) 0	17 ± 12	2 (6)	0
Burgdorf et al,[99] 2008	50/47 (94) 70 ± 10	Europe	— 0.15	3 (6)	35 ± 19	—	6 (12) 3 (6)
Eshtehardi et al,[24] 2009	41/35 (85) 65 ± 11	Europe	1.7 0.3	0	23 ± 10	2 (5)	1 (2.4) 0
Regnante et al,[94] 2009	70/67 (95) 67 ± 11	United States	— 0.4	1 (1.4) 1 (1.4)	12	2 (2.9)	2 (2.9) 0
Opolski et al,[100] 2010	31/29 (93.5) 67 ± 11	Europe	0.5 —	0	31.38 ± 16.5	0	1 (4) 0

Study	N, Age	Location						
Sharkey et al,[36] 2010	136/130 (96) 68 ± 13	United States	— —	3 (2)	27.6 ± 24	7 (5)	17 (12.5) 0	
Schneider et al,[101] 2010	324/296 (91) 68 ± 12	Europe	— —	7 (2.2)	—	—	—	
Parodi et al,[25] 2011	116/106 (91) 73 ± 10	Europe	2.9 —	2 (1.7)	24 ± 15.6	2 (1.7)	11 (9.6) 7 (6)	
Previtali et al,[102] 2011	132/125 (98) 67 ± 11	Europe	— —	1 (0.8) 1 (0.8)	13	2 (1.5)	1 (0.7) 0	
Eitel et al,[66] 2011	256/227 (89) 69 ± 12	Europe/North America	— —	4 (1.5) 3 (1.1)	At 1 to 6		4 (1.6) 2 (0.8)	
Citro et al,[58] 2012	190/175 (92) 66 ± 11.4	Europe	—	5 (2.8)	—	—	—	
Samardhi et al,[103] 2012	52/51 (98) 64 (43–89)	Australia	— —	0	32.66	0	0	
Looi et al,[26] 2012	100/95 (95) 65 ± 11	New Zealand	3.4 (F); 0.1 (M) —	1 (1) 1 (1)	36 ± 20	7 (7)	4 (4) 0	
Cacciotti et al,[104] 2012	75/73 (97.3) 71.9 ± 9.6	Europe	1.3	0	26.4 ± 24	1 (1.3)	2 (2.6) 2 (2.6)	
Song et al,[105] 2012	137/101 (74) 59	Korea	2	0	68.4	0	12 (9) 0	

Abbreviations: —, not reported; CV, cardiovascular.

standard acute heart failure medications, including angiotensin-converting enzyme inhibitors, β-blockers, diuretics, and vasodilators.[90,91] In patients with low cardiac output syndrome and cardiogenic shock, mechanical support with an intra-aortic balloon pump may be preferred to intravenous inotropic agents that can have deleterious effects, given the potential role of catecholamine excess in the TTC pathophysiology.[35] In cases of LV outflow tract obstruction and hypotension, intravenous short-acting β-blockers (propranolol) and fluids should be used.[92] In presence of LV thrombus or significant apical akinesia, intravenous heparin followed by oral anticoagulation is recommended, until the thrombus and ventricular dysfunction have resolved.

Anxiolytic agents along with treatment of physical stressors (ie, seizure, pain, and asthma) should be considered in acute and long-term management of the precipitating trigger event.[93] With respect to the occurrence of torsades de pointes ventricular tachycardia, drugs that might cause QT prolongation should be avoided (eg, ibutilide).[93]

Even if there is not evidence to support long-term pharmacologic treatment with angiotensin-converting enzyme inhibitors and β-blockers after LV systolic function recovers,[36,94] it is reasonable to continue empiric therapy with β-blockers with the objective of preventing recurrences.[95]

PROGNOSIS

TTC patients have generally a good short-term prognosis, with a rapid improvement of LV systolic function in a period of days to few weeks.[5,36] The incidence of out-of-hospital mortality is currently unknown, even if TTC could probably be considered another important cause of sudden cardiac death. Owada and colleagues,[96] in an autopsy study (91 patients; 85% men) of sudden cardiac death, reported that 19.8% of patients had cardiac dysfunction related to stress. In-hospital mortality rates range from 0 to 8% (Table 2).[5,22–26,36,58,66,94,97–105] Several complications have been reported during the acute phase of TTC: (1) acute heart failure (18%–45%),[35,106] with or without pulmonary edema; (2) cardiogenic shock (3%–10.3%); life-threatening arrhythmias (14.6%), such as third-degree atrioventricular block; and ventricular tachycardia, mostly torsades de pointes due to QT prolongation, ventricular fibrillation (1.5%), and cardiac arrest; (3) dynamic LV outflow tract obstruction (10%–15%) and acute mitral regurgitation due to transient valve dysfunction; and (4) apical thrombus formation, cardioembolic stroke,

LV rupture, and RV involvement with pleural effusions and pericarditis.[28,35] The long-term prognosis, however, is generally favorable. The overall long-term mortality rate ranges from 0 to 17%, with a lower rate of cardiovascular death (range 0–7%). The TTC recurrence rate ranges from 0 to 11.4% (see Table 2).[5,22–26,36,58,66,94,97–105] Recently, in the Nationwide Inpatient Sample discharge database of 24,701 patients with TTC (89% women) from the period from 2008 to 2009, in-hospital mortality rate was 4.2% (>80% dead patients had underlying critical illness), with higher mortality rates men than women (8.4% vs 3.6%, $P<.0001$) and similar to those of myocardial infarction. Race and increased age were not associated with in-hospital mortality.[107,108]

REFERENCES

1. Prasad A, Lerman A, Rihal CS. Apical ballooning syndrome (Tako-Tsubo or stress cardiomyopathy): a mimic of acute myocardial infarction. Am Heart J 2008;155:408–17.
2. Sato H, Taiteishi H, Uchida T. Takotsubo-type cardiomyopathy due to multivessel spasm. In: Kodama K, Haze K, Hon M, editors. Clinical aspect of myocardial injury: from ischemia to heart failure. Tokyo: Kagakuhyouronsha; 1990. p. 56.
3. Dote K, Sato H, Tateishi H, et al. Myocardial stunning due to simultaneous multivessel coronary spasms: a review of 5 cases. J Cardiol 1991;21:203–14.
4. Bybee KA, Kara T, Prasad A, et al. Systematic review: transient left ventricular apical ballooning: a syndrome that mimics ST-segment elevation myocardial infarction. Ann Intern Med 2004;141:858–65.
5. Elesber AA, Prasad A, Lennon RJ, et al. Four-year recurrence rate and prognosis of the apical ballooning syndrome. J Am Coll Cardiol 2007;50:448–52.
6. Nef HM, Mollmann H, Kostin S, et al. Tako-Tsubo cardiomyopathy: intraindividual structural analysis in the acute phase and after functional recovery. Eur Heart J 2007;28:2456–64.
7. Lyon AR, Rees PS, Prasad S, et al. Stress (Takotsubo) cardiomyopathy—a novel pathophysiological hypothesis to explain catecholamine-induced acute myocardial stunning. Nat Clin Pract Cardiovasc Med 2008;5:22–9.
8. Wittstein IS, Thiemann DR, Lima JA, et al. Neurohumoral features of myocardial stunning due to sudden emotional stress. N Engl J Med 2005;352:539–48.
9. Nef HM, Mollmann H, Troidl C, et al. Abnormalities in intracellular Ca2+ regulation contribute to the

pathomechanism of Tako-Tsubo cardiomyopathy. Eur Heart J 2009;30:2155–64.

10. Ueyama T, Kawabe T, Hano T, et al. Upregulation of heme oxygenase-1 in an animal model of Takotsubo cardiomyopathy. Circ J 2009;73:1141–6.

11. Paur H, Wright PT, Sikkel MB, et al. High levels of circulating epinephrine trigger apical cardiodepression in a beta2-adrenoceptor/gi-dependent manner: a new model of takotsubo cardiomyopathy. Circulation 2012;126:697–706.

12. Pison L, De Vusser P, Mullens W, et al. Apical ballooning in relatives. Heart 2004;90:67–9.

13. Cherian J, Angelis D, Filiberti A, et al. Can takotsubo cardiomyopathy be familial? Int J Cardiol 2007;121:74–5.

14. Kumar G, Holmes DR Jr, Prasad A, et al. "Familial" apical ballooning syndrome (Takotsubo cardiomyopathy). Int J Cardiol 2010;144:444–5.

15. Spinelli L, Trimarco V, Di Marino S, et al. L41Q polymorphism of the G protein coupled receptor kinase 5 is associated with left ventricular apical ballooning syndrome. Eur J Heart Fail 2010;12:13–6.

16. Small KM, Forbes SL, Rahman FF, et al. A four amino acid deletion polymorphism in the third intracellular loop of the human alpha 2C-adrenergic receptor confers impaired coupling to multiple effectors. J Biol Chem 2000;275:23059–64.

17. Limongelli G, D'Alessandro R, Masarone D, et al. Takotsubo Cardiomyopathy. Do the genetics matter? Heart Fail Clinics, in press.

18. Vriz O, Minisini R, Citro R, et al. Analysis of beta1 and beta2-adrenergic receptors polymorphism in patients with apical ballooning cardiomyopathy. Acta Cardiol 2011;66:787–90.

19. Paur H, Wright PT, Sikkel MB, et al. High levels of circulating epinephrine trigger apical cardiodepression in a β2-adrenergic receptor/Gi-dependent manner: a new model of Takotsubo cardiomyopathy. Circulation 2012;126:697–706.

20. Bamshad MJ, Ng SB, Bigham AW, et al. Exome sequencing as a tool for Mendelian disease gene discovery. Nat Rev Genet 2011;12:745–55.

21. Akashi YJ, Goldstein DS, Barbaro G, et al. Takotsubo cardiomyopathy: a new form of acute, reversible heart failure. Circulation 2008;118:2754–62.

22. Abdulla I, Kay S, Mussap C, et al. Apical sparing in tako-tsubo cardiomyopathy. Intern Med J 2006;36:414–8.

23. Kurowski V, Kaiser A, von Hof K, et al. Apical and midventricular transient left ventricular dysfunction syndrome (tako-tsubo cardiomyopathy): frequency, mechanisms, and prognosis. Chest 2007;132:809–16.

24. Eshtehardi P, Koestner SC, Adorjan P, et al. Transient apical ballooning syndrome—clinical characteristics, ballooning pattern, and long-term follow-up in a Swiss population. Int J Cardiol 2009;135:370–5.

25. Parodi G, Bellandi B, Del Pace S, et al. Natural history of tako-tsubo cardiomyopathy. Chest 2011;139:887–92.

26. Looi JL, Wong CW, Khan A, et al. Clinical characteristics and outcome of apical ballooning syndrome in Auckland, New Zealand. Heart Lung Circ 2012;21:143–9.

27. Schneider B, Athanasiadis A, Sechtem U. Gender-related differences in takotsubo cardiomyopathy. Heart Fail Clin, in press.

28. Pilgrim TM, Wyss TR. Takotsubo cardiomyopathy or transient left ventricular apical ballooning syndrome: a systematic review. Int J Cardiol 2008;124:283–92.

29. Deshmukh A, Kumar G, Pant S, et al. Prevalence of Takotsubo cardiomyopathy in the United States. Am Heart J 2012;164:66–71.

30. Citro R, Previtali M, Bovelli D, et al. Chronobiological patterns of onset of Tako-Tsubo cardiomyopathy: a multi center Italian study. J Am Coll Cardiol 2009;7(54):180–1.

31. Bossone E, Citro R, Eagle KA, et al. Tako-tsubo cardiomyopathy: is there a preferred time of onset? Intern Emerg Med 2011;6:221–6.

32. Manfredini R, Citro R, Previtali M, et al. Monday preference in onset of takotsubo cardiomyopathy. Am J Emerg Med 2010;28:715–9.

33. Manfredini R, Eagle KA, Bossone E. Acute myocardial infarction and tako-tsubo cardiomyopathy: could time of onset help to diagnose? Expert Rev Cardiovasc Ther 2011;9:123–6.

34. Manfredini R, Gallerani M, Salmi R, et al. Circadian rhythms and the heart: implications for chronotherapy of cardiovascular diseases. Clin Pharmacol Ther 1994;56:244–7.

35. Gianni M, Dentali F, Grandi AM, et al. Apical ballooning syndrome or takotsubo cardiomyopathy: a systematic review. Eur Heart J 2006;27:1523–9.

36. Sharkey SW, Windenburg DC, Lesser JR, et al. Natural history and expansive clinical profile of stress (tako-tsubo) cardiomyopathy. J Am Coll Cardiol 2010;55:333–41.

37. Park JH, Kang SJ, Song JK, et al. Left ventricular apical ballooning due to severe physical stress in patients admitted to the medical ICU. Chest 2005;128:296–302.

38. El-Sayed AM, Brinjikji W, Salka S. Demographic and co-morbid predictors of stress (Takotsubo) cardiomyopathy. Am J Cardiol 2012;110:1368–72.

39. Schneider B, Athanasiadis A, Stöllberger C, et al. Gender differences in the manifestation of takotsubo cardiomyopathy. Int J Cardiol 2011. [Epub ahead of print].

40. Sharkey SW, Lesser JR, Menon M, et al. Spectrum and significance of electrocardiographic patterns, troponin levels, and thrombolysis in myocardial

infarction frame count in patients with stress (tako-tsubo) cardiomyopathy and comparison to those in patients with ST-elevation anterior wall myocardial infarction. Am J Cardiol 2008;101:1723–8.

41. Madhavan M, Borlaug BA, Lerman A, et al. Stress hormone and circulating biomarker profile of apical ballooning syndrome (Takotsubo cardiomyopathy): insights into the clinical significance of B-type natriuretic peptide and troponin levels. Heart 2009;95: 1436–41.

42. Ahmed KA, Madhavan M, Prasad A. Brain natriuretic peptide in apical ballooning syndrome (Takotsubo/stress cardiomyopathy): comparison with acute myocardial infarction. Coron Artery Dis 2012;23:259–64.

43. Nguyen TH, Neil CJ, Sverdlov AL, et al. N-terminal pro-brain natriuretic protein levels in takotsubo cardiomyopathy. Am J Cardiol 2011;108:1316–21.

44. Kurisu S, Sato H, Kawagoe T, et al. Tako-tsubo-like left ventricular dysfunction with ST-segment elevation: a novel cardiac syndrome mimicking acute myocardial infarction. Am Heart J 2002;143:448–55.

45. Neil C, Nguyen TH, Kucia A, et al. Slowly resolving global myocardial inflammation/oedema in Tako-Tsubo cardiomyopathy: evidence from T2-weighted cardiac MRI. Heart 2012;98:1278–84.

46. Kosuge M, Ebina T, Hibi K, et al. Simple and accurate electrocardiographic criteria to differentiate takotsubo cardiomyopathy from anterior acute myocardial infarction. J Am Coll Cardiol 2010;55: 2514–6.

47. Bybee KA, Motiei A, Syed IS, et al. Electrocardiography cannot reliably differentiate transient left ventricular apical ballooning syndrome from anterior ST-segment elevation myocardial infarction. J Electrocardiol 2007;40:38.e1–6.

48. Ogura R, Hiasa Y, Takahashi T, et al. Specific findings of the standard 12-lead ECG in patients with "Takotsubo" cardiomyopathy: comparison with the findings of acute anterior myocardial infarction. Circ J 2003;67:687–90.

49. Mitsuma W, Kodama M, Ito M, et al. Serial electrocardiographic findings in women with Takotsubo cardiomyopathy. Am J Cardiol 2007;100:106–9.

50. Syed FF, Asirvatham SJ, Francis J. Arrhythmia occurrence with takotsubo cardiomyopathy: a literature review. Europace 2011;13:780–8.

51. Parodi G, Salvadori C, Del Pace S, et al. Left bundle branch block as an electrocardiographic pattern at presentation of patients with Tako-tsubo cardiomyopathy. J Cardiovasc Med (Hagerstown) 2009;10:100–3.

52. Citro R, Rigo F, Ciampi Q, et al. Echocardiographic assessment of regional left ventricular wall motion abnormalities in patients with tako-tsubo cardiomyopathy: comparison with anterior myocardial infarction. Eur J Echocardiogr 2011;12:542–9.

53. Hurst RT, Askew JW, Reuss CS, et al. Transient midventricular ballooning syndrome: a new variant. J Am Coll Cardiol 2006;48:579–83.

54. Reuss CS, Lester SJ, Hurst RT, et al. Isolated left ventricular basal ballooning phenotype of transient cardiomyopathy in young women. Am J Cardiol 2007;99:1451–3.

55. Citro R, Caso I, Provenza G, et al. Right ventricular involvement and pulmonary hypertension in an elderly woman with tako-tsubo cardiomyopathy. Chest 2010;137:973–5.

56. Jaguszewski M, Fijalkowski M, Nowak R, et al. Ventricular rupture in Takotsubo cardiomyopathy. Eur Heart J 2012;33:1027.

57. Parodi G, Del Pace S, Salvadori C, et al. Left ventricular apical ballooning syndrome as a novel cause of acute mitral regurgitation. J Am Coll Cardiol 2007;14(50):647–9.

58. Citro R, Rigo F, Previtali M, et al. Differences in clinical features and in-hospital outcomes of older adults with tako-tsubo cardiomyopathy. J Am Geriatr Soc 2012;60:93–8.

59. Meimoun P, Passos P, Benali T, et al. Assessment of left ventricular twist mechanics in Tako-tsubo cardiomyopathy by two-dimensional speckle-tracking echocardiography. Eur J Echocardiogr 2011;12: 931–9.

60. Meimoun P, Malaquin D, Benali T, et al. Transient impairment of coronary flow reserve in tako-tsubo cardiomyopathy is related to left ventricular systolic parameters. Eur J Echocardiogr 2009;10:265–70.

61. Galiuto L, De Caterina AR, Porfidia A, et al. Reversible coronary microvascular dysfunction: a common pathogenetic mechanism in Apical Ballooning or Tako-Tsubo Syndrome. Eur Heart J 2010;31:1319–27.

62. Sanz J. Evolving diagnostic and prognostic imaging of the various cardiomyopathies. Ann N Y Acad Sci 2012;1254:123–30.

63. Assomull RG, Prasad SK, Lyne J, et al. Cardiovascular magnetic resonance, fibrosis, and prognosis in dilated cardiomyopathy. J Am Coll Cardiol 2006; 48:1977–85.

64. Eitel I, Behrendt F, Schindler K, et al. Differential diagnosis of suspected apical ballooning syndrome using contrast-enhanced magnetic resonance imaging. Eur Heart J 2008;29:2651–9.

65. Friedrich MG. Tissue characterization of acute myocardial infarction and myocarditis by cardiac magnetic resonance. JACC Cardiovasc Imaging 2008;1:652–62.

66. Eitel I, von Knobelsdorff-Brenkenhoff F, Bernhardt P, et al. Clinical characteristics and cardiovascular magnetic resonance findings in stress (takotsubo) cardiomyopathy. JAMA 2011;306:277–86.

67. Nakamori S, Matsuoka K, Onishi K, et al. Prevalence and signal characteristics of late gadolinium

enhancement on contrast-enhanced magnetic resonance imaging in patients with takotsubo cardiomyopathy. Circ J 2012;76:914–21.

68. Rolf A, Nef HM, Mollmann H, et al. Immunohistological basis of the late gadolinium enhancement phenomenon in tako-tsubo cardiomyopathy. Eur Heart J 2009;30:1635–42.

69. Naruse Y, Sato A, Kasahara K, et al. The clinical impact of late gadolinium enhancement in Takotsubo cardiomyopathy: serial analysis for cardiovascular magnetic resonance imaging. J Cardiovasc Magn Reson 2011;13:67.

70. Athanasiadis A, Schneider B, Sechtem U. Role of CMR. Heart Fail Clinics, in press.

71. de Gregorio C, Grimaldi P, Lentini C. Left ventricular thrombus formation and cardioembolic complications in patients with Takotsubo-like syndrome: a systematic review. Int J Cardiol 2008; 131:18–24.

72. Leurent G, Larralde A, Boulmier D, et al. Cardiac MRI studies of transient left ventricular apical ballooning syndrome (takotsubo cardiomyopathy): a systematic review. Int J Cardiol 2009;135:146–9.

73. Haghi D, Athanasiadis A, Papavassiliu T, et al. Right ventricular involvement in Takotsubo cardiomyopathy. Eur Heart J 2006;27:2433–9.

74. Akashi YJ, Takano M, Miyake F. Scintigraphic Imaging in Tako-Tsubo Cardiomyopathy. Herz 2010;35:231–9.

75. Abe Y, Kondo M, Matsuoka R, et al. Assessment of clinical features in transient left ventricular apical ballooning. J Am Coll Cardiol 2003;41:737–42.

76. Obunai K, Misra D, Van Tosh A, et al. Metabolic evidence of myocardial stunning in takotsubo cardiomyopathy: a positron emission tomography study. J Nucl Cardiol 2005;12:742–4.

77. Feola M, Rosso GL, Casasso F, et al. Reversible inverse mismatch in transient left ventricular apical ballooning: perfusion/metabolism positron emission tomography imaging. J Nucl Cardiol 2006; 13:587–90.

78. Burgdorf C, von Hof K, Schunkert H, et al. Regional alterations in myocardial sympathetic innervation in patients with transient left-ventricular apical ballooning (Tako-Tsubo cardiomyopathy). J Nucl Cardiol 2008;15:65–72.

79. Cimarelli S, Sauer F, Morel O, et al. Transient left ventricular dysfunction syndrome: patho- physiological bases through nuclear medicine imaging. Int J Cardiol 2010;144:212–8.

80. Bastarrika G, Thilo C, Headden GF, et al. Cardiac CT in the assessment of acute chest pain in the emergency department. AJR Am J Roentgenol 2009;193:397–409.

81. Halpern EJ. Triple-rule-out CT angiography for evaluation of acute chest pain and possible acute coronary syndrome. Radiology 2009;252:332–45.

82. Goldstein JA, Chinnaiyan KM, Abidov A, et al. The CT-STAT (Coronary Computed Tomographic Angiography for Systematic Triage of Acute Chest Pain Patients to Treatment) trial. J Am Coll Cardiol 2011;58:1414–22.

83. Litt HI, Gatsonis C, Snyder B, et al. CT angiography for safe discharge of patients with possible acute coronary syndromes. N Engl J Med 2012;366: 1393–403.

84. Truong QA, Bayley J, Hoffmann U, et al. Multimarker strategy of natriuretic peptide with either conventional or high-sensitivity troponin-T for acute coronary syndrome diagnosis in emergency department patients with chest pain: from the "Rule Out Myocardial Infarction using Computer Assisted Tomography" (ROMICAT) trial. Am Heart J 2012;163:972–9.

85. Hoffmann U, Truong QA, Schoenfeld DA, et al. Coronary CT angiography versus standard evaluation in acute chest pain. N Engl J Med 2012;367: 299–308.

86. Nance JW, Schoepf UJ, Ramos-Duran L. Tako-tsubo cardiomyopathy: findings on cardiac CT and coronary catheterisation. Heart 2010;96:406–7.

87. Kim DH, Bang DW, Park HK. Atypical basal type takotsubo cardiomyopathy: MDCT findings correlated with echocardiography. Int J Cardiol 2010; 141:e28–30.

88. Otalvaro L, Zambrano JP, Fishman JE. Takotsubo cardiomyopathy: utility of cardiac computed tomography angiography for acute diagnosis. J Thorac Imaging 2011;26:W83–5.

89. Kim ST, Lee H, Paik SH, et al. Apical-sparing variant of stress cardiomyopathy: integrative analysis with multidetector row cardiac computed tomography in dual-energy mode. J Cardiovasc Comput Tomogr 2012;6:140–2.

90. McMurray JJ, Adamopoulos S, Anker SD, et al. ESC Guidelines for the diagnosis and treatment of acute and chronic heart failure 2012: the Task Force for the Diagnosis and Treatment of Acute and Chronic Heart Failure 2012 of the European Society of Cardiology. Developed in collaboration with the Heart Failure Association (HFA) of the ESC. Eur Heart J 2012;33:1787–847.

91. Bietry R, Reyentovich A, Katz S. Clinical management of Takotsubo cardiomyopathy. Heart Fail Clin, in press.

92. Yoshioka T, Hashimoto A, Tsuchihashi K, et al. Clinical implications of midventricular obstruction and intravenous propranolol use in transient left ventricular apical ballooning (Tako-tsubo cardiomyopathy). Am Heart J 2008;155:526.e1–7.

93. Kurowski V, Radke PW, Schunkert H, et al. Patient care in the acute phase of stress induced cardiomyopathy (Tako-Tsubo cardiomyopathy)–and thereafter? Herz 2010;35:245–50.

94. Regnante RA, Zuzek RW, Weinsier SB, et al. Clinical characteristics and four-year outcomes of patients in the Rhode Island Takotsubo Cardiomyopathy Registry. Am J Cardiol 2009;103:1015–9.

95. Summers MR, Prasad A. Takotsubo cardiomyopathy: definition and clinical profile. Heart Fail Clin, in press.

96. Owada M, Aizawa Y, Kurihara K, et al. Risk factors and triggers of sudden death in the working generation: an autopsy proven case-control study. Tohoku J Exp Med 1999;189:245–58.

97. Tsuchihashi K, Ueshima K, Uchida T, et al. Transient left ventricular apical ballooning without coronary artery stenosis: a novel heart syndrome mimicking acute myocardial infarction. Angina Pectoris-Myocardial Infarction Investigations in Japan. J Am Coll Cardiol 2001;38:11–8.

98. Hertting K, Krause K, Harle T, et al. Transient left ventricular apical ballooning in a community hospital in Germany. Int J Cardiol 2006;112:282–8.

99. Burgdorf C, Kurowski V, Bonnemeier H, et al. Long-term prognosis of the transient left ventricular dysfunction syndrome (Tako-Tsubo cardiomyopathy): focus on malignancies. Eur J Heart Fail 2008;10:1015–9.

100. Opolski G, Pawlak MM, Roik MF, et al. Clinical presentation, treatment, and long-term outcomes in patients with takotsubo cardiomyopathy. Experience of a single cardiology center. Pol Arch Med Wewn 2010;120:231–6.

101. Schneider B, Athanasiadis A, Schwab J, et al. Clinical spectrum of tako-tsubo cardiomyopathy in Germany: results of the tako-tsubo registry of the Arbeitsgemeinschaft Leitende Kardiologische Krankenhausärzte (ALKK). Dtsch Med Wochenschr 2010;135:1908–13 [in German].

102. Previtali M, Repetto A, Camporotondo R, et al. Clinical characteristics and outcome of left ventricular ballooning syndrome in a European population. Am J Cardiol 2011;107:120–5.

103. Samardhi H, Raffel OC, Savage M, et al. Takotsubo cardiomyopathy: an Australian single centre experience with medium term follow up. Intern Med J 2012;42:35–42.

104. Cacciotti L, Passaseo I, Marazzi G, et al. Observational study on Takotsubo-like cardiomyopathy: clinical features, diagnosis, prognosis and follow-up. BMJ Open 2012;2.

105. Song BG, Oh JH, Kim HJ, et al. Chronobiological variation in the occurrence of Tako-tsubo cardiomyopathy: experiences of two tertiary cardiovascular centers. Heart Lung 2013;42:40–7.

106. Madhavan M, Rihal CS, Lerman A, et al. Acute heart failure in apical ballooning syndrome (TakoTsubo/stress cardiomyopathy): clinical correlates and Mayo Clinic risk score. J Am Coll Cardiol 2011;57:1400–1.

107. Brinjikji W, El-Sayed AM, Salka S. In-hospital mortality among patients with takotsubo cardiomyopathy: a study of the National Inpatient Sample 2008 to 2009. Am Heart J 2012;164:215–21.

108. Roe MT, Messenger JC, Weintraub WS, et al. Treatments, trends, and outcomes of acute myocardial infarction and percutaneous coronary intervention. J Am Coll Cardiol 2010;56:254–63.

Index

Note: Page numbers of article titles are in **boldface** type.

A

Adrenergic stress hypothesis, of takotsubo cardiomyopathy, 208
Anagrelide, takotsubo cardiomyopathy induced by, 229
Angiography, cardiac CT, in takotsubo cardiomyopathy, 258–259
    coronary, in takotsubo cardiomyopathy, 129, 141–142, 179–180, 255
Angiotensin-converting enzyme inhibitor therapy, in takotsubo cardiomyopathy, 182
Anticoagulation therapy, in takotsubo cardiomyopathy, 182
Aortic aneurysms, rupture or dissection of, patterns of onset of, 149
Apical ballooning syndrome. See *Takotsubo cardiomyopathy.*
Arrhythmias, in takotsubo cardiomyopathy, 130, 131, 140, 141, 184

B

ß-blocker therapy, in takotsubo cardiomyopathy, 181–182, 194
Bevacizumab, and takotsubo cardiomyopathy, 238–239
Biomarker and laboratory evaluation, in takotsubo cardiomyopathy, 180
Broken heart syndrome. See *Takotsubo cardiomyopathy.*

C

Calcium homeostasis, in takotsubo cardiomyopathy, 198–200
Cardiac catheterization, in takotsubo cardiomyopathy, 114–115
Cardiogenic shock, in takotsubo cardiomyopathy, 183
Cardiomyopathy, stress. See *Takotsubo cardiomyopathy.*
    takotsubo. See *Takotsubo cardiomyopathy.*
Cardiotoxicity, 5-fluorouracil and, 237–238
    rituximab and, 236–237
Cardiovascular diseases, acute, patterns of onset of, 148–149
Catecholamine, in takotsubo cardiomyopathy, 133, 151–152, 189–193, 200–203, 225, 226–228
CD36 deficiency, and takotsubo cardiomyopathy, 214

Chemotherapy-induced takotsubo cardiomyopathy, **233–242**
Chonobiology, insights of, into takotsubo cardiomyopathy, **147–156**
Coagulation factors, in takotsubo cardiomyopathy, 209
Combretastatin, takotsubo cardiomyopathy induced by, 228, 239–240
Congestive heart failure, in takotsubo cardiomyopathy, 128–130

D

Drugs, inducing takotsubo cardiomyopathy, **225–231**
    withdrawal of, takotsubo cardiomyopathy induced by, 229

E

Echocardiography, in takotsubo cardiomyopathy, 115, 116, 123, 124, **157–166**, 174, 179, 233, 234, 253–254, 256
Electrocardiography, in takotsubo cardiomyopathy, 112–114, 115–116, 123, 124, 127–128, 129, 139–140, **157–166**, 174, 179, 234–235, 253–254, 256
Endomyocardial biopsy, in takotsubo cardiomyopathy, 180
Estrogen deficiency, and takotsubo cardiomyopathy, 208
Estrogen supplementation, in takotsubo cardiomyopathy, 182–183

F

Fluorouracil, takotsubo cardiomyopathy induced by, 228
5-Fluorouracil, and cardiotoxicity, 237–238
Fragile X syndrome, and takotsubo cardiomyopathy, 211–214

G

Gadolinium, in takotsubo cardiomyopathy, 173–174

H

Heart-hand syndrome, and takotsubo cardiomyopathy, 214

Heart Failure Clin 9 (2013) 267–269
http://dx.doi.org/10.1016/S1551-7136(13)00010-X
1551-7136/13/$ – see front matter © 2013 Elsevier Inc. All rights reserved.

Printed and bound by CPI Group (UK) Ltd, Croydon, CR0 4YY

03/10/2024

01040346-0017